Doing psychological research

Gathering and analysing data

NICKY HAYES

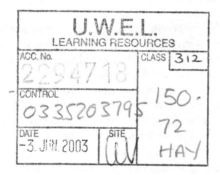
Open University Press
Buckingham • Philadelphia

Open University Press
Celtic Court
22 Ballmoor
Buckingham
MK18 1XW

email: enquiries@openup.co.uk
world wide web: www.openup.co.uk

and
325 Chestnut Street
Philadelphia, PA 19106, USA

First Published 2000

A catalogue record of this book is available from the British Library

ISBN 0 335 203795 (pb)

Library of Congress Cataloging-in-Publication Data
Hayes, Nicky
    Doing psychological research: gathering and analyzing data/Nicky Hayes.
        p. cm.
    Includes bibliographical references and index.
    ISBN 0-335-20379-5 (pbk.)
        1. Psychology—Research—Methodology. I. Title.

  BF76.5.H39 2000
  150′.7′2—dc21   00-037515

Typeset by Graphicraft Limited, Hong Kong
Printed in Great Britain by St Edmundsbury Press,
Bury St Edmunds, Suffolk

To my nephew Christopher, with my love

Contents

List of figures

List of tables

List of worked examples

List of formulae

Introduction

The psychologist and the hamster

Many years ago, as a psychology student, I learned all about operant conditioning, which was very fashionable at the time. I learned how a hungry small rodent in a Skinner box would wander around the box, active because it was hungry, and would eventually press a lever, which would give it a food reward. Gradually, I learned, the animal would come to associate the two events – the pressing of the lever and the receipt of food – at which point it would approach the lever when it was hungry, and begin pressing. It all seemed very straightforward and logical.

In those days it was compulsory for BSc psychology students to undertake some coursework involving animals – not vivisection, but usually some kind of learning experiment. I was rather reluctant to do this, but wasn't able to articulate why: the idea of ethical objections to 'harmless' animal coursework had not yet been voiced, and I only understood later where my own reluctance came from. Eventually, therefore, I found myself in the animal lab with two hamsters, charged with the task of seeing that they obtained their food by means of the Skinner box. The hamsters had previous experience, so didn't have to learn the task from scratch. They had been reduced to four-fifths body weight to make sure they would be hungry, as per the textbook, and my task was to place them in the box, and record how they behaved.

The first hamster, it appeared, had been reading the same books as I had. It explored a bit, and then began pressing the lever, breaking off every now and again to nose into the food box. This rapidly produced the predicted response, and that hamster would hammer away on its lever throughout the experimental session, pausing now and then to eat, then going straight back to pressing its lever. So far, so good. I came away with a nice clear frequency chart, and an even clearer conviction that doing an animal experiment as coursework was just pointless. After all, we knew what was going to happen.

The second hamster, however, had other ideas. It wandered over to a corner of the box, curled up, and went to sleep. That *wasn't* in the textbooks. According to everything I had learned, a hungry animal should get more active, not less. Occasionally it would wake up a bit, and wander around some more. I held my breath whenever it approached the lever, but no, the excitement of perambulating was evidently too much, and it would go back to the corner for another little lie-down.

That set the pattern of its experimental sessions. I think that hamster pressed the lever about five times in total during a twenty-minute 'training' session, and of course, that wasn't enough to get any reward. Its body weight was re-checked, and it was definitely hungry; but there was no way that hamster was going to press that lever twenty times just for one measly food pellet. After four days, the experimenter (not me, I was just the assistant) dropped it from the study.

That hamster taught me an awful lot. I still hold the view that using animals for coursework studies is unnecessary and undesirable, and I was very pleased to see that practice disappear over the next decade or so. On a personal level, though, I learned a great deal about the practicalities of real research. Like many young people, I was inclined to see the world as being much more straightforward than it really is, and I believed that both people and animals acted for the most part in ways which would conform to straightforward, logical rules. That hamster showed me that reality was rather different. Even small rodents sometimes don't act predictably. So it wasn't surprising that people, too, don't always act according to expectations.

The need to do research

All psychology qualifications involve learning how to do psychological research. Sometimes it seems a bit of a waste of time. Why spend time conducting elaborate studies of things that seem obvious? But, as that hamster showed me, actually doing research is very different from just learning about it. If we only learned about psychological research, without actually doing it ourselves, we'd end up with a perfectly logical, highly idealised idea about how people work. But it's unlikely that our ideas would correspond very closely to reality. Real life is more tricky than that.

Actually, what I have said applies to other sciences as well as to psychology. Psychologists often have a very idealised view of the physical sciences – being slightly envious of the fact that their subject matter doesn't talk back. But when you actually get down to doing real research, you find that the physical world, too, doesn't always operate as predicted. During the years, I have worked with metallurgists, physicists and chemists, and I have always been amused by the contrast between the psychologist's idealised view of that type of research, and the uncertain, probabilistic realities of doing it. Real life is *really* tricky!

That said, psychology does have to take some special precautions. We all feel as though we have some understanding of other people. After all, we deal with them all the time, and we are learning about others from the moment that we're born. But that very experience shapes our beliefs and assumptions, in ways that we aren't aware of. It is much too easy to conduct a psychological study which only allows us to find out what we expect to find – not to mention the fact that our research participants have expectations too, which influences their own behaviour. A great deal of what we have to learn about psychological research is about ways of acknowledging these influences, and dealing with them – either positively, as factors which will enrich our knowledge, or negatively, by trying to rule them out.

The power of the paradigm

Scientific research doesn't take place in a vacuum. Ever since human societies first began, people have developed explanations for why the world is like it is. What we know as science operates with a particular set of explanations, which are largely accepted by the scientific community of the time. Those explanations change over time – sometimes dramatically, sometimes gradually – but at any given moment they set the framework for making sense of scientific findings. In the Middle Ages, it was the phlogiston theory which was used to make sense of observations about heat and light, and the Theory of the Humours which made sense of observations about human personality. These theories rested on assumptions about how the world worked, and what counted as evidence, which were very different from modern ones.

Modern paradigms are very different. We make very different assumptions about how the physical world works, and about the functioning of the human body. But, like their predecessors, modern researchers look at their research findings in terms of the accepted **paradigm** of their own scientific community.

The hamster, you may recall, was dropped from the experiment. No way was its behaviour going to contaminate the actual learning experiment which was going on. And that was another lesson I learned: just how powerful a paradigm can be. The experimenter concerned was operating within a very specific experimental framework, which made very definite assumptions about how the world worked, how animals behaved, and the nature of causality. Taking that hamster's behaviour seriously would have challenged that framework of ideas at its most basic level. And it was unthinkable that a whole scientific community's assumptions and ideas should be challenged by the behaviour of just one small hamster.

Modern psychology is very different from the psychology of those days. At that time, psychology consisted of one or two large, dominant paradigms, with minor challenges coming in from other directions. Nowadays, in common with the changes in society as a whole, the discipline is far more pluralistic. Psychological research takes a lot of different forms, and there is more than one generally accepted **methodology**. In this book, we are going to look at several different ways of going about psychological research. Each of these approaches has developed over time, and each has contributed in its own way to the whole sum of modern psychology.

Although any one psychological investigator usually operates within a single main paradigm, psychology itself contains more than one. The fundamental assumptions of approaches such as discourse analysis are very different from those of the hypothetico-deductive experimental tradition, and rest on very different ideas about the nature of knowledge. We will, in this book, be taking samples from several approaches to psychological knowledge. Taken as a whole, they represent some very different ways of going about collecting evidence about what people do. And as a result, I hope that you will be able to gain a full and well-rounded picture of the range and depth of psychological research.

Nicky Hayes

Acknowledgements

I would like to express my thanks to the following for their support and/or helpful advice during the preparation of this text: Nigel Lemon, Mike Stanley, Charles Antaki, Judith Greene, Karen Henwood, Carol Sherrard, Jonathan Smith, Christine Sefton, and many students.

Approaches to
psychological research

The scientific method
The evolution of psychological research

There are quite a number of things which make psychology rather a special sort of science. One of them is its very broad range – from the action of single nerve fibres, to the beliefs of large social groups. Another is the scope of its application: psychology has something valuable to contribute in just about any area of human endeavour – something which psychologists themselves are only just beginning to grasp. And the third is the diversity of its research methods. Psychologists draw on a much wider range of research methods than any other science: from precisely measured and highly controlled laboratory investigation to large-scale action research projects in organisations.

What brings all of these together, as part of the same academic discipline, is the way that psychological knowledge is based on a rigorous and careful collection of evidence – in short, on scientific research. All applied psychologists, no matter what area they are working in, apply psychological knowledge which is based on rigorous and careful research; all research psychologists aim to ensure that the methods they are using are systematic and relevant to the phenomenon they are investigating.

It is psychology's underpinning of scientific investigation which draws psychology, and psychologists, together. And it is for that reason that a sound knowledge of psychological research is an essential part of any psychology student's education in the discipline. This book is designed to provide a basic grounding across the range of psychological research.

In the first part of this book, we will be looking at the process of gathering **data**. Psychological data can take lots of different forms, and the type of data you gather really depends on what type of psychological event you are interested in – and the level of analysis you are concerned with. You might be studying how the brain works, but if you're interested in looking at how people recover from brain injuries, then the type of data you collect is at a different level from the data you need if you are interested in how individual brain cells function. Similarly, if you are interested in why some people always seem to succeed while others usually fail, you'll need to collect a different type of data than you would if you were looking at the social skills which make someone popular with their peers.

Levels of analysis

These examples are all about different **levels of analysis**. If we are trying to understand human beings, we can't do it just by focusing on one level, and ignoring the rest. That was the mistake that the behaviourists made – they believed that associative learning would tell them everything they needed to know about human psychology, since (they thought) human experience really consisted of chains of stimuli and responses. So they believed that a full understanding of **stimulus–response learning** would be the key to understanding human behaviour in all its different forms.

But it doesn't work like that. Understanding the basic elements of a cake only tells us what the cake is made of. It doesn't tell us what it is used for, or who is likely to eat it, or why it was made in the first place. There are what we call **emergent properties** which come into being as soon as different elements are combined. They are called 'emergent' because they emerge from the combination: they aren't there in the elements. The symbolic nature of a birthday cake, for example, isn't there in the elements of flour, sugar, etc. It only emerges as a property once those elements have been transformed into a cake.

Similarly, understanding how human beings learn doesn't tell us everything about human beings – there are other levels of analysis which are just as important, like the study of cognitive mechanisms, of social interaction, of cultural beliefs, of developmental processes, and so on (see Figure 1.1). Any one researcher usually operates at just one level of analysis, but most psychologists are aware that psychology is a broad discipline, and that psychological investigations can take place at any level.

The aim of this book is to introduce the main ways that psychologists go about doing research. There are two sides to this: firstly, collecting the information – the data – that we need; and secondly, making sense out of it, so we can understand what it means. So in the second part of this book, we will go on to look at how psychologists make sense of the data that they have obtained. There are two broad distinctions here: quantitative analyses, which involve analysing data using numbers and statistics, and qualitative analyses, which involve

---

What do these three terms mean?
levels of analysis
stimulus–response learning
emergent properties

Figure 1.1 Levels of
analysis in psychology

cultural and historical
socio-political
subcultural
social cognition
social networks and groups
interpersonal interaction
intentions and motives
cognitive processes
habits and learned associations
emotions
genetic/evolutionary
physiological
neurological
biochemical

analysing data by looking at their content and meaning. Part II will allow us to explore a number of different ways of doing both quantitative and qualitative analyses.

The idea, then, is that the book should give you a pretty fair idea of some of the many ways that psychologists go about gathering data. No individual psychologist would use all of these methods – instead, a psychologist chooses research methods which are appropriate to the topic that is being investigated, and the level of analysis in which the investigation is located. But equally well, it is a rare psychologist who only uses one research method in their work, and no more. Having a range of research techniques to draw on is important for any psychologist, because only that way can we make sure that the methods we are using are appropriate for the problem that we are investigating.

The scientific method

Psychology, as we have seen, adopts a scientific approach to its knowledge base. But as you will have gathered by now, there are a lot of different ways of doing science. Although you will often hear researchers talk about 'the scientific method', the truth is that there isn't just one single way of going about doing science. Scientists approach their work in different ways, depending on the material that they are investigating. Some scientists, such as chemists, are able to manipulate substances in the laboratory. Others, such as astronomers, don't have that option. Some scientists operate by deduction based on observations; while others are able to set up changes to conditions and see what happens as a result.

Figure 1.2 The hypothetico-deductive research cycle

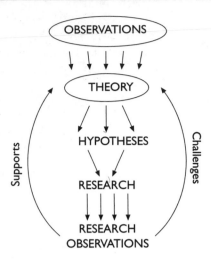

Hypothetico-deductive research

The approach which is most commonly accepted as typical of 'the scientific method' is also known as the **hypothetico-deductive** approach. It involves testing hypotheses – predictions about what will or won't happen if a particular theory is true – and making deductions from the results of those tests. Figure 1.2 shows the cycle of the research process which occurs in hypothetico-deductive research.

The first stage in hypothetico-deductive research, then, is the formulation of a theory. A theory is an explanation for a set of observations, which have usually been obtained from other research, but might also have been picked up informally. If it is a scientific explanation, it will be possible to use that theory to make a number of predictions about what will or won't happen in a given situation, if the theory is true. A prediction of this kind is known as a **hypothesis**.

The hypothetico-deductive approach involves setting up a research process which allows a researcher to test a hypothesis – that is, to see whether the prediction really does come true when it is checked out in reality. The research process might be an experiment, an observation, a survey, a case study, or some other recognised way of gathering and evaluating data. By testing the hypothesis, it then provides some more observations. If these turn out to be the kind that the theory predicted, we take them as support for the theory. If not, then assuming that the research was well designed and carried out rigorously, we take them as challenging the theory and suggesting that some other explanation is needed.

In reality, of course, it takes more than just one set of challenging results to challenge a whole theory. Scientists work within a generally accepted framework of ideas, known as a **paradigm**, and it needs quite

---

What do these three terms mean?

hypothetico-deductive research

paradigm

inductive research

a lot of challenging observations to come up before a whole paradigm is rejected. But the cyclical nature of hypothetico-deductive research means that data are continually being collected, and theories are continually being refined as the body of observations grows.

Inductive research

Inductive research, on the other hand, doesn't begin with a theory and the construction of testable hypotheses. Instead, it begins with the collection of data, so that the research has a set of observations to interpret. Much of our knowledge of how the brain works, for example, began with psychologists and neurologists collecting data about odd things which happened when brains were stimulated or damaged, and using those observations to formulate theories about what was going on.

The process of inductive research, then, begins with data collection and uses the information derived from the data to formulate a theory. As you might imagine, it is particularly useful when psychologists are beginning to investigate a new area, and it provides a theoretical framework which can then, if it seems appropriate, be investigated using the hypothetico-deductive approach. Figure 1.3 illustrates the inductive approach to research.

Figure 1.3 The inductive research cycle

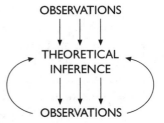

The inductive and hypothetico-deductive approaches can both involve a variety of research methods for collecting the data, and a variety of analytical techniques, although some are more suitable than others. Experiments, for example (Chapter 3), assume a hypothetico-deductive approach, while grounded theory (Chapter 11) assumes an inductive one. But observations (Chapter 4) can be used in either hypothetico-deductive or inductive research, and so can most other research techniques.

Positivism and anti-positivism

These approaches to research have relevance for another distinction which is sometimes made by social scientists, and has become increasingly relevant in modern psychology. This is the distinction between

Table 1.1   Four features of the positivist approach to science

1. It emphasises particular assumptions about causality: that causality is inferred by the human senses when particular events are seen as occurring together in space and time, and that causes are replicable.

2. It emphasises a belief that the observer is completely independent of what is being observed.

3. It holds an ideal of scientific knowledge as being value-free, and as occurring independently of culture and the social context.

4. It maintains that all sciences can and should be conducted by the same overall methodology.

positivist approaches to science, and anti-positivist ones. **Positivism** is an approach that distinguishes between the 'positive' data of sensory experience, and what is referred to as 'transcendental' (that is, going beyond the data) speculation of various kinds. Positivism insists that only that which can be directly observed and measured counts as knowledge, while any other kind of information or approach to evidence is seen as being unscientific. Accordingly, positivist approaches to social science reject the idea of mind as an important influence in understanding social behaviour, and tend to ignore symbolic or communicative levels of explanation. Some basic assumptions of positivist research are summarised in Table 1.1.

The term is often used interchangeably with the term **empiricist**, because they have quite a lot in common. Empiricist approaches take the view that valid knowledge comes only from the kind of experience which can be directly perceived through the senses; other kinds of knowledge are seen as inferior and misleading. In the social sciences, positivism tends to be linked with the hypothetico-deductive approach to science, which we will be looking at later in this section; although some researchers see it as possible to use hypothetico-deductive approaches in other contexts.

The positivist approach takes as its model the methods used in the 'hard-core' sciences of physics and chemistry, and much of the opposition to positivism in social science stems from the idea that human beings are fundamentally different from metals or chemical elements. Human beings have thoughts, ideas and cultural expectations, which influence their behaviour so much that there are some who see positivist ideas as being completely inappropriate in human or social sciences. These researchers adopt an anti-positivist approach.

Anti-positivism is sometimes known as 'interpretivism', or 'the social action approach'. It originated from a number of German philosophers and social scientists writing at the end of the nineteenth

What do these three terms mean?

empiricism

anti-positivism

phenomenological

The following are all studies of vision or visual perception carried out by psychologists. Arrange them in order of the level of analysis which they adopt.

A study of the perception of line drawings in traditional African societies

A study of the perception of vertical lines in kittens reared in a restricted environment from infancy

A study of the way that brain cells fire in response to lines at different angles

A study of the smallest amount of light which the human eye can detect when fully dark-adapted

A study of colour perception and colour naming among people of different cultures

A study investigating how human vision can adapt to upside-down goggles

A study of perceptual closure, showing that we see complete shapes even if we are shown partial ones

A study of visual illusions produced by simple line drawings

A study showing that some people give false judgements of line lengths if the correct judgement would set them against the group

A study of eye-colour inheritance in particular families

A study showing that prejudiced people perceive more exaggerated differences in drawings of people from different ethnic groups than non-prejudiced people do

A study showing that the wording of a question can affect whether a line drawing is perceived as a rabbit or a duck

century, who emphasised that it was important to distinguish between the human/cultural sciences and the natural sciences, on the grounds that the two were concerned with fundamentally different forms of knowledge. The natural sciences were concerned with finding causal explanations for external events, while the human sciences were concerned with grasping the meaning of the individual's experience of and in the world.

The approach put forward by Weber and other like-minded social scientists of the time became known as **Verstehen** (which is German for 'understanding'). This involved an interpretive treatment of social and cultural events, adopting an approach which concerned itself with understanding rather than with simple 'objective' approaches to causality in human behaviour. As such, it represented a direct contrast to the increasing emphasis on quantification, prediction and causality which was developing among positivist social scientists, and the development of Verstehen became an initial stage of anti-positivism as a movement.

Anti-positivists see social reality as consciously and actively created by individuals. Rather than being something which has an 'objective' existence, it is directly produced by the people who participate in it. Accordingly, to treat social life, or human beings, as 'things' to be studied is seen as misleading: it is forcing it into a category which it simply doesn't belong to. Human social life, according to the anti-positivists, is not an objective event: it consists of meanings and of intentional participation. Studying it as if those meanings didn't exist, or were just a by-product of behaviour, produces a distorted picture.

Anti-positivism emphasises a **phenomenological** approach to understanding people. That means that in order to catch the meaning of a social event, we need to look at it through the eyes of the people actively involved – to see it as they see it. This means in turn that the social scientist must be receptive to people's own ideas and explanatory frameworks; it means that it is inappropriate to formulate hypotheses in advance, because that is imposing an explanation beforehand; and it also means that the idea of the sociologist being the 'expert', and having superior knowledge of the social event being studied is inappropriate.

These two approaches to science are both reflected in modern psychological research. There are psychologists who stick rigidly to one side or other of the debate; but psychology is a pretty pragmatic discipline, and most psychologists are eclectic – that is, they use a mixture of approaches depending on what seems to be most suitable for what they are doing.

Nomothetic, idiographic and hermeneutic research

One of the most tricky aspects of psychological research is the way that what the psychologist is investigating is able to think, change its behaviour, and interpret social meanings. For this reason, different areas of psychology adopt different methods for their research. All of them emphasise the importance of rigour and systematic investigation; but they go about doing that investigation in the way that is most appropriate for the phenomenon that they are exploring. Despite the diversity, though, it isn't just an amorphous mass. We can identify three major perspectives in psychological research, which are generally referred to as nomothetic, idiographic and hermeneutic.

The **nomothetic** approach is concerned with identifying general laws about human behaviour (the name comes from the Greek word 'nomos', meaning 'law'). The idea is that discovering laws about human behaviour will allow researchers to make predictions about how people are likely to behave in a given circumstance. As a result, psychologists who engage in nomothetic research often use statistical methods which allow for, and average out, human variation. They take group measurements, looking for general differences between groups rather than individual idiosyncrasies. They also have to pay a great deal of attention to issues such as **sampling**, which we will be looking at in Chapter 2.

In contrast to nomothetic research, **idiographic** research is concerned with exploring uniqueness – what makes a person distinctively individual. So idiographic research concerns itself with fewer cases, and looks at them in more depth. Sometimes, this means detailed interview studies probing an issue in detail; sometimes it means single case studies using a variety of different approaches to explore a particular type of experience. Idiographic researchers don't rule out the identification of general principles; but they go about looking for them in a different way. The idea is that gaining a thorough and more subtle understanding of just a few people will lead to more general understanding of others.

The third approach to research is known as the **hermeneutic** approach. Hermeneutic research is concerned with meaning – the meanings in social living, the meanings we place on our experience, the meanings we encounter during everyday life. Meanings occur on a number of levels: conscious, unconscious, personal, social, cultural and socio-political. Hermeneutic researchers investigate how people interpret their experience, and how various forms of symbolism are used to convey meaning in human life.

Each of these perspectives goes about studying human beings in a slightly different way. They ask different questions, and utilise different research techniques. For example, the nomothetic approach tends to emphasise the general similarities of human beings, and looks for cause-and-effect mechanisms in human behaviour. The idiographic approach, by contrast, emphasises uniqueness, exploring the way that each individual person, or each social situation, is distinctive and special. The hermeneutic approach takes a third route: examining the symbolic nature of much human experience, and attempting to understand human behaviour in those terms. It is primarily concerned with the meanings of human behaviour, and the way that our understanding of those meanings shapes and colours human interactions.

What do these three terms mean?

nomothetic

idiographic

hermeneutic

The evolution of psychological research

The three different perspectives in psychological research have largely come about because of the way that psychological methodology has evolved. Psychology has gone through many different phases in its history, and each of these has left its mark on psychological methodology. In the earliest days of psychology, for example, psychologists used qualitative methods almost exclusively, and some areas of psychology such as clinical neuropsychology continued to use it throughout the whole of the twentieth century.

For many psychologists, though, the behaviourist influence which dominated experimental psychology in the middle of the twentieth century left a powerful legacy of prejudice against qualitative methods. The behaviourist school was intolerant of many aspects of psychological knowledge. In fact, it was a classic example of a **modernist** theory, promoting what it regarded as the one 'scientific' approach for all of psychology, ignoring the past, and rejecting all other approaches as inadequate or unscientific.

For example, the behaviourists dismissed psychological research into the workings of the mind – what we now know as cognitive psychology – because they argued that the mind could not be observed directly, and was therefore not open to scientific investigation. The existence of the mind, they argued, was always inferred from behaviour, and it was behaviour which psychologists should be studying.

> **What do these three terms mean?**
>
> *behaviourist*
>
> *cognitive*
>
> *methodology*

As the century progressed, psychologists gradually managed to break free from this approach. They demonstrated that it was perfectly possible to study mental attributes scientifically (although they did call them 'cognitive' attributes, rather than 'mental' ones, to avoid association with the behaviourists' earlier diatribes against 'unscientific' research). By the 1980s, cognitive psychology had become a thriving, even dominant, part of the psychological mainstream.

The behaviourist legacy worked on many levels, though. Obvious influences like that could be recognised and challenged. But their methodological approach was more insidious. Even after behaviourism was no longer regarded as a major influence in psychology, the behaviourist view that only numbers and quantitative analysis were appropriately 'scientific' remained. It didn't matter that lots of the other sciences used qualitative methods of analysis: the behaviourists had taken physics as their ideal science, on which psychology should be modelled, and for them this implied that all scientific analysis should take the form of numbers.

This wasn't the case across the whole of psychology: psychologists studying brain functions or other clinical projects often used qualitative analysis, and so did studies of child development. But mainstream psychology became dominated by the idea that only numerical results

---

Rigid assumptions

The behaviourist insistence that only quantitative data counted as valid created a stranglehold on many research projects. One of the most dramatic examples was the effect it had on the research into Genie, the child who was found at thirteen years of age without any language experience. The researchers conducted a tremendously detailed study, collecting many hours of video- and audio-taped recordings, and looking at the way that Genie's linguistic and social development was progressing as she became accustomed to her foster-family. There were many dramatic changes, as she gradually learned the basis of social functioning, and developed some language abilities. But the data the researchers collected were all qualitative, and they had very few options for converting them into numerical data which could be analysed statistically (Curtiss 1977).

As a result, the researchers were unable to demonstrate 'scientifically' how the project was progressing, and how much they were learning from it. In a modern research project, they would have had no problem demonstrating Genie's progress, but this was the late 1960s when the behaviourist influence was at its height. The funding for the research project was ended because of the perceived lack of results, and Genie was returned to the care of the social service department. They placed her in a situation where she was again subjected to physical and social abuse. All the linguistic and social progress she had made during the two years of the research project disappeared. She deteriorated rapidly, and died a couple of years later.

---

were really scientific, and that other types of information shouldn't really be regarded as valid at all.

Over time, however, the narrow 'quantitative only' approach became whittled away, as psychological researchers recognised that there was more to understanding research outcomes than numbers alone. Cognitive researchers began to use techniques such as **protocol analysis**, which is a form of qualitative analysis that we will be looking at in Chapter 13, to explore the ways that research participants reasoned as they carried out problem-solving tasks; and other psychologists too began to ask their research participants questions and take into account how they were thinking about what they were doing.

There were several major sources which encouraged these developments. One of them was the advent of explicitly feminist psychological research in the late 1980s. The feminists challenged the conventional received wisdom of psychological methodology, arguing that it was positivistic and sterile, and emphasising the importance of human

EXERCISE 1.2   Nomothetic, idiographic or hermeneutic?

Sort the following examples of psychological studies according to whether they are most likely to adopt a nomothetic, idiographic or hermeneutic approach.

A biographical study of a famous athlete

A study of the age of onset of menopause in modern women

A phenomenological investigation of six elderly gardeners and their relationship with their gardens

A study looking at how retired people are portrayed in TV dramas

A study of exam stress focusing on a small set of high-achieving, high-anxiety students

A case study of a woman's experience of pregnancy

An exploration of mythical beliefs about examinations

A study of the exam revision practices of A-level students

An experimental investigation of the effects of massed or spaced practice among basketball players

An investigation of the perceived images of various sports held by teenagers

An exploration of images of women in magazine advertisements

An investigation of time spent in hobbies by men aged between 40 and 60

What do these three terms mean?

feminist research

ethical issues

real-world research

---

meanings and experience for psychological research. The exemplars given by feminist researchers showed those psychologists who were open to the new ideas how such research could be both rigorous and meaningful, without having to depend on statistical number-crunching for its rigour and academic acceptability.

There were other pressures, too, which were developing in psychological research. One of them was for an increased recognition of ethical issues, and the way that these required researchers to stop regarding their research participants as material to be manipulated, and to begin regarding them as human beings with the right to make their own choices. This recognition of choice led investigators to begin seeing research participants in a different way, and that led to a need for data-analysis techniques which could respect research participants as human beings with ideas, opinions and emotions.

The growing interest in ethical issues also led to the development of guidelines and principles for psychological researchers. The conscious rejection of a researcher's entitlement to manipulate the 'subject' without their consent led many to re-evaluate their research questions, and to adopt alternative methodologies such as account analysis, since these were more able to express respect for the participant.

Research funding, as always, played its part too. Psychological research projects became increasingly funded by agencies and commercial bodies, rather than by research councils, and this meant that researchers needed to demonstrate the real-world applicability of their research projects. Even the research councils began to emphasise commercial and social relevance to research funding, and, as a result, psychologists became increasingly interested in approaches to research which could be shown to be meaningful and relevant. There was a growing interest in ecological validity and real-world research, and that was accompanied by a recognition that qualitative methods were often more suited to real-world research projects than quantitative approaches.

By the 1990s, psychologists as a whole were beginning to recognise explicitly that qualitative methods could also be a valid approach to data analysis. A number of books and papers appeared on the subject, and various groups set about challenging the prejudice against this type of research on the part of the psychological 'establishment' – journal editors, PhD examiners and the like. The time was evidently right for such a development, because the progress was very evident. As we are seeing in this book, qualitative methods are now acknowledged as the other side of the psychological tool-kit. They work together with, and complement, quantitative analytical techniques, and in the rest of this book we will be exploring both.

Modern psychology, in my view, is reaching a very healthy situation. It has become able to encompass both research extremes, and a wide range of choices in between. In the first part of this book, we look at psychological research methods; but in the second, we will be looking at both quantitative and qualitative ways of analysing research data. For a student of psychology, just as much as for a research psychologist, the important thing is that the form of analysis should be appropriate to the data that have been collected and to the topic which is being investigated. And to ensure that is the case, all psychologists need be aware of a range of research methods and analytical techniques, which they can adopt if their material requires it.

In the next chapter, we will be looking at some of the specific issues which arise when we gather data as part of psychological research. We'll be looking at the constraints of sampling; at problems of ecological validity and the ways that people act in accordance with what they believe the researcher wants of them; and, in particular, at the ethical challenges thrown up by psychological research.

Self-assessment questions

1. *What is meant by the term 'levels of explanation', and how is it relevant to psychological research?*

2. *When might an inductive approach to psychological research be more appropriate than a hypothetico-deductive one?*

3. *What is meant by a positivist approach to research?*

4. *How do nomothetic, idiographic and hermeneutic research differ?*

5. *What problems can arise from adopting a strictly quantitative approach to psychological research?*

Concepts in use

1. *How might the concept of levels of explanation be useful to a group of research psychologists studying exam stress?*

2. *Describe a practical situation where the hypothetico-deductive approach would be the most appropriate way of conducting a piece of psychological research, and a practical situation where an inductive approach would be preferable.*

3. *Taking the particular topic of emotion, describe how a positivistic approach to studying it would be different from an anti-positivist approach.*

4. *Give a specific example of a nomothetic research study, a specific example of an idiographic research study, and a specific example of a hermeneutic research study. If you like, you can draw your examples from your knowledge of existing psychological research.*

5. *Imagine that you are conducting a major research project investigating people's leisure activities. Give an example of one part of the project in which quantitative data would be most appropriate, and one part in which qualitative data would be preferable.*

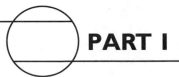

PART I

Gathering data

The aim of this book is to provide a reasonably comprehensive introduction to the basis of psychological research. To this end, it is divided into two parts. Part I is concerned with gathering data, while Part II addresses the way that we go about analysing it.

Part I begins by exploring some of the general issues about data collection, and the way that different approaches to scientific research lead us to collect data in different ways. From there, we will go on to look at different research methods, and at the types of things we need to be careful of when we are carrying them out. We will be looking at experiments, exploring issues of experimental control, variables, field and laboratory experiments. We will also look at observational studies, exploring issues concerned with behavioural sampling and recording, and with different types of observation, such as laboratory and ethological observations, epidemiology, and diary methods.

The section will continue with a look at how questionnaires are used in psychology, exploring the tricky matters of questionnaire design and the effects of different types of questions. This will lead us into psychometrics, where we will look at the process of test construction and the important issues of reliability, validity, and standardisation. Interviewing is another essential research method for modern psychologists, and we will be looking at interview schedules, interviewer effects, and the different types of interview such as structured and rapport interviewing.

Those methods are largely independent of one another; but often, psychologists will use case-study methods to gather data, applying several different techniques to understanding one particular case. This leads us into the process of triangulation, in which a psychologist can use several different types of measurement. We'll also be looking at idiographic measures – measures which are not for comparing people with one another, but for looking in depth at one person's own characteristics. And we will be looking at the research method known as meta-analysis, which psychologists use to make sense out of a series of different, independent studies which have all been investigating a particular phenomenon.

By the end of Part I, the reader should have obtained a fair idea of the range of methods in psychology, and a reasonable methodological 'tool-kit' which can be applied to student research projects of different kinds. There is, of course, more specialised information available on each of these methods, and following up the references given in the text will lead someone requiring more advanced or detailed knowledge into the relevant literature. These references are provided in full at the end of the book.

2

Gathering data for psychological research

Sampling
The participant as agent
Ethics and practicality

In this chapter, we will be looking at some of the issues which arise when we are aiming to gather data from human beings. These issues range from the problems of sampling groups of research participants, to looking at the kinds of problems which occur because our participants are thinking, co-operative human beings, to looking at the ethical considerations which need to be addressed in modern psychology.

As we will be seeing in the next few chapters, there are a number of different techniques that psychologists use to gather data, ranging from experiments to case studies and diary methods. Sometimes we use these as **idiographic** techniques, which means, as we saw in the last chapter, that their focus is on describing individuality – the distinctive characteristics of one person or one particular group. More often, though, psychological research is **nomothetic** – that is, it is trying to look at what groups of people have in common, in the hope that this will allow us to identify general principles, or laws, about human behaviour. In that type of research, it is vitally important that the group of people who are being studied are reasonably typical of other people too. And that brings us into the extremely important area of sampling.

Sampling

Sampling is the process of collecting the set of research participants who will provide the data for a psychological research project. You might wonder why we refer to such a collection of people as a **sample**, rather than as a 'set', or 'group', or any other such word. But there is a good reason for this. It's because it really is a sample – a small amount obtained just for testing purposes. It isn't the whole amount of people who the study might possibly apply to – that simply wouldn't be practical. Rather, we obtain a sample of people, and try to make sure that they are reasonably typical of the type of people that we are interested in.

The whole group that we are interested in is known as the **population**. A population, in psychological terms, means all of the relevant individuals for that particular topic of interest. If we were interested in teenage drinking habits, for example, our population would be teenagers. If we were interested in the psychology of retirement, our population would be people of retirement age or older. If we were interested in forms of dyslexia, our population would be all people who might be categorised as dyslexic.

Obviously, when you are carrying out psychological research, you can't test the whole population. Even if you thought you had tested every single dyslexic in a particular country, there would still be some who you had missed out – and then there would be dyslexics from other countries as well. And in any case, nobody would have a research budget large enough for that size of research project. So psychologists carrying out nomothetic research try to obtain a sample from the population – a set of people to participate in their research who will be reasonably representative of the rest.

Representative sampling

So far so good; but it's the idea of a **representative sample** that really causes the trouble. Just taking anyone from the population can mean that the sample becomes biased. For example, suppose you wanted to know what the general public thought about the idea of extra-sensory perception (ESP). You want to ask the general public rather than academics or students, so you decide to obtain your sample by advertising in mainstream newspapers. That would make it more typical of the general public than just asking students or academics, but it still wouldn't guarantee that your sample was truly representative of the population as a whole – mainly because it would be the people who were most interested in the topic who would be most likely to respond to your advert. And it is very likely indeed that they would include a higher proportion of 'believers' in ESP than was typical of the general population.

As a result, we need to obtain samples in other ways, in order to tackle the idea of representativeness. There are two ways that psychologists try to make sure that samples are typical of their populations. One is through size, and the other is by using specific sampling techniques.

What do these three terms mean?
population
representative sample
extreme scores

The size of the sample is important, because small groups are much more open to distortion than large ones. In a small group, each individual has quite a lot of influence on the overall pattern which results from the scores. Someone who is near the extreme in a particular measure can pull the total scores up or down a great deal if there are only a few people in the group. In a large group, having someone near the extreme doesn't matter nearly as much because the effect of all of the other scores will mean that the influence of that single score isn't so big.

Having said that, what counts as a large sample in psychological research has changed a great deal over the past thirty years. In the 1970s and before, a sample of 40 or so participants was considered to be 'large'. Nowadays, it would be considered to be quite small, because psychologists are able to deal with sample sizes in the thousands, or even tens of thousands. The difference isn't because the participants have changed, but because the technology has. In the 1970s and before, calculations were mainly done by hand, or using hand-calculators. It was possible to book computer time on large mainframe computers for important projects, but these were rare and involved large research budgets. Later in that decade, and through the 1980s, computers became much more widespread, until all research psychologists became able to analyse samples with very large numbers. As a result, ideas about small and large samples gradually changed.

The other side of obtaining representative samples, which really needs to go hand in hand with adequate sample sizes, is the use of specific **sampling techniques**. The four main kinds are summarised in Table 2.1, but they are discussed in more detail in Chapter 5, so if you

Table 2.1 Specific sampling techniques

random sampling	Everyone in the population has an equal chance of being selected.
quota sampling	The population is sorted into categories, with a proportionate number of people being taken from each category. So the sample comes to resemble the population in terms of the proportion of category numbers it contains.
stratified sampling	The population is divided into layers, or strata, (the most common of which is social class) with an appropriate number of participants from each layer.
opportunity sampling	The researcher uses whatever participants are available at the time that the research is being conducted.

(See chapter 5 for more details about these sampling techniques.)

What do these three terms mean?

random sampling

opportunity sampling

quota sampling

are interested in finding out more about them than is given in the table, you should turn to that chapter and read that section – there isn't much point in saying it all again here.

Overall, though, random sampling is considered to be by far the most desirable sampling method because, assuming that the sample is large enough, it is most likely to contain all of the characteristics of the population. The last one on the list – opportunity sampling – is the least desirable because it is the most open to bias and distortion;

But is it really random?

One of the traditional approaches to random sampling, described in the older textbooks, was to take the population list and select an arbitrary number using a chance technique or calculated according to the size of the population and the sample size required. The arbitrary number would then be applied throughout the population to see who would participate. For example, if the number was eight, then every eighth name on the list would be selected. In recent years, though, researchers have argued that this is not truly random sampling, since taking every eighth name automatically means that people who come ninth, eleventh or anywhere else in the sequence are excluded. So they don't have an 'equally likely' chance of being selected.

The issue is really about when the definition of random sampling is applied, during the sampling process. In the 1960s and 1970s, it was assumed that the definition – that every member of the population had an equally likely chance of being selected – applied only at the beginning of the sampling process. Once it had begun, then the technique which had been adopted would automatically exclude some people – in this example, those who did not appear tenth, twentieth, etc. on the list; but the important thing was that they had an equally likely chance of being selected at the beginning. More recently, though, some writers have taken the view that the random principle should apply throughout the sampling process, rather than just at the beginning. So where a sample used to be considered random if participants were selected on the basis of an arbitrary ranking, nowadays more elaborate procedures are required.

In reality, of course, it makes very little difference. To most psychologists, the question of randomness isn't important in itself. It is important as a means to an end – because it allows the researcher to feel more confident that the sample they have obtained is typical of the population. A random sample was considered important because it was not likely to introduce a systematic bias into the sampling data. Neither approach is likely to do that, and even those proposing the more recent argument admit that, in practice, any statistical difference between the two techniques is negligible.

but in practice it is used by a great many researchers. It is surprising (and slightly worrying), for example, to read through the journals and discover just how many psychological research reports are based on data from undergraduate psychology students. It also begs the question of whether they are really typical of people in general.

We will be coming back to the idea of the representative sample in Chapter 5, and also in Chapter 14, when we look at some of the fundamental principles underlying the use of statistical techniques in psychology. Many, if not most, of the statistical techniques which psychologists use are based on the assumption that the samples which are being used in the research are reasonably typical of their populations. They take that information into account, and go on to make inferences about how likely those results are to occur. So typicality, or representativeness in sampling, is a fundamental aspect of psychological research, and one which influences how we carry out most kinds of psychological study.

Sampling isn't vital in all psychological research, though. There are some kinds of study in which it is much less of an issue. Studies which adopt an idiographic approach – we discussed idiographic studies in the last chapter – are generally concerned with exploring the experiences of specific individuals; and in those cases, obtaining groups of people who are typical of the population as a whole is largely irrelevant. Similarly, hermeneutic studies are concerned with meanings and symbols, and are often less concerned with typicality than nomothetic research. So it is important to remember that although representative sampling is fundamental to some kinds of psychological research, not every psychological research project is aiming to obtain results which provide general laws or principles which will apply to large groups of people.

The participant as agent

What may be even more important in psychological research is the way that some research methods don't take into account how human beings are active agents, rather than just passive experimental material. Psychological methodology in the first half of the twentieth century, and particularly behaviourist methodology, was modelled on a highly idealised view of what physics research was like – experimenting on inert matter, getting consistent results time after time, and so on. Anyone who has discussed these things with real research physicists knows that the reality of physics research isn't actually anything like that definite, but the idealised model is very pervasive throughout science, and it was this which psychologists aimed to emulate.

The problem, though, is that psychology's subject matter isn't inert. Gradually, through the 1960s and 1970s, psychologists came to recognise how the fact that their research material is people rather than minerals makes a great deal of difference to their research. We looked at some of the outcomes of this realisation in the last chapter, when we looked at idiographic and hermeneutic research methodologies. But even within the standard nomothetic research paradigm, there were challenges which occurred.

Some of those challenges to psychological methodology came up when psychologists began to recognise the importance of demand characteristics and self-fulfilling prophecies in psychological research. These processes raise questions about how typical the results obtained by experimenters are, and lead us into all sorts of questions about how far we can really trust our research findings. They do this not by challenging the way the data have been handled, but by challenging the **validity** of the information which has been collected in the first place.

Validity, as we will see in Chapter 6, is all about whether something really measures what it is supposed to measure. For many decades, psychologists assumed that they could study human beings by treating them as experimental 'subjects'. They assumed that they were passive, simply doing what was expected of them, and not influencing the outcomes in any personal way at all. Any behaviours which they observed when conducting their experiments would purely be the result of the experimental variable that they were manipulating, and nothing else.

> **What do these three terms mean?**
>
> *demand characteristics*
>
> *self-fulfilling prophecies*
>
> *validity*

Demand characteristics

That assumption was challenged by two major findings, both of which occurred at about the same time. The first of these resulted from a research project conducted by Martin Orne, in 1962. Orne was trying to see whether he could discover any differences in behaviour between people who had been 'hypnotised' – that is, people who believed that they had been hypnotised – and those who were simply pretending to be. Orne asked them to do a variety of tasks, and found that it wasn't possible to distinguish between the two groups at all. But more importantly, he found that people who believed they were taking part in a psychological experiment acted in ways that were entirely different from the way that they would act in everyday life.

In one part of the study, participants were asked to add up columns of numbers presented to them on a sheet of paper. When they had finished the sum, they then had to tear up the paper, throw it away, and add the numbers on a second sheet. When they had finished that, they were to tear it up and do a third, and so on. Orne found that in the normal run of things, people would do one or two of these sheets, and then refuse to do any more. But if they believed that they were

EXERCISE 2.1   What's what?

Match the examples in list A to the appropriate technical terms in list B.

List A	*List B*
A professional runner included in a sample of research participants in a study of jogging and exercise	*demand characteristics*
Choosing your research participants by picking numbers from a hat, in which a number is included for every member of the population you are studying	*ethical guidelines*
Conducting an observational study of children's playground activities, in which the observers don't actually know what the object of the study is	*self-fulfilling prophecy*
Studies which emphasise a particular individual's experience, and so do not require special attention to be given to sampling	*representative sample*
Those features of a research project which provide people with cues as to how they ought to behave	*quota sampling*
Choosing research participants in such a way as to obtain six people from each major population category	*random sampling*
A group of research participants who are typical of the wider population which is being studied	*extreme score*
A statement about what is likely to happen, which comes true purely because it has become known to the researchers or participants in a study	*idiographic studies*
Ways of carrying out experiments so that every research participant gets exactly the same set of experiences	*double-blind control*
Ideas about how psychological studies should be carried out which are primarily concerned with what is right and wrong in psychological research	*standardised procedures*

taking part in a psychological experiment, they would continue indefinitely. One participant continued for over six hours, and eventually had to be stopped by the experimenter, who wanted to go home!

What this study did was to raise a number of questions about what Orne called the **demand characteristics** of the psychology experiment. People who are taking part in an experiment do so in a spirit of co-operation, and they want their results to be helpful to the experimenter – in much the same way that people who take part in hypnosis demonstrations don't want to 'spoil it' for the hypnotist (stage hypnotists are very good at spotting the ones who might take a different view, and not selecting them for the demonstration). As a result of this, they are overly co-operative, and this can mean that a psychology researcher ends up with data which are nothing at all like the data which would be obtained from people acting more normally.

Demand characteristics are features of the psychological study to which the participant responds, often unconsciously. Researchers often assume that their participants are naïve, doing what they are told without speculating as to what it is they are supposed to do. But people are often curious about what is going on, and very ready to pick up on subtle cues, from the design of the study itself, the setting in which it takes place, and the researcher in person. The psychology experiment (or observation, or other type of study) is an unusual situation, and people often respond to it by being on their 'best behaviour' and acting in the ways that they believe they are supposed to act.

Self-fulfilling prophecies

What do these three terms mean?
non-verbal cues
expectations
experimenter effects

Sensitivity to subtle cues also extends to sensitivity to the messages which are coming from the researcher. People pick up minute non-verbal cues which indicate what the experimenter expects to happen, and respond to these unconsciously. In fact, the cues which experimenters unconsciously communicate can even extend to animals, as emerged in the second study which dramatically challenged assumptions about psychological methodology.

In 1963, Rosenthal and Fode published a paper which showed that experimenter expectations could even communicate themselves to laboratory rats. They took two groups of rats, identical in all respects as far as they could establish, and allocated them to groups of students for experimental purposes (in those days, psychology students were expected to carry out at least one animal study, and this was often about maze-learning in laboratory rats). One group was told that their rats came from a special strain which was bred to be 'maze-bright', so they could be expected to learn the maze very quickly. The other students were told that their rats were 'maze-dull', and wouldn't be likely to learn very fast.

Although there was no difference between the rats in the first place, they performed quite differently in the experiment. The supposedly 'maze-bright' rats learned quickly, and completed the learning in just a couple of days. The supposedly 'maze-dull' rats took much longer to learn their task. Yet the only difference was in the expectations of the experimenters. Those expectations had become **self-fulfilling prophecies**, which had come true simply because they existed.

There wasn't anything magical about this. When Rosenthal and Fode looked at how it had happened, they found that those with 'maze-bright' rats had handled them more, given them more experience of the maze, and been more patient with early errors. Those with 'maze-dull' rats had been quite the opposite, so it wasn't really surprising that the first group learned more quickly. But what was much more important was the fact that the students were entirely unconscious of their treatment of the animals. They assumed that they had simply handled the animals professionally and objectively.

Rosenthal followed this up by a **field experiment** with school children, reported by Rosenthal and Jacobsen in 1968. A set of children were all given a standard intelligence test, and their teachers were told that it was a new test, able to detect 'spurters' – late-developing children who could be expected to start showing unusual gains in their schoolwork. Nothing was said to the children, but the teachers were allowed to overhear a conversation in which several children were explicitly named as being of this kind. When the researchers returned to the school a year later, they found those children had indeed improved dramatically. The teachers expected more of them, and as a result treated them differently, giving them more attention and encouragement. The children responded to these changed expectations with more interest and better work.

Experimenter effects

What Rosenthal had shown, then, was that the outcomes of psychological experiments could be dramatically affected by the expectations held by the experimenter. These **experimenter effects** could mean that an experimenter could unconsciously produce the outcomes they expected from an experiment, purely as a result of people responding to their subtle differences in behaviour. Researchers quickly showed that there were many kinds of experimenter effects occurring in psychological studies. People responded not just to the experimenter's expectations, but also to their gender, their ethnic background, their age and even their size! All of these affect the outcomes of a study. Moreover, experimenter effects were not limited to experiments. They occurred with observational studies, case studies and other types of psychological research, as well.

Clever Hans

Perhaps the most famous example of experimenter effects in psychology was the case of a counting horse, known as 'Clever Hans'. This horse could solve arithmetical puzzles that were presented to it, by striking the ground with its hoof the correct number of times. It was tested over and over again, and it was almost always correct. The owner made a living by exhibiting it as a sideshow attraction.

Eventually, Clever Hans came to the attention of a psychologist, Oskar Pfungst, who began to investigate what was going on. By a series of systematic experiments, ruling out one variable after another, Pfungst eventually discovered that the horse was taking its cues from the unconscious non-verbal signals given off by its owner – who was as mystified by its abilities as anyone else. But as the horse counted, the owner would be tense, hoping that it would reach the correct number; and when it did so he would relax, unconsciously, but enough so that the horse could detect it. (Horses are very sensitive to signs of tension, as any experienced rider will testify.) The horse would take that relaxation as a sign to stop its 'counting'. But the owner was entirely unaware that he was 'cueing' the horse, and it was not until Pfungst demonstrated that Hans could not do his sums unless he could see or feel his owner, that the mystery was uncovered.

What do these three terms mean?

standardised instructions

standardised procedures

double-blind control

There were a number of strategies designed to counteract experimenter effects, such as the use of **standardised instructions**, to make sure that the researcher always gave exactly the same instructions to each research participant; and the use of **standardised procedures** to make sure that every participant was treated in exactly the same way. These had some drawbacks, though, because if they were not well done, they managed to introduce a kind of robotic quality to many experimental procedures, and people responded differently to that, too.

The most common way of challenging this type of experimenter effect is to use what is known as a **double-blind control**. This is a situation where neither the participant nor the experimenter knows what is expected of them – they are 'blind' to the hypothesis. In this way, the experimenter cannot influence the results in one particular direction. Double-blind controls have become compulsory in all tests of new drugs, because the effect demonstrated by Rosenthal and later researchers was so powerful.

However, double-blind controls raise their own ethical problems. In the case of new drug testing, this particularly concerns the way that such trials always involve comparing the real drug with a **placebo** – an inert substance which looks like the drug but has no real effect – in order to separate the effect of the drug itself from the effects of being

EXERCISE 2.2   **Applying ethical guidelines**

Imagine that you are a psychology student, and want to conduct the following study:

The project involves asking someone, in a naturalistic setting, to show you how they shuffle a pack of cards. When they have shown you the first time, you ask them to show you again, and you continue this until they refuse to show you any more. You do the same thing with nine other people, making sure that it seems as if it is a causal conversation; and notice how many times each one will carry out the task before they get fed up.

Then you approach another ten people, again individually, and tell them you are conducting a psychological experiment about shuffling cards. Ask them to show you how they shuffle cards. Then ask them to show you again, and continue this until they refuse to do it any more. Do the 'psychological experiment' people continue for longer than the 'natural setting' group do?

Use the ATP ethical guidelines for psychology students to evaluate the proposed study. Ask yourself each of the following questions as if this were a study you wanted to carry out for your course assessment:

- What is the most ethical way of carrying out this study?
- Am I sufficiently competent to carry it out?
- Will I have informed the participants of all that they need and would expect to know before taking part?
- Will the participants have willingly agreed to take part?
- How will I ensure that all research records are confidential and anonymous, and will remain so?
- How will I ensure that my research is carried out professionally, and in a way that protects the rights of those involved?

When you have answered each of these, address the first question in the ATP guidelines:

- Should I be conducting this kind of study at all?

Explain your conclusions.

given medical treatment of any kind. But AIDS campaigners and others have argued that where the drug which is looked for might be a possible cure for a fatal disease, giving somebody a placebo amounts to sentencing them to certain death. Medical research is still struggling with the ethical problems which this raises.

Ethical issues in psychological research

There are other, less dramatic but also important, ethical concerns which arise from double-blind controls and other such manipulative strategies in psychological research. These reflect the growing import-ance of respect for the research participant which has emerged during the past two or three decades. Psychological studies before the 1970s were traditionally very manipulative, treating their participants as 'subjects', deceiving them, giving them little or no say in whether they would participate or not, and in some cases even causing physical or mental distress. Nowadays, however, the situation is very different.

There were a number of reasons for the change. One of them was the growing influence of the social responsibility of science movement, which challenged the idea of 'value-free' science on the grounds that science is always located within a social context and has social implica-tions. Psychology's explicit claims to be a science meant that it was not exempt from this type of influence.

Another reason was the wider economic context. The growth of consumer society brought with it a growing emphasis on the rights of the individual; and this too led to increasing pressure for psychology to clean up its act when it came to the way that it treated people. Concern with morals and ethics has arisen throughout modern society: it has become part of the current *Zeitgeist*. And it has been helped within psychology by the influence of the humanistic school, and also by the direct challenges to 'objective' and manipulative methodologies raised by feminist researchers and others.

The result is that professional psychologists in almost all countries are now bound by ethical codes of conduct; and psychological research is obliged to follow a strict set of ethical guidelines. In the USA, these guidelines are provided by the American Psychological Association. In the UK, they come from the British Psychological Society (BPS), and are summarised in Table 2.2. The UK also has special guidelines for psychology students carrying out research projects, which were drawn up by the Association for the Teaching of Psychology (ATP) and are stated in Table 2.3. The BPS guidelines are regulations, and they form part of the Code of Conduct to which all professional psychologists should adhere. The student guidelines, on the other hand, take the form of a series of questions which any student should be able to answer about a project they are about to carry out. They are intended to guide students into considering the ethical issues which are raised by any psychological study.

Overriding all of these specific points is the question of respect for the psychological participant. That respect is manifest in a number of different ways: by the way that it is no longer acceptable to deceive people, or at least not without their permission; by the care that has

---

What do these three terms mean?

research participant

social responsibility of science

ethical guidelines

Table 2.2 Ethical guidelines for research with human beings

1. Investigators must always consider ethical implications and psychological consequences for research participants.

2. Investigators should inform participants of the objectives of the research and gain their informed consent.

3. Withholding information or misleading participants is unacceptable. Intentional deception should be avoided.

4. Participants must be fully debriefed, so they can complete their understanding of the nature of the research

5. Investigators must emphasise the subject's right to withdraw from the experiment at any time.

6. All data obtained must be treated as confidential unless otherwise agreed in advance.

7. Investigators must protect participants from physical and mental harm during or arising from investigations.

8. Studies based on observation must respect the privacy and psychological well-being of the people studied.

9. Investigators must exercise care in giving advice on psychological problems.

10. Investigators share responsibility for ethical treatment, and should encourage others to rethink their ideas if necessary.

Source: Adapted from British Psychological Society (1990).

Table 2.3 Ethical guidelines for students carrying out psychological research

Students who are about to carry out a psychological research project need to evaluate it using the following questions:

- Should I be conducting this kind of study at all?
- What is the most ethical way of carrying out this study?
- Am I sufficiently competent to carry it out?
- Have I informed the participants of all that they need and would expect to know before taking part?
- Have the participants willingly agreed to take part?
- How do I ensure that all research records are confidential and anonymous, and will remain so?
- How do I ensure that my research is carried out professionally, and in a way that protects the rights of those involved?

Source: Association for the Teaching of Psychology Ethical Guidelines for Psychology Students.

to be taken to ensure that people do not experience any form of distress; through the emphasis on the participant's right to know what is going on; and through the emphasis on their entitlement to withdraw from the study at any time if they feel so inclined.

Although initially a few researchers argued that the restrictions made it impossible to conduct psychological research properly, most researchers have actually found little difficulty in conducting psychological research which can conform readily to their ethical responsibilities. There is, after all, an argument that manipulating people may not be the best way of learning about their behaviour anyway; and many researchers are of the view that the ethics movement has enriched psychological methodology rather than weakened it.

Different research methods, of course, raise different ethical questions. When we look at each of the different research methods in this book, we will consider their distinctive ethical implications, and the things that researchers using those methods need to be particularly aware of. But no research method which deals with people is free of ethical implications, and any research which involves people needs to be conducted in a proper and defensible way. In most universities nowadays, research psychologists submit research outlines to an ethics committee which appraises the ethical implications of the project and ensures that all of these considerations have been met.

Animal studies

We will not be looking at animal experiments in this book. They raise their own ethical implications, and have their own set of ethical guidelines, which are summarised in Table 2.4. But this is essentially a book about research methodology for psychology students, and the days when all psychology students were obliged to carry out an animal study are, thankfully, long gone. Any student who aims to carry out such research would need to do so under very close supervision, and in those universities which do allow it, it is usually the case that the student only designs the study, and it is carried out by experienced and approved animal researchers. Animal studies are not for those who are only learning, because the risk of harm or distress to the animal caused by inexperience or lack of knowledge is much too great.

In any case, of course, there is a much smaller proportion of modern psychology which rests on animal data. Psychological research has become much more rounded, methodologically speaking, than it used to be, and so it is more capable of investigating the complexities of human social and cognitive experience. Under behaviourism, such experience was entirely discounted, since it was thought that everything came down to stimulus–response learning in the end. That, of course,

Table 2.4 Ethical guidelines for psychologists conducting research on animals

---

1. The law
Researchers are obliged to abide by the laws protecting animals, as outlined in the Universities Federation for Animal Welfare handbook.

2. Ethical considerations
If the animals are confined, constrained, harmed or stressed in any way the investigator must consider whether the knowledge to be gained justifies the procedure . . . experiments must not be done simply because it is possible to do them. Alternatives to animal experiments should also be considered.

3. Species
Wherever research involves confining animals or the use of procedures likely to cause pain or discomfort, the researchers should bear in mind that members of some species may suffer less than others, and should choose the species accordingly.

4. Number of animals
Laboratory studies should use the smallest number of animals necessary. This can often be greatly reduced by good experimental design and the use of appropriate statistical tests.

5. Endangered species
Members of endangered species should not be collected or manipulated in the wild except as part of a serious attempt at conservation.

6. Animal suppliers
Animals should be obtained only from reputable suppliers and full records kept of their provenance and laboratory history.

7. Caging and social environment
Caging conditions should take into account the social behaviour of the species: an acceptable density of animals of one species may constitute overcrowding for a different species, while in social animals caging in isolation may have undesirable effects.

8. Fieldwork
Fieldworkers should disturb the animals they study as little as possible, since even simple observations on wild animals can have marked effects on their breeding and survival.

9. Aggression and predation, including infanticide
The fact that pain and injury may come to animals in the wild is not a defence for allowing it to occur in the laboratory. Wherever possible, field studies of natural encounters should be used in preference to staged encounters, and if the latter are thought to be necessary, the use of models or animals behind glass should be considered.

10. Motivation
When arranging schedules of deprivation the experimenter should consider the animal's normal eating and drinking habits and its metabolic

Table 2.4   *continued*

requirements. Also, differences between species must be borne in mind: a short period of deprivation for one species may be unacceptably long for another.

11. Aversive stimulation and stressful procedures
Procedures that cause pain or distress to animals are illegal in the UK unless the experimenter holds a Home Office licence and the relevant certificates. The experimenter should be satisfied that there are no alternative ways of conducting the experiment without the use of aversive stimulation. If alternatives are not available the investigator has the responsibility of ensuring that any suffering is kept to a minimum.

12. Surgical and pharmacological procedures
Such procedures should only be performed by experienced staff, and it is a particular responsibility of senior staff to train and supervise others. Experimenters must be familiar with the technical aspects of anaesthesia, and appropriate steps should be taken to prevent post-operative infection in chronic experiments. In pharmacological procedures experimenters must be familiar with the literature on the behavioural effects and toxicity of the drugs being used.

13. Anaesthesia, analgesia and euthanasia
The experimenter must ensure that animals receive adequate post-operative care, and that, if there is any possibility of post-operative suffering, this is minimised by suitable nursing and the use of local anaesthetics where appropriate. Regular monitoring of the animal's condition is essential, and if at any time an animal is found to be suffering severe and enduring pain it must be killed (also a requirement of a Home Office licence). Established procedures must be strictly followed for euthanasia, since methods vary from species to species.

14. Independent advice
If an experimenter is ever in any doubt about the condition of an animal, a second opinion should be obtained, preferably from a qualified veterinarian, and always from someone not directly involved in the experiments concerned.

15. Further enquiries
Any researcher uncertain about any aspect of their research with animals should direct enquiries to the appropriate professional bodies.

Source: Adapted from the British Psychological Society Code of Conduct and Ethical Principles for Psychologists

was why the behaviourists considered studies of animal learning to be so important. But few modern psychologists would agree with this point of view, so the relevance of such studies to our understanding of people is now much smaller.

Ethological animal studies, of course, are another matter. Ethological studies are studies of behaviour in the natural environment, and those follow many of the principles of observational studies which we look at in Chapter 4. In fact, Chapter 4 does deal with animal observations as well as human ones, and should provide enough of a basic understanding of these issues for someone who is conducting that sort of study. But such studies should only be conducted by students under close supervision, since the risk of disturbing the animals concerned purely through inexperience is high.

How far one can generalise from animal observation to human psychology is, of course, a matter for debate, and one which has generated heated arguments. It is not really practical to explore them here, but I have looked at some of these arguments in another book (Hayes 1995) if you are particularly interested. For the rest of this one, however, we will be looking at how psychologists go about carrying out research with human beings, beginning with the thorny challenges of experimental methods.

 ### Self-assessment questions

1. *Why does the representativeness of a sample matter in a psychological study?*

2. *What are the main kinds of sampling techniques?*

3. *How can the effects of extreme scores be minimised in a psychological study?*

4. *What is meant by the phrase 'the participant as agent'?*

5. *In psychological methodology, what is the difference between a 'subject' and a 'research participant'?*

 ### Concepts in use

1. *How might the concept of demand characteristics be useful to a group of research psychologists studying attractiveness?*

2. *Describe a practical situation in which a self-fulfilling prophecy is likely to be taking place. How could you study this situation psychologically?*

3. *Taking the particular topic of co-operation, describe how a behaviourist approach to studying it would be different from a broader psychological approach.*

4. *Describe three different studies conducted by psychological researchers before 1980, which illustrate a disregard of ethical issues. Choose your examples so that each one illustrates disregard of a different ethical criterion from the BPS ethical guidelines.*

5. *Parapsychologists investigating different aspects of ESP have to be careful to control for experimenter expectations. Why is this? How might experimenter expectations influence experimental findings in this context?*

3

Experiments

Designing experiments
Experimental variables
Types of experiments
Ethics of experimentation

In this chapter, we are looking at the research method known as the **experiment**. Experiments have rather a special place in psychology, because they are the only research methods which directly explore causality – in other words, because they can allow us to sort out whether something is really causing something else to happen. Other research methods may suggest that something is causing something else, but they can't really tell us for sure that it is.

The problem, though, is that investigating causality isn't that straightforward, particularly when you are trying to investigate causality in human beings or animals. There are all sorts of ways that people (and animals) can be influenced, and also ways in which their own understanding of what is going on influences how they act. So experiments in psychology need to be rather elaborately designed, if they are really going to identify causes.

Hypothesis testing

One of the most important aspects of experiments as a research method is the way that they are always designed to test a **hypothesis**. Experimental studies generally adopt the **hypothetico-deductive** approach to research which we looked at in Chapter 1. This means that they aim to investigate a **theory** – some kind of general explanation for why something happens. The aim of an experiment, ideally, is to gain evidence which will support that theory, or which will challenge it.

So one of the first things we need to do if we are about to conduct an experiment is to sort out the hypotheses which it will be investigating. Any one theory can give rise to several different hypotheses, which, as we saw in Chapter 1, are predictions about what is likely to happen in particular circumstances if the theory is true. An experimental investigation proceeds by testing out an experimental hypothesis (or sometimes more than one), to see if it holds up in real life.

This means that an experimental hypothesis takes the form of an 'if–then' prediction: '*if* the theory is true, *then* under these conditions, this will happen'. It is about identifying a specific implication of the theory, which can be explored or tested. So, for example, *if* it is true that overcrowding leads to aggression, *then* if I ask children to play in a small and crowded room, they should play more aggressively. Or, *if* noise stops people concentrating, *then* if I ask people to concentrate in a noisy room, they will not do it very well. In summary, then, when we do an experiment, we begin by identifying an experimental hypothesis, and then we set up situations which will allow us to test it.

Incidentally, at the same time we tend to identify a **null hypothesis** for the study. Effectively, the null hypothesis summarises what is likely to be the case if the theory isn't true. But it has to be very precisely phrased, because it serves an important role when we come to analysing our findings, and making sure that they haven't just come about because of chance or coincidence. We will be exploring the null hypothesis when we look at the basic principles of quantitative analysis in Chapter 14.

Once we have identified our hypothesis – or hypotheses if there are more than one – we are in a position to carry out the experiment. We know the prediction we want to test, and we know why we want to test it. So we set up a practical way of testing that prediction. In an experiment, this takes the form of at least two **conditions** – one where we do something which we hope will produce a result, and the other which is almost the same in every other respect, but doesn't include that crucial something. If the thing we have set up really does produce a different result, and we are sure that nothing else is influencing our findings, then we conclude that we have identified causality – the thing we were looking at really does cause the result to happen.

This, as I said before, makes experiments rather special. Other research methods in psychology can gather data in various ways, but experiments are the only method we have of isolating causes. There are good and bad sides to this, of course. The good side is the way that it allows us to tease out specific factors, and to be much more definite about what we are investigating; but the bad side is that concentrating on single causes can often blind us to the complexities of human experience, and the way that we generally have several different causes for any one human experience, all happening at once and working together. Nonetheless, a sound knowledge of experimental design is a fundamental part of the psychologist's research tool-kit.

Designing experiments

An experiment, then, is a research technique in which events or circumstances are deliberately manipulated in order to make something happen. But being certain that something has really happened isn't as obvious as it might seem. People have a wonderful ability to see what they expect to see, and to forget what things were like before. If you set up an experiment to investigate aggression and overcrowding, for example, it would be very easy for your experimenters to exaggerate how aggressive the children in the overcrowded room were being. And that could happen without anybody concerned realising what they were doing: it's a completely unconscious process.

We get round this problem by designing the experiment in such a way that it will give us 'baseline' information, that we can use for comparison, as well as information from the condition that we are interested in. Sometimes, we obtain that 'baseline' information by having the same people do the study in different conditions. One of those conditions will be designed to give us a measure of 'normal' behaviour, and that is known as a **control condition**. The control condition needs to be carefully arranged to make sure that the information which it gives us will really show up any differences between the research participants' 'baseline' ways of behaving, and how they act during the experimental condition.

Sometimes it isn't practical for the same people to participate in a control condition and an experimental condition, so we obtain our 'baseline' comparison information from a different group of people instead. This is called a **control group**. The problem with control groups, though, is that everyone is different. People have different backgrounds, different abilities, different ideas, different skills and different ways of reacting to situations. So control groups have to be carefully selected to make sure that the information they give us really can be compared with the information from the experimental group.

Randomisation

If we have a reasonably large number of people in each of the groups, we can try to make sure individual differences are not important by **randomising** which participants are in each group. This means sorting out who is in the experimental group and who is in the control group by using a method in which any research participant has an equal chance of being in either group. It doesn't matter what the method is – it could even be tossing a coin – as long as any research participant is equally likely to end up in any group once the selection is finished.

As long as there are enough research participants in the study, random allocation of them to the conditions of the experiment should

EXERCISE 3.1   Experimental control

Match the experimental problems in list A to the control procedures which would sort them out, in list B.

List A

1. The experimenter carrying out a drugs test knows which drug is expected to produce faster reaction times.

2. In a study involving several different experimental groups, the experimenter describes the task more clearly to some participants than to others.

3. The participants taking part in one condition of an experiment which involves solving maths problems are much better at maths than those taking part in the other condition; but the experimenter only has one set of problems available to use.

4. An experimenter has set up a complicated experiment involving different kinds of rewards given to children for reading books, but has no way of knowing how much the children would have been reading books anyway.

5. One of the conditions of an experiment takes place on a Friday morning, while the second condition takes place late on Friday afternoon. Participants mainly choose to take part in the morning session.

6. In a study of reading skills, some participants seem to be improving at the experimental task as a result of practice.

7. The participants in an experiment are very keen that the experiment should come out the way that the researcher wants it to.

8. In a complex experiment involving several different tasks, there is some variation between different experimenters as to the order in which the participants complete them.

9. The temperature of the experimental room varies from very hot to quite cold, in an experiment requiring close concentration from the participants.

10. An experiment investigating driving errors after the consumption of alcohol has better drivers in one condition than it has in the other.

List B

control group

standardised procedures

double-blind control

matched-participant design

standardised instructions

random allocation of participants to conditions

counterbalancing

repeated-measures design

standardised conditions

single-blind control

mean that any individual differences are averaged out between the two conditions. Some people, as we will see later in this chapter, believe that random allocation of research participants to conditions is essential in a true experiment; but not all researchers agree with this.

Repeated-measures designs

There are other ways of controlling for individual differences. The strongest way is to use the same research participants in the different conditions of our experiment. It is stronger, because that way we can make absolutely sure that individual differences and people's past experiences don't affect the study: because we are not comparing two different people. We compare the same person's score in each condition. This type of experimental design is known as a **repeated-measures design**, though you may also find it referred to in other books as a **related-measures design**, or a **correlated-subjects design**.

If we are using a repeated-measures design, we need to take great care that the way that we do the experiment doesn't affect our results. If we always ran the control condition first, for example, and then the experimental condition, we might find that our research participants were simply tired, or bored, or fed up, by the time they did the experimental condition. The same would apply if we always ran the experimental condition first, and then the control condition. Their results would be different, purely because of **order effects**.

EXERCISE 3.2   **Persuading the public**

Design an experiment which will enable you to compare how effective two different forms of publicity are in persuading people to switch to a more environmentally friendly lifestyle.

When you have done so, answer the following:

1. What is your null hypothesis?

2. What is your experimental hypothesis?

3. What is your independent variable?

4. What is your dependent variable?

5. Which possible confounding variables will you need to control, and how will you go about doing so?

We can control order effects by varying the sequence in which people do the different conditions of the experiment. We do this by **counterbalancing** them, so that half of the research participants do the control condition first, and the other half do the experimental condition first. If we have three conditions in the experiment – for example, if we have two different experimental conditions and a control condition – we need to arrange our conditions so that each condition comes first for a third of the participants. It gets even more complicated when we have three or more experimental conditions, but the basic principle is always the same: that the order in which each condition is presented to the participant must be balanced properly.

One of the most common ways of making sure variables are properly counterbalanced is to use what is known as an **ABBA design**. This doesn't mean singing or harmonising in tune (not a strong point for many psychologists). Rather, it refers to the way that the two conditions of an experiment are generally referred to as Condition A and Condition B. In an ABBA design, one trial of condition A is followed by two trials of condition B, and then by another one of condition A. In this way, order effects, particularly those caused by fatigue or boredom, are balanced out, because condition A has been both first and last – when the participant is freshest, and when she is most tired.

Sometimes, though, we can find **practice effects**, where someone gets better at a task as they learn how to do it. If it seems likely that most of the practice effects will happen during the first trial, and not during the second, third or fourth, then the ABBA design isn't enough on its own. In most cases of this type, the researcher will make sure that a second group of research participants experiences the conditions in the order BAAB, just to balance out this problem.

You might occasionally come across mention of an ABBA design in which each research participant only carried out two trials. In that case, what it means is that one group experienced condition A before condition B, while the second group experienced condition B before condition A. That isn't a pure ABBA design really, but the term has come to be used as shorthand for both types of counterbalancing.

A repeated-measures design, then, allows us to draw stronger conclusions about causality because it controls for individual differences; but it also means that we have to take special precautions to make sure that our research participants aren't unduly affected by practice effects or order effects. People learn during experiments, and often what they learn can have an influence on how they perform. We can sometimes control this by using counterbalancing and similar techniques. Sometimes, though, that just isn't possible and we have to turn to a design which involves comparing different people instead.

What do these three terms mean?

order effects

counterbalancing

ABBA design

Independent-measures designs

Independent-measures designs involve different people doing each condition of the study. This, as we have seen, can cause problems if there are systematic differences between the two groups of people, but there are ways that we can make sure that those differences are minimised as much as possible. We have already looked at one way, which is to use large groups and allocate them randomly to the two conditions, on the ground that the more people who are involved, the more individual differences should be averaged out.

Even when you have different groups, you still need to make sure that you have similar types of people in each group. For example, if your experimental group consisted of young people aged between 16 and 20 years, then you would need to make sure that your control group did too – after all, there wouldn't be much point using a control group of grandmothers aged between 50 and 70, would there?

Matching participants

But another option is to match up the two groups even more closely than that. A **matched-participant design** (these used to be called 'matched-subject designs', but we don't call people 'subjects' any more) does involve different people in the different conditions, but those people have been matched on important background factors which could be relevant to the study. For example, if five people in the experimental group were office workers, then five of the people in the control group would also need to be office workers, and really they should also be of the same sex, age and educational backgrounds.

In practice, matching participants is really quite difficult. It can also be quite expensive, because it takes time and money to locate people with the perfect characteristics. But a matched sample doesn't have to be matched for every possible characteristic – just those ones which are likely to affect the study. If it's an experiment which involves linguistic skills, then it's important that the experimental group and the control group should be matched for level of education, because differences in education could make a lot of difference. But if the experiment is about colour preference in different situations, educational level is less likely to be a factor, and if it's about physical skill learning then educational level would be even less so – although school experience with sports or PT would be relevant.

Matching participants, then, involves identifying personal characteristics which could influence the study, and making sure that those are the ones which are matched. It isn't often as simple as just matching for age and sex. In fact, it is quite common for modern psychological

---

Children's reading problems

Bryant and Bradley (1985) discussed the question of identifying relevant factors for matching in their book *Children's Reading Problems*. They pointed out that when researchers were investigating dyslexia, they tended to match their research participants with children who had the same mental age (calculated by looking at their age and intelligence scores). But Bradley and Bryant argued that this was not really adequate for comparison, because having reading problems could affect a child's life in a lot of ways, and there was no way of telling whether differences between the groups came from the dyslexia or from other factors.

In their own studies, Bryant and Bradley included another group, which was matched for reading age. Having a control group matched for intelligence, and one matched for reading age as well, allowed them to tease out even quite subtle effects, and also to explore which effects were really caused by the reading problems themselves.

---

studies to have several different control groups, each allowing the researchers to look at different aspects of the problem that they are studying. They are usually referred to as **comparison groups**, rather than control groups, but their purpose is the same.

What do these three terms mean?

independent-measures design

matched-participant design

comparison groups

Matched-participant designs can be tricky to arrange, but they have most of the advantages of a repeated-measures design, so they are worth doing if it is at all possible. The usual way of organising them is to arrange the complete set of research participants available for the experiment into pairs, matching them up as closely as possible. Then one person from each pair is allocated to the control group, and the other to the experimental group.

The ideal matched-participant design, of course, would consist of pairs of identical twins, with one twin from each pair in the control group and one in the experimental group. This is the strongest type of design of all, because it has the advantages of a repeated-measures design, but very few of the disadvantages. Since identical twins are so similar in so many respects, they are regarded as being the perfect matched sample. In fact, many researchers consider that results from twin studies of this sort can be treated as identical to those obtained from repeated-measures designs. There is some dispute about this, which is really all about how identical such twins really are; but it is usually regarded as acceptable to use statistical techniques for repeated-measures designs to analyse a twin study comparing identical twins.

Experimental variables

All experiments involve a number of variables. A variable, as its name implies, is something which varies – in other words, which changes its value. Table 3.1 gives examples of some different variables which might be involved in psychological experiments. If we look at these examples carefully, the first thing we notice is that they don't all vary in the same way. Some of them vary continuously – that is, in between their two extremes they can have lots of intermediate values. Lighting levels are a good example of this. It can be pitch dark, or it can be dazzlingly bright. But there are also lots of values in between: very dim, fairly dim, moderately bright, and so on. We could measure these values precisely, if we had the right equipment.

Table 3.1   Variables

1. The number of correct answers on a test

2. Experience in playing darts

3. Lighting levels

4. The selected picture from a set of four

5. Identification of countries by their silhouette shapes

6. The age of an experimenter

7. The sex of a research participant

8. Preference for different types of music

9. The temperature of a room

10. The colour of a book cover

Some of the variables in Table 3.1, though, can only vary in a much more restricted way. There are only four possible values of the variable which is the picture which has been chosen from a set of four. And, unless we are dealing with a very unusual population medically, there are only two values for gender. It is still something which can vary – whether someone is male or female – but it doesn't vary very much. It is a variable with a restricted set of possible values.

Measuring variables

Some variables are more difficult to measure than others. With the right scientific equipment, we can get accurate measures of lighting levels or temperature. But very few people have accurate records of the exact number of hours they have spent playing darts in their lives; and in any case, some experience is qualitatively different from other time. The experience of playing in high-ranking competition, for example, is very different from playing casually with friends. So a simple measure of experience which just tried to calculate it by the number of years someone had played darts would be over-simplistic: measuring any kind of experience isn't all that easy.

We can use this type of variable in psychological experiments, but only by constructing a measuring scale which can combine objective information and other, more subjective factors. If we were developing a measuring scale for experience in playing darts, we would probably need to use the judgements of experienced darts players, to make sure that it was appropriate. In the end, our scale would probably combine objective information, like the number of years someone has been playing, with more subjective factors, like the quality of training or other experience that they have received.

Operational definitions

Sometimes, measuring a variable can involve making an **operational definition** of the subject under study. An operational definition is a way of defining something which isn't quite perfect, but which will do for the purposes of the research project. Taking the number of years of play as a measure of experience in playing darts would be an example of an operational definition. We would recognise that it isn't a perfect way of measuring experience, but, depending on the study that we were doing, it might be adequate for our experimental purpose.

Operational definitions are used a lot in psychological research: they do allow us to get on with things, but they can also sometimes raise problems of **validity**. Validity, in essence, is to do with how well something really measures what it is supposed to measure. Psychologists assess validity in a number of different ways, and we will be looking at these more closely in Chapter 6. But it is worth bearing in mind that validity applies to just about any measure that we use in psychology – not just psychometric measures.

Some variables are much more subjective. For example, preference for different types of music is a personal thing, and it varies widely from one person to another. But there are still lots of ways that a variable like that can be used in psychological studies. The type of music itself can be a variable, in the same way that the specific picture chosen from a set of four is. And people can express preferences in many different ways – for example, by rating a type of music on a scale from 1 to 10, or by ranking several different types of music in order of preference. So even though a variable may be subjective, it is still possible for us to look at the way that it varies, and to measure it if we need to. We will be looking at levels of measurement, and the sorts of measures we use for different kinds of variables, in Chapter 14.

Types of variable

Altogether, there are four types of variable which can be involved in an experiment. Two of them are directly influenced by the experiment: the independent variable and the dependent variable. They are the main purpose of the experiment. But there are other types of variable which can interfere with the study, and these are known as confounding variables and contaminating variables.

The condition which is being manipulated by the experimenter in order to cause an effect is known as the **independent variable**. It's called 'independent' because once it has been set up by the experimenter it isn't affected by what else happens in the experiment, and it's called a variable because it varies. For example, if we were looking at the effect of overcrowding on aggression, we would vary the amount of crowding, and see what effects it had. The amount of crowding would be the independent variable. Or if we were looking at the effects of noise on concentration, we would vary the amount of noise. The amount that the independent variable varies is set up by the experimenter, and doesn't depend on what happens during the experiment.

The **dependent variable**, though, does depend on what happens in the experiment. The dependent variable is the one which we measure to see if the independent variable has caused an effect. It's called 'dependent' because – if the experimental hypothesis holds true – its value depends on the independent variable. Two conditions of the independent variable should produce two different values of the dependent variable. So the outcome of an experiment is assessed by comparing measures of the dependent variable in the experimental condition, with measures of the dependent variable in the control condition.

The other two types of variable are ones we don't really want. A **confounding variable** is a variable which affects one condition of your independent variable, but not the other. For example, if we were doing a study of concentration in learning, and we ran the experimental group on one day and the control group the next, we might find differences in the weather which would affect concentration. If the experimental group did the experiment on a sunny day, they might not concentrate as well as a control group which was doing it on a cloudy day. In that case, the weather would be a confounding variable which affected the outcome of the study.

Confounding variables can produce two types of error in our results.

What do these three terms mean?

variable

independent variable

dependent variable

If they exaggerate the difference between the experimental and the control group, they can make us believe, wrongly, that the experimental hypothesis has been supported – or, more accurately, that we should reject the null hypothesis. This is known as a **Type I error** – a false positive result. Alternatively, they might act in such a way as to minimise any differences between the experimental and control group, making us think there weren't any real differences between them when there should have been. That is known as a **Type II error** – a false negative. We will be looking at these types of error again in Chapter 14.

The other type of variable involved in an experiment is the type which affects how 'pure' our results are – in other words, how certain we can be that we really have isolated all of the possible other factors which might have influenced the results. These are known as **contaminating variables**. They don't necessarily operate in a systematic way, as confounding variables do. Instead, they could be randomly distributed across the conditions of the experiment, or they might only come into effect on some occasions and not others. If they were truly randomly distributed across the study, they probably wouldn't affect it too much; but they confound our results because we can't be sure whether they have been properly controlled or not.

For many studies, contaminating variables are something which can be minimised as much as possible, and then ignored, on the grounds that they are equally likely to affect both conditions. But in some types of psychological research, it is absolutely vital that we know we have controlled these things. Parapsychological research, for example, raises so many strong feelings among critics and advocates that the least bit of possible weakness in the study is enough for it to be regarded as invalid. So psychologists investigating parapsychological phenomena have to be meticulous in their control of any possible contaminating variables. Psychologists who are working in other areas, though, can often afford to be a little more tolerant of contaminating variables.

Confounding and contaminating variables can often be very subtle. For example, sometimes they are caused by the experimenter themselves. People pick up slight variations in tone and body language very easily, and they can often detect what an experimenter is expecting to happen. The guesses they make about this then affect how they act in the experiment. So the experimenter's own expectations can produce **experimenter effects** which need to be controlled.

Sometimes, too, research participants are overly anxious to please, and to do what they think the experimenter wants them to do. These are known as **volunteer effects**, and they have to be controlled as well. There are a number of different techniques which psychologists use to minimise the effect of confounding and contaminating variables in

Table 3.2 Control procedures

Standardised procedures are needed to ensure that all groups carry out the study in exactly the same way, in order to rule out contaminating or confounding variables like the amount of practice someone has, or the sequence in which they carry out different tasks.

Standardised instructions may also be needed, ensuring that exactly the same wording is given to all the participants, in order to rule out the possibility that some participants might receive clearer instructions than others.

Standardised conditions are needed to ensure that all groups have the same experiences while carrying out the study, in order to rule out contaminating or confounding variables like the size of the room, or the amount of background noise they are experiencing.

The **single-blind technique** is when the researcher knows the hypothesis but the subjects don't. It is used to control volunteer effects.

The **double-blind technique** is when neither the subjects nor the experimenter is aware of the hypothesis of the experiment. It is used to control experimenter effects.

Randomisation involves ensuring that a possible confounding or contaminating variable is equally likely to affect all experimental conditions, so that any effects it has will not introduce a systematic bias into the results.

experiments, and some of the main ones are listed in Table 3.2. But it is important to remember that the people who take part in an experiment are actively trying to make sense of their experiences, and if they don't know why they are doing something, they will draw their own conclusions – which may be wildly off the mark, or may be exactly right. People don't remain mentally passive and inert, no matter how much experimenters might wish they would!

Types of experiment

Experiments can come in several guises. Actually, if we want to get strictly technical about it, many of the projects which are referred to as experiments aren't really experiments at all. We can distinguish roughly five different types of experiment which are in common use in psychology. They are listed in Table 3.3, and we will be looking at each of them in turn. They all have elements in common – effectively, that they look at outcomes which have occurred as a result of changes

Table 3.3 Types of experiment

Laboratory experiments
The experimenter manipulates variables under controlled conditions, in the psychological laboratory, using randomised allocation of the participants to the experimental conditions.

Quasi-experiments
The experimenter manipulates variables under controlled conditions, in the psychological laboratory, but randomised allocation of participants to conditions is not possible.

Field experiments
The experimenter manipulates variables in a natural setting, and is therefore not able to control all possible contaminating or confounding variables.

Natural experiments
The experimenter does not manipulate the variables, but studies a situation in which a single variable has changed through natural or socio-political causes.

Single-case experiments
The experimenter manipulates variables under controlled conditions, but draws the data from one single case rather than from a group of participants.

in one particular variable. But although they are all often referred to as 'experiments', they don't always match up to the full criteria used in psychology to define an experiment.

This is partly because the definition of what constitutes an experiment has drifted a little during the past century. Early definitions of an experiment focused on the manipulation of a variable to produce a distinct and specified effect – an experiment was the manipulation of an independent variable to produce changes in a dependent variable. But as laboratory experimentation came to be regarded as the hallmark of a true research psychologist, the emphasis shifted onto the idea of control – the idea that an experiment must also involve ensuring that all other variables are ruled out or held constant, as much as possible.

More recently, the concept of control has become even more tightly refined, and it now includes the principle of **random allocation** of participants to the separate groups in the experiment. A 'true' experiment, in psychological terms, is one in which participants are randomly allocated to the conditions of the study. Any other study is deemed to be a quasi-experiment, rather than an experiment. (It's worth remembering, though, that these more recent definitions don't actually apply in physics or the other physical sciences. Psychologists are much more picky about this sort of thing than many other scientists.)

Laboratory experiments

A laboratory experiment, then, is the 'pure' type of experiment used by psychologists. It involves manipulating an independent variable, under controlled conditions, to produce changes in a dependent variable, in a situation where participants have been randomly allocated to the experimental conditions.

Laboratory experiments have the advantage that they can offer conditions which lend themselves well to tight control of variables and highly accurate measurement. Laboratory equipment allows researchers to deliver precise stimuli – lights, words, colours, sounds, images or other types of information. It enables them to detect minute responses, such as changes in brain activity or heart rate, pupil dilation, simulated driving errors, sleep behaviours, or whatever else is being investigated. It often allows experimenters to observe behaviour unobtrusively, through closed-circuit TV monitors or two-way mirrors. And it provides an environment where sound, temperature, lighting and other environmental factors are held constant.

Laboratory experiments don't inevitably involve huge banks of technology, of course. Many of them are quite simple in the equipment that they use, and might involve nothing more complex than a couple of paper-and-pencil exercises. But the important thing is that they are undertaken in a controlled setting, without interference from extraneous and unexpected variables.

There's a downside to this, of course. As we saw in Chapter 2, people respond to the situations that they find themselves in, and finding themselves in highly controlled, artificial environments can mean that they actually behave quite differently from the way they would act in their everyday lives. This is a problem with **ecological validity**, which can be overcome to some extent by an imaginative researcher, but never completely (we will be looking at types of validity in Chapter 6). It is one of the reasons why most researchers tend to use laboratory experiments in conjunction with other methods of investigation when they are researching a specific topic.

Another problem that laboratory experiments have is with **construct validity**. Sometimes, the process of narrowing down a variable in order to get a precise measurement means that it no longer really represents the kind of thing it was originally designed to explore. A good example of this came in the early experimental studies of reading, in which laboratory researchers tried to control for variables such as meaning and different word lengths by looking at the recognition of individual words. But that turns out to be a completely different process from the way that we read meaningful text; so those studies weren't really much help in understanding the whole reading process. Too much control or too much refining of variables can be a problem.

We have already looked at the third problem which laboratory experiments have, which is the way that they aim to isolate single causes. This is an advantage if what we are looking at really is only caused by one variable; but most human activity is much more complex than that. Exploring a study purely by using experiments can blind researchers to the complexity of the phenomenon which is being examined, and the ways that several different variables all work together to produce the end result. In the past, this has sometimes led to researchers making overly simplistic claims about what 'causes' a behaviour or activity. Nowadays, researchers are a bit more circumspect, and recognise that there are more complex issues involved. When we look at quantitative analysis, we will be looking at some of the statistical tests designed to deal with multiple factors; but we are as yet a long way from having a methodology which can really allow us to explore complex causality.

Deciding to conduct a laboratory experiment, then, involves a trade-off between precise measurement, the identification of single causes, and the advantages and perils of over-control and artificial situations. And sometimes, we are in a situation where conducting a pure laboratory experiment just isn't possible. We may still want to explore causality, but we have to compromise on one or more of the features of the 'true' experiment.

Quasi-experiments

Perhaps the most common of these situations is the **quasi-experiment**, which can be conducted in the laboratory, under controlled conditions, but which for some reason doesn't involve random allocation of participants to conditions. A study of gender differences, for example, doesn't allow the experimenter to allocate the participants randomly to one condition or the other. They are already assigned to one of the conditions before they come to the laboratory, and there isn't much the experimenter can do about it.

There are other conditions where quasi-experiments have to be used, such as when an experimenter needs to find a matched sample. We looked at some of the problems involved in matching samples earlier in this chapter. A matched sample, by definition, isn't assigned randomly to the conditions of the experiment. It is arranged so that one from each pair goes into each condition. So in technical terms, an experiment which involves matched samples is actually a quasi-experiment rather than a true experiment. But it is an experiment in all other respects – the control of variables, the manipulation of the independent variable and measurement of the dependent variable, and so on. All the other issues which apply to laboratory experiments apply to quasi-experiments too.

Field experiments

What do these three terms mean?

field experiments

quasi-experiments

single-case experiments

Field experiments, by contrast, are experiments which are a lot different from the laboratory situation. These are experiments which, for one reason or another, take place in the natural environment of the people being studied. That might be a hospital, a school, a community district, or any other place where people are to be found.

Field experiments, almost by definition, can't involve the same level of control as laboratory experiments do. But they have other advantages, not least of which is the question of ecological validity. By conducting their research in the natural environment, experimenters can be much more sure that they are really looking at the thing that they are interested in. The downside to this, of course, is that it isn't possible to control all of the other variables which might affect the study. In any real-life situation, there are going to be a great many other things going on; and minimising their influence is quite a challenge.

The trade-off with field experiments, therefore, is between close control, or rather the lack of it, and the advantages offered by a far more realistic situation. Participants are much more likely to be aware of the situation and the nature of the experiment, because of the various ways that information is transmitted in everyday life; so that type of factor will need to be taken into account. Conducting a field experiment requires considerable design expertise on the part of the researcher, and they can be expensive to carry out; but they offer many benefits too.

Natural experiments

Occasionally, we come across a real-life situation which appears to offer us a real-life experiment. This happens when one particular variable in a situation is changed for one group of people, but not for a similar group. One example might be the introduction of a new practice in a hospital ward, while other, similar wards continue in the same way as they did before; or the introduction of a new management system for a particular department in an organisation. These situations offer researchers an opportunity to look at the kinds of outcomes produced by the new practice, and to use the other group or groups for comparison. They are not true experiments, because the variables are not controlled by the experimenter; but they act in much the same sort of way.

Natural experiments can vary in scale, from small-scale studies conducted in families or classrooms, to huge-scale social phenomena. Psychologists interested in education, for example, are able to study the massive natural experiment conducted in the German educational system, whereby half of the country experienced over forty years of an educational system designed to promote a capitalist society, while the other half experienced a communist-oriented educational system. Before the division the educational base of the two halves of the country were the same; afterwards, the emphasis of the two educational systems was very different. And now, of course, they have come back together again.

Sometimes, too, natural experiments can be studied retrospectively, with researchers looking back in time to identify outcomes from particular cases. These are known as **retrospective studies**, or sometimes as **ex post facto research**. There are a lot of problems with that type of approach, not least of which is our tendency to select out the bits of information we find most relevant and to ignore or never learn about other information which might also be relevant. Studies of maternal deprivation, for example, were treated as if they were natural experiments by several researchers in the late 1950s and early 1960s, but the selective collection of data meant that they were deeply flawed. The general consensus seems to be that retrospective natural experiments are only really of much value when they deal with very small, specific areas of human behaviour which are fully documented. And even then they can be misleading if important other factors are overlooked.

Single-case experiments

Single-case experiments are not the same as case studies. Case studies involve looking at a particular phenomenon which has occurred or is occurring, and analysing the different psychological factors and mechanisms which are involved in, or contributing to, that phenomenon. We will be looking at them in more detail in Chapter 8. But single-case experiments are very different, in that they involve an active manipulation of variables to produce an effect.

Perhaps the classic example of a single-case experiment in psychology is the extensive range of memory studies which Ebbinghaus conducted using himself as the research participant. By cutting out extraneous variables using nonsense syllables, and systematically varying factors such as exposure time, number of trials, and so on, Ebbinghaus was able to identify a number of factors in memory, such as forms of remembering, which still hold true today.

The other main area where single-case designs are commonly used in psychological research is the area of clinical neuropsychology. If we are studying a distinctive individual with a unique kind of brain injury, it often makes sense to conduct small experiments to see what kind of variables can influence their performance. These studies don't involve large groups of people, since that sort of comparison would be meaningless. Instead, the comparisons are the other data drawn from the same research participant. While most psychological experiments adopt a nomothetic approach, and look at large samples of participants, single-case experiments are examples of experimental research which uses an idiographic approach (see Chapter 1 if you have forgotten what idiographic and nomothetic mean!).

Ethical issues in experimental research

Carrying out experimental research with human beings raises a great many ethical issues. In the past, many psychologists took the view that since they were scientists and in pursuit of truth, they could do pretty much what they liked. So psychology's history contains some pretty awful instances, such as the Minnesota starvation studies, in which volunteers were deliberately starved of food for several months in order to identify the psychological consequences of food deprivation. There were other studies, too, of drug effects, effects of electric shocks, and so on. From the 1960s onwards, the emphasis shifted on to psychological deception, with research participants being tricked into behaving in all sorts of ways.

This type of experiment is entirely unacceptable nowadays. Researchers operate under strict ethical guidelines, and anything which might cause a research participant pain or distress is out of the question. But, in addition, modern ethical guidelines recognise the rights of the research participant as an autonomous, active individual who has chosen to participate in the study, and whose participation gives them certain rights – the right to be fully informed about the study, the right to withdraw if they so choose, the right to make informed choices, and so on. The main ethical guidelines in use in Britain were summarised in Table 2.3, in the previous chapter; and you can see if you look back through them that many of them derive from this new attitude of respect for the research participant.

All of this doesn't make experimental studies impossible; but it does constrain researchers into conducting them in rather more responsible ways. As we have seen, quite a lot of experimental methodology does involve deception – the use of single-blind or double-blind controls, for example – to avoid confounding variables; but modern researchers make sure that any deception included in a study is only short-term, and only used with the participant's permission. And many researchers have given up using manipulative techniques like that altogether. The concern with ethical issues has, in many cases, produced a much more imaginative approach to experimental methodology.

Other researchers, too, have turned to different research methods to gather their data. The experiment is an important part of the psychologist's tool-kit, but it has never been the only one. In the next few chapters, we will be looking at some of the other ways that psychologists collect information about other people: how and why they act as they do.

Self-assessment questions

1. *How do modern researchers define an experiment?*

2. *What does it mean when we say that we have made an operational definition of a variable for research purposes?*

3. *What is the difference between a Type I error and a Type II error?*

4. *How may volunteer effects influence experimental outcomes?*

5. *What are the main problems with using retrospective studies as a research method?*

Concepts in use

1. *Recently there have been ethical objections to the use of double-blind controls when testing drugs which might represent a cure for AIDS. What ethical problems are raised by this practice?*

2. *Researchers exploring racist attitudes among members of the general public need to be very careful to avoid experimenter effects. What types of experimenter effect might arise in that kind of study?*

3. *What were the main problems which occurred as a result of the use of retrospective studies to explore issues of maternal deprivation?*

4. *Describe a practical situation which forms a natural experiment. How might you go about studying that situation for its psychological implications?*

5. *Make a list of the design problems you would be likely to encounter if you were wanting to conduct an experimental study of management style in university departments.*

4

Observational studies

About observations
Types of observation
Collecting data in observational research
Ethics of observational research

A great deal of psychological research takes the form of observational studies of one kind or another. In observational research, we try to work out what is going on by looking at what happens, and recording it in such a way that we will be able to analyse the relevant factors involved in the situation.

About observations

Experiments, as we saw in the last chapter, can establish causality by manipulating circumstances and producing effects. But other forms of research, including observation, can really only show that two things occur together. If you observe that, say, children in small playgrounds play more aggressively than children in large playgrounds, you haven't necessarily shown that there is a causal link between them. All you may really have shown is that the two things correlate – that they both happen together. The real cause might lie in something quite different (like, say, the effects of poverty or social deprivation). Observations, like most of the other research methods available to psychologists, can only detect **correlation**, not causality.

Choosing what to observe

Observation may seem easy before you have tried it, but conducting a fully rigorous scientific observation is not as easy as it might seem. One of the first challenges is being very clear about exactly what it is that you are observing. Try going to your local shopping centre or bus station, sitting on a bench, and writing down what you can see.

You'll quickly find that there is far too much going on; which is why we automatically pay attention to some things and not to others. And, of course, what we do observe will be affected by who we are and what we expect to find.

An environmental psychologist, for instance, might pay particular attention to the way that people move in and out of different areas, and how they use the space that they are in (chatting, sitting down, window-shopping, etc.). A social psychologist, on the other hand, might be interested in the different kinds of social behaviour that are going on: for example, how close people stand to each other, whether they touch (holding hands, linking arms) or avoid contact with others, the expressions on their faces, etc. That social psychologist could be sitting side by side with the environmental psychologist, looking at the same scene, yet they would both be observing something quite different. Because of this, it's important to be very clear about exactly what your study is trying to investigate, and why.

The statistics that are used to analyse observational studies are also different from those used for experiments. The main difference is that observational studies are more likely to involve **correlation tests**, which look at how closely two variables relate to one another, than tests to see how different two sets of variables are. We will be looking at correlation tests in Chapter 18.

Types of observation

Observational studies can take many different forms. Some are conducted in special environments, set up to allow careful monitoring and precise recording. Others are conducted in more 'natural' environments, such as homes, offices, parks or shopping centres. Some observational studies are highly structured, with the researchers being interested in very specific behaviours and regulating carefully the way that the information is collected. Others are more relaxed, allowing the observer to exercise their own judgement and record what seems to be important.

Laboratory observations

A great many observational studies are conducted by psychologists in the laboratory. Psychologists who are conducting sleep research, for example, don't go into people's homes and sit and watch them sleeping. We wouldn't learn very much if we did! Instead, the participants in a sleep research study go to the laboratory and stay there for the night, being observed while they sleep. This allows the psychologists concerned to observe them in detail, and in more than one way.

One way, of course, is just to watch people while they are sleeping, and a sleep research lab is equipped with cameras and microphones to record movements and any sounds they might make. Observations can be much more detailed than that, though. A sleep psychologist will also observe and record the changes in the participant's brain wave patterns as they go through the different periods of sleep. Before the person goes to sleep, electrodes are attached to the skull, and they pick up the electrical activity happening in that part of the brain. They feed this information to a polygraph – a machine which records the information coming from several different sensors – and a record is kept of that activity through the night. In this way, a sleep psychologist is able to observe the brain's activity and other aspects of physical functioning – not just what that person looks like in bed.

Not all **laboratory observations** are so technical. Some research psychologists use observational laboratories which are really only rooms that have been wired for sound and video, so they allow researchers to see and hear the participants without being obvious about it. Rooms might be used as playrooms, if a psychologist is studying something like how children act with one another while they are playing; or as interview rooms or therapy rooms. But they are different from ordinary rooms, because of the way they allow hidden observers to see and record what is happening.

Most research laboratories of this type have special observation rooms which are equipped with **two-way mirrors**. A two-way mirror is a kind of window between two rooms, which is specially made so that if the room is brightly lit it acts just like a mirror, and reflects light back into the room. But it also lets some light through, and if observers sit on the other side of the window, in a darkened room, they can see through the mirror as if it were a window. The observers in the next room can see what is going on, but the people in the room itself only get the normal reflection of an ordinary mirror. So, for instance, a mother and child could be playing together in the observation room, and a researcher interested in mother–child interaction would be able to observe and record their behaviour without having to be in the same room with them.

Ethological observations

The main alternative to laboratory observations in psychology are **ethological observations**. These are observations of behaviour in the natural environment. Ethological observations often have higher **validity** than laboratory observations, because the participants in the study act more naturally than they would if they were in unfamiliar territory. But they are more difficult to carry out, partly because it is less easy to obtain systematic recordings of what the people or animals being studied are doing at any given time.

What do these three terms mean?
observational study
polygraph
two-way mirror

Perhaps the biggest challenge of all in ethological observation is observing unobtrusively. It's very difficult for anyone to act naturally when an observer is sitting there noting down everything they do! Anyone would be bound to be self-conscious in that situation, and even animals react to the presence of observers. So the observer needs to make sure that their behaviour doesn't affect the other person too much.

The most usual way that ethological observers do this is by getting their participants so used to their presence that after a while they don't notice the observer, or at least they don't take any notice of the observer (which isn't always the same thing!) The observer sits quietly in an unobtrusive place, being as uninvolved as possible in what is going on. After perhaps an initial period of curiosity, their presence becomes familiar, and those being observed carry on with what they were doing. Many observational studies are carried out in this way.

The observer observed

A word of warning: just because those being observed don't react to the observer's presence any more, it doesn't mean that the observer has been forgotten. That applies to animals, too: in 1974 I was conducting an observational study of some chimpanzees from behind a thick glass window at Chester Zoo. For the first few days, the chimps would throw mud at the strange face at the window (staring is a threat gesture for chimpanzees as well as humans). One chimpanzee, Jeannie, didn't throw any mud. Instead, on the first day, she settled down in a hollow facing my window and observed me for the whole time I was observing the troop. After that day, she acted as if she had entirely forgotten about my existence. Within a week the mud-throwing and other protests from the other chimpanzees had ceased. They had become used to my presence, and acted as if I wasn't there.

About five weeks later – when my presence had become completely familiar to all of the chimpanzee troop – I was late into the Zoo one morning, and had to stand at the side of the enclosure, unprotected by the glass, to conduct my observations. At one point I observed Jeannie, over on the far side of the chimpanzee island, pulling up a chunk of mud from the bank. A bit later, she walked over towards me, hiding one hand behind her back, and then settled down as if sitting idly, doing nothing in particular. Suspicious, I checked my watch. Ten minutes later – when I had indeed forgotten all about it – that chunk of mud came flying through the air towards me! So much for my impression that my presence had become unnoticed. It was clear that, although I was usually ignored by the animals, one chimpanzee at least was still very much aware that I was there!

Participant observation

A third way of conducting observational research is through **participant observation**. Participant observers conduct research into social groups or situations by joining in with those situations, and becoming members of the group that they are studying. This allows them to get to know the people concerned, and to find out what is going on from the point of view of the participants.

Perhaps the main difficulty of participant observation is that of recording the data. Most researchers solve that problem by keeping a regular diary and noting down the significant events of each day in it. Some are lucky enough to be able to use tape-recorders or video cameras to keep records of what has happened, or to have these available to back up their diary notes. But there are ethical problems with keeping notes on people secretly, and these become even more important – to the point where it is considered unacceptable unless there are very strong reasons for it – when a study involves secret taping or filming. We will be looking at ethical issues of observational research later in this chapter.

Sometimes, too, systematic record-keeping simply isn't possible. The social psychologist Bruno Bettelheim survived a period of time in a Nazi concentration camp. He was unable to make notes, but, being a psychologist of his time, was very familiar with a range of mnemonic techniques, and he carefully memorised salient factors and events which would allow him to analyse what was happening in the camp. His study still provides us with important insights into the way that the whole horrifying process operated (Bettelheim 1943).

Other, less dramatic problems with data collection also happen. Sometimes, data recording is just entirely inappropriate, or even undesirable. For instance, Holdaway (1982), in an account of a participant observational study on police behaviour, reported how his notes were of necessity incomplete, as at times events would occur which would be experienced as an abuse of privilege. For example, he did not record a distraught young mother's comments on her marriage at a time when her young infant had just died. Indeed, to have done so could have been regarded as ethically questionable in itself.

Most participant research, though, isn't of that nature. In psychology, it is usually conducted by researchers who find that they have an opportunity to investigate something which would otherwise have been inaccessible. For instance, the investigation of cult beliefs by Festinger, Riecken and Schachter (1956) arose because the investigators found that they had the opportunity of seeing what happened when a specific prophecy failed. They joined a cult which believed that the world was scheduled to end on a specific date, and got to know the cult members. Because of this, when that date arrived and passed without incident, they were able to talk with the cult members and see how their beliefs had been adjusted in the face of such clear disconfirmation. A more 'objective' or distant observational technique would not have allowed them access to that information.

Obviously a study of that kind couldn't work if the investigators were known to be psychologists studying the group. So there are ethical issues involved here. However, it is generally considered that a certain amount of deception is inevitable in this type of research, because some kinds of information simply cannot be gathered in any other way. What is essential, though, is that the individual's privacy and confidentiality are respected by the researcher.

Participant observation of psychiatric life

One of the most famous participant observations in psychology was the investigation of the treatment of schizophrenics, carried out by Rosenhan, in 1973. Rosenhan and several of his colleagues were admitted to psychiatric hospitals and diagnosed with schizophrenia, on the basis of one symptom – they said they heard voices that were not there. Their hospital admissions gave them the opportunity to study what conditions were really like for patients in the hospitals; and also to look at the process of psychiatric diagnosis.

Among other things, they observed that behaviour which was perfectly normal in the world outside was treated with deep suspicion by the hospital staff. One patient kept a diary, which the nursing staff regarded as very questionable. 'The patient engages in writing behaviour' was entered in his hospital notes, with the clear implication that this was part of his psychiatric condition.

Epidemiology

What do these three terms mean?

participant observation

data

epidemiology

Epidemiology is a kind of observational technique which is used most often in medical or environmental health research, rather than by psychologists. But it is a technique which psychologists use too, when it is relevant to what they are looking at. Some researchers believe that it has a great deal more potential for psychological research than is generally believed. For example, in 1987, Farr argued that epidemiological studies of the distribution of social representations could do a great deal to clarify our understanding of the social behaviour of cultural and subcultural groups within modern societies. Social representations are the shared beliefs held by groups of people, and they vary widely from one culture to another, and within societies as well. Taking an epidemiological look at how that variation happens could tell social psychologists a great deal.

EXERCISE 4.1   **Observing shoppers**

An environmental psychologist is conducting an observational study of the ways that people use an urban shopping mall. There are three parts to the study. The first concerns who uses the shopping mall and at what times. The second concerns what parts of the shopping mall are used and by how many people at a time. And the third concerns what people actually do when they are in the shopping mall.

Taking each of these parts of the study separately, outline:

(a) an initial set of observational coding categories which might prove useful for a pilot study

(b) some of the practical issues which will need to be considered in carrying out the research

(c) any ethical problems which might arise from carrying out this project.

Epidemiology is a form of indirect observation. We don't observe the behaviour directly. Instead, we observe and monitor its occurrences – when, where and how often it happens. For example, an environmental psychologist might be interested in the relationship between a local environment and children's traffic accidents. To explore this, the psychologist would be most likely to begin with an epidemiological study which identified the occurrences of traffic accidents in that particular locality. In the classic epidemiological model, each accident would be categorised in some way and plotted on a map.

The categories would express those aspect of the accidents that the researcher was interested in – it might be something like the age of the child involved; or the type of activity that the child was involved in (coming out of school, playing, walking to the shop, etc.); or the time of year; or the degree of severity of the accident. The map would allow the researcher to explore the distributions of these accidents, and see whether they clustered together – for example, whether a particular accident 'black spot' tended to involve younger or older children, or was more likely to produce accidents during the summer holidays, and so on.

In practice, a great deal of epidemiological research uses complex statistical analysis to identify clusters of events, rather than physically plotting them on a map. But the essential concept is the same, and many psychologists find that using a simple epidemiological mapping technique can often be a useful way of taking a different look at their

What do these three terms mean?

hypotheses

ethological observation

selective perception

data, or seeing aspects of it which wouldn't be apparent any other way. Health psychologists, in particular, often find that epidemiological techniques can be invaluable as a first step in tracking down a particular problem and developing hypotheses which can be used as the basis of future research.

Epidemiology, then, is a much more indirect form of observation than the other three methods which we have looked at in this chapter. Its source material may be other studies, documents, or even official statistics. But it is, nonetheless, a method of observing what is going on, even if that observation is at a slightly higher level of abstraction.

Collecting data in observational research

One of the first difficulties that we encounter when collecting observational data is that observations, unless they are carried out very carefully, are extremely vulnerable to **selective perception**. When we first begin to observe anything, we are faced with a flood of information, and it is simply not possible for anyone to analyse all of it. So we focus in on the things that we are interested in, and that can mean that we lose a great deal of information in the process. It's very easy to fail to notice things that we don't really think are important. Our perceptual system filters them out without us being aware that it is happening.

In addition, because we all tend to notice things that we expect to find, and we all have our own ideas about what causes what in society, it's very easy to be misled during the observational period. As Neisser (1976) showed, our perception is an active cycle of **anticipatory schemas** – our expectations, ideas and plans for action – directing what we look for in the environment and how we go about looking for it, which in turn selects what we actually do notice, which then informs our anticipatory schemas (see Figure 4.1). All of this means that we

Figure 4.1 Neisser's perceptual cycle

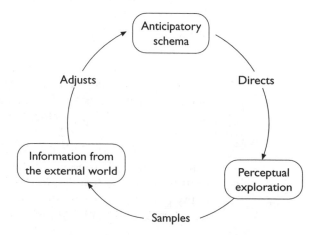

have a powerful tendency to see what we expect to see, or, at the very least, to see things which fit generally with the type of phenomenon that we were expecting.

As a result, psychologists conducting observational studies need to be very careful. There are several precautions we can take if we are conducting observational studies. One possibility is to structure the form of the observation very carefully, so that there is very little room for personal bias or involvement from the observer. Typically, these observations will take the form of behavioural coding, or time-sampling, or both.

Behavioural coding

What do these three terms mean?

behavioural coding

time-sampling

structured observation

A **behavioural coding** system involves using a series of categories of behaviour, and fitting all of the observations which are made into one of those categories. They have usually been worked out before the main study begins, on the basis of similar studies or pilot tests. It is important that the categories are reasonably comprehensive, covering most of the behaviour likely to be shown by the subject of the observation. At the same time, it is also important that there are not too many categories for the observer to manage. Table 4.1 gives an example of a possible set of behavioural coding categories for observing children at play, while Table 4.2 gives an example of a different set which has been used by psychology students for observing the behaviour of small pet animals. You can see that the two sets of categories are very different. The behavioural coding that we use has to reflect our own interests and the purpose of the study we are conducting.

Sometimes, the categories are applied by the observer as they watch what is going on. Whenever it is practical, though, a video-recording is likely to be made of the whole thing, so that the behavioural coding can be done later. Video-recordings have advantages in this way, but they also have disadvantages, in that the camera doesn't have the same range as human vision, and things may happen which the tape doesn't pick up.

Time-sampling

Time-sampling is another type of structured observation, and it is often used together with observational coding to record what is happening among a group of people or animals over a period of time. Using this method, the observer does not try to record everything all the time. Instead, at preset intervals – say, every five minutes – the observer scans the scene and notes down what everyone is doing. What happens in between the observational sampling times is ignored,

Table 4.1 Observing children at play

Social interaction (positive)	
Interaction (neutral)	
Interaction (negative)	
Social play	
Manipulating objects	
Play with objects	
Pretend play using objects as props	
Pretend play without objects	
Exploration of surroundings	
Exploration of objects	
Physical activity with objects	
Physical activity without objects	
Verbalising	
Social talk	
Conversation	

but the assumption of this technique is that, over a period of time, it will give a reasonably accurate picture of typical activities. Usually, researchers use a quiet 'beeper' or some other device to remind them that it is time to make the recording.

For example, if we were observing the behaviour of visitors to a Science Activity Centre, we might use a time-sampling approach to get

Table 4.2 Coding animal behaviour

Molecular movements (movements of part of body only)			Molar movements (whole-body movements)		
Functional	Exploratory	Other	Functional	Exploratory	Other

Note: This set of coding categories has been used for behavioural observations of small domestic pets, such as hamsters or gerbils.

a pattern of how exhibits are used by visitors during the day. Doing this would allow us to build up a systematic record of which exhibits attracted the most attention, and it would also indicate to us whether an exhibit was typically used by groups or by individuals, whether spectators looked on while somebody else tried out the action, and a number of other factors which would be helpful in evaluating the exhibits.

Multiple observers

Sometimes, using behavioural coding or time-sampling is not appropriate for the type of observation which is being carried out. An alternative precaution in that situation is to use independent observers. This has two advantages – first, that one observer might notice something which another one has missed; and second, that it allows the researcher to become aware of the amount of agreement between observers. It's a standing joke among traffic police that twenty witnesses to an accident will have seen twenty different accidents. Observers often interpret what they have seen completely differently, and our memories of the event are often adjusted until they fit with our interpretations. But equally, that means that data which different observers agree on can be seen as reasonably valid.

> **What do these three terms mean?**
>
> *inter-observer reliability*
>
> *expectations*
>
> *correlation*

If there is more than one person observing the same thing but independently (so that each doesn't know what the others are noting down), then it is possible to compare their different observations and see how far they agree. **Inter-observer reliability** is the amount of agreement between the different observers' reports of the same phenomenon. If it is high (say, with a correlation of .8 or more), then the observations are considered to be reliable, and acceptably accurate. If it is low, there are two possible explanations: either there is a great deal going on – too much for one person to take it all in – and the observers have each been watching different things; or the observers are being influenced by personal bias or expectations. In either case, though, knowing the inter-observer reliability score gives useful information to the researcher about the nature of the observations which have taken place.

Ethics of observational research

Observations, as we have seen, can vary from the highly structured, laboratory-based 'objective' observations, to participative ventures in which the distinctions between observer and observed are minimised. But all types of observation, in common with all other types of research in psychology, raise ethical problems of some kind.

Observational studies should always have the full consent of the person being observed. In a formal observational study, the normal system is that the research participant is shown the observation room beforehand, so that they know what is going on. People are normally very willing to co-operate with this set-up, even in highly personal situations, such as family therapy. But they have to be given the option of refusing the observation if they want: people are entitled to have their personal privacy respected.

There are also issues raised by the question of feedback. Modern thinking about the ethical responsibilities of researchers emphasises the need to give observational study participants full feedback about the study, and to share research findings with them. Failing to do so is seen as adopting a manipulative stance, in which the person is used by the researcher without regard to their own rights as a self-determining person. So a researcher needs to be conscientious about keeping in touch with participants, and giving them the information when it becomes available.

EXERCISE 4.2   **Classifying observational studies**

What type of observational study is represented by each of these examples?

Observing children playing in a special playroom through a two-way mirror

Exploring the use of a bus station by making observational records every five minutes

Observing a chimpanzee colony in a zoo

Video-taping a family therapy session for subsequent expert analysis

Observing children playing in a school playground

Exploring the way that street accidents are distributed in a particular district

Observing athletes in their training sessions

Using electrical recordings to study the different phases of sleep

Observing family interactions in a science exploratory centre

Rosenhan's study of psychiatric diagnosis

Using a polygraph to note people's reactions to emotional stimuli

Observing the farmyard behaviour of ducklings with their mothers

Covert observation

Other issues are raised by the question of covert observation. Studies which involve observing people in public places are sometimes regarded as exempt from the need for feedback and consent, since the behaviour which is being observed takes place in public and can be freely observed by anyone else. It is argued that the person would expect to be observed in that sort of situation in any case, so the information which is being collected is public.

Covert observation of private behaviour, though, is much more ethically dubious. It always involves some element of deception, and this raises very strong feelings. According to Banister (1994), publication of such findings has even been called an 'act of betrayal', since it makes behaviour public which was previously kept secret. On the other hand, this type of observation can sometimes highlight serious social issues. For example, the study of 'canteen cultures' in a police force conducted by Holdaway in 1982 revealed racist attitudes and behaviours which would not have been uncovered using other research methods.

A research proposal which includes covert research, therefore, needs to be scrutinised very carefully, with the benefits the study will bring being weighed very carefully against the elements of deception and responsibility to the participants. It is at this time that the criteria for ethical decision-making summarised by Reynolds (1982) and described in Table 4.3 come into play. Ethical decisions are rarely cut and dried, and in professional research it is often necessary to make judgements about the value of the study. Which is, of course, why such decisions are given to ethics committees, rather than being left to the judgement of the individual researcher.

> **What do these three terms mean?**
>
> *covert research*
>
> *action research*
>
> *real-world research*

Table 4.3 Ethical decisions about covert research

1. **Utilitarian, cost–benefit criteria**	Do we learn more from the research than we could do from research carried out differently, and if we do, is it worth it?
2. **The effects on the participants**	What will the outcome of our research be for the participants involved? Clearly, if covert observation has no effect whatsoever, this is different from research in which the covert intervention produces change.
3. **Issues of individual integrity**	Have we had to engage in personal dishonesty and manipulation, and if so, to what extent may this be offset by humanitarian consideration?

Source: Reynolds (1982).

Passive observation and action research

Passive observation, as we've seen, presents some problems in terms of the way that both people and animals respond to being observed. Many psychologists, any number of philosophers, and even some physicists argue that the act of observation changes what is being observed. It is not possible, they say, to observe without the observing process influencing the target of the observation. We won't be considering the physicists' problem here – if you are interested, look up references to Schrödinger's cat: I can recommend Gribbin (1995). But certainly human beings and animals do react very strongly to the presence of an observer.

As we have seen, most observational researchers try to deal with this problem by minimising the effect that the observer has on the people or animals being observed. But the alternative is to recognise the effect that the process of observation is having and to take that into account as part of the study. This approach is known as **action research**, and in many cases it is the only practical option for research carried our in real-world settings. Effectively, action research is where the researcher becomes an active agent in what is going on, not just a passive observer. We will be looking at it in detail in Chapter 11.

The distinction between action research and passive observation may seem very clear, but in real research it is much more blurred than that. In Judy Dunn's (1988) ethological observations of pre-school children, for example, the same researcher would visit the family for each observational period (the study spanned several years, because it was concerned with how social awareness changed as the children grew older). The observer would sit quietly, observing the children, and staying as uninvolved as possible.

Nonetheless, this was a human situation, involving human beings, with their own curiosity and interests. So sometimes the children would address the researcher directly. In that situation, she would always reply. Although there was a slight chance that she would affect the findings by replying as she did, the research team knew that was by far the lesser of two evils. To avoid answering at all would be much more unnatural, and would have made the children very curious about this peculiar visitor – exactly what the researchers wanted to avoid.

Most forms of research involve some kind of compromise of this kind. Indeed, modern ethical considerations are such that it is generally considered unacceptable for people to be observed for a psychological study if they have not given their consent beforehand, so the ideal of an 'invisible' observer, having no effect at all on the study, is rather unrealistic. It is up to the researchers designing any particular study just how far they wish to go along the continuum between the passive observer and action research. And it is up to their particular ethics committee to evaluate just what type of ethical issues that raises, and how it should be addressed.

In the next chapter, we will be looking at the use of questionnaires to gather data. This research method often accompanies, or emerges from, a detailed observational study. But it too presents its own unique set of challenges for the researcher.

Self-assessment questions

1. *What is the difference between correlation and causality?*

2. *Outline some of the problems involved in conducting laboratory observations.*

3. *What are the main methods of conducting observational research?*

4. *Briefly describe the advantages and disadvantages of participant observation as a research method.*

5. *Describe the processes involved in carrying out an epidemiological study.*

Concepts in use

1. *A psychologist wishes to conduct a covert research study exploring sexism in trainee management programmes. What ethical problems might be raised by this study?*

2. *How might you go about conducting an observational study of student revision habits?*

3. *What coding categories might you use when conducting an observational study of football crowds? Why would you choose those particular categories?*

4. *What type of data collection might you use for a study which involves monitoring changes in EEG patterns during sleep? What problems might you encounter regarding collecting the data?*

5. *A city council wishes to obtain information about the ways that members of the public use the local parks. It has been decided that ethological observation might be the most suitable research method. What issues would you need to consider when designing an appropriate study?*

5

Questionnaire studies

Stages of questionnaire design
Administering questionnaires
Ethical issues of questionnaire research

Questionnaire studies are a valuable tool for the research psycho-logist. Although they don't permit a researcher to look at things in much depth, they do make it possible to collect information from very large numbers of people – far more than could reasonably be studied using experimental or observational research designs.

One of the most useful ways that questionnaire-type studies are applied in psychology is when a completely new area of research is being opened up. It is not at all uncommon for someone who is inter-ested in a new area to begin by conducting a questionnaire study about it, and then to use the results of that study to generate hypotheses which can then be investigated by more in-depth research.

Questionnaires are also used when psychologists want to investigate how widespread a phenomenon is. For example, when a research team wanted to investigate just how common the experience of nightmares was, the obvious way to go about it was to conduct a questionnaire study, asking about sleepwalking, sleeptalking, nightmares, and other dream-related experiences. The questionnaire study allowed them to gain an idea of how widespread these experiences were, and what proportion of the population was likely to have them.

That doesn't mean, however, that questionnaires can be used to research every topic in psychology. Questionnaires are very vulnerable to **response bias** – to people adjusting their responses so as to give the 'right' sort of answer to the researcher. Because of that, they need to be carefully planned and designed. But if that is done properly, they can provide useful information – of certain types. Table 5.1 outlines some of the main types of information which can be gained from questionnaires.

Questionnaires can collect **factual information**, such as information about people's habits, their depth of knowledge on particular issues, or immediate sources of stress. They can also be used to tell us about past behaviour: patterns of domestic behaviour, educational or work

What do these three terms mean?

response bias

sampling technique

ambiguous questions

Table 5.1 Types of information from questionnaires

Facts and knowledge	Motives
Past behaviour	Opinions and attitudes
Likely future behaviour	

experiences, musical preferences, and so on, and this can allow us to collect information about changes during specified time periods, or, for that matter, about consistency during the same periods. Information can also be gleaned from sensitive questioning about what people are likely to do in the future, e.g. in terms of their social habits, their ideals and ambitions, and their expectations.

Those types of information are concerned with what people experience as facts or knowledge. But questionnaire studies can also give us some insight into people's **motivation** – why they act as they do, and what motivates them to take action, or to interact with particular people or behave in particular ways. This is a rather less reliable type of information, partly because our insights into our own motives are not in themselves very reliable. But information of this type can be helpful nonetheless. And questionnaires can also be used to identify people's attitudes and opinions about circumstances, events or people, including an assessment of the strength of those opinions. We will be looking in more detail at attitude measurement, and at psychometrics, in Chapter 6.

Stages of questionnaire design

Designing a good questionnaire isn't a simple task, although on the surface it can often seem so. The main problems lie in making sure that you produce a questionnaire which really does allow you to find out about your topic, given the fact that the people you are asking are all individuals, with very different prior experiences, attitudes and understandings. A good questionnaire has to allow for these differences, and at the same time has to make itself crystal clear to every member of its target population.

Questionnaires are designed to elicit information from people, in a manner which will allow the researcher to make generalisations about the topic. But people designing a questionnaire often feel that they already know the sort of answer that they expect people to come up with – and that's a large part of the problem. Learning to design a good questionnaire is partly learning to expect people to want to respond in unpredictable ways – they almost always do! But, at the same time, if they are faced with a limited range of choices, they will tend to co-operate and choose one of them.

EXERCISE 5.1	Using questionnaires to study AIDS

Imagine that you have been asked to conduct a questionnaire study of AIDS-related behaviours among an older population of people aged between 35 and 50. There is some anxiety that most campaigns designed to raise awareness of AIDS have been targeted at younger people, and that the 35–50 age group is also very much at risk. As a result, it is important to gather data about the number of sexual encounters these people have, their use of condoms, and other relevant information.

1. Formulate three hypotheses about AIDS-related behaviours in the 35–50 age group which your study could address.

2. Identify two topics or pieces of information which you would want to find out about for each hypothesis. This will give you the subject matter for six questions.

3. Look at each question subject, and decide whether it would be better addressed using an open or a closed question format.

4. What are the main ethical issues you will need to address when designing and carrying out this type of study?

The questionnaire fallacy

This leads to a major source of error, known as the **questionnaire fallacy**. The questionnaire fallacy occurs when researchers assume that they have acquired a picture of what human beings actually do, whereas in reality their limited choice of responses has not made that possible. The questionnaire fallacy is a major problem in marketing and social research, where questionnaires are the dominant – and sometimes the only – way of collecting information. It is less of a major problem in psychological research, partly because questionnaires are usually supplemented by other research methods. But it can affect psychological questionnaires just as much as it does marketing ones, if they are badly designed and, in particular, if they are not piloted rigorously enough.

What do these three terms mean?

questionnaire fallacy

piloting

ecological validity

Design stages

Producing a good questionnaire involves several distinct stages, which are listed in Table 5.2. Each of these stages is important. Designing a competent research questionnaire involves following this sequence

Table 5.2 Stages of questionnaire design

1. Working out the aims of the questionnaire
2. Selecting appropriate question styles
3. Designing the questions
4. Piloting the questionnaire
5. Revising the questionnaire
6. Administering the questionnaire
7. Analysing the data
8. Reporting the study

carefully, in order to make sure that all of the various factors have been taken account of.

The first stage involves working out the **aims** of the questionnaire. At this point – before you do anything else – you need to write down the main purpose of the study, and the hypotheses which the questionnaire's information will allow you to investigate. Only when you have done this will you be able to sort out what type of information you need to obtain; without that, you won't be able to decide on either appropriate question styles or question content. Table 5.3 lists a number of useful questions which you can use to guide this stage in your planning.

Table 5.3 Identifying questionnaire aims

Why are you conducting this study in the first place?

What are your hypotheses for this study?

What type of information is it that you need to obtain?

Who should be responding to the questionnaire, to give you that information in the best way?

What is the purpose of obtaining the information?

Who will use the information you come up with?

What will they need to know?

The second stage involves using the information you have obtained from stage 1 to select appropriate **question styles**. You need to begin by considering the types of information which you need to fulfil your research aims, and to look for styles of question which will provide you with that type of information. Figure 5.1 shows a number of different question styles, which provide a range of different types of information as data.

Figure 5.1   Styles of
questions

QUESTIONS INDICATING AGREEMENT OR DISAGREEMENT

1. Do you believe that a nuclear deterrent is effective?

   YES   NO

2. Do you believe that there is life after death?

   YES   NO   DON'T KNOW

3. I believe that corporal punishment should be made illegal

   **Strongly —— Agree —— Don't —— Disagree —— Strongly
   agree   know   disagree**

QUESTIONS PROVIDING ALTERNATIVE ANSWERS

4. What do you think is the most important factor to consider when buying
   food?

   (a)   *Value for money*
   (b)   *Hygienic processing*
   (c)   *No chemical additives*
   (d)   *Good flavour when cooked*
   (e)   *Easy to prepare*

5. Which of the following do you believe to be most important to the
   general welfare of the world? Please rank them in order, giving 1 to the
   most important, 2 to the next and so on:

   (a)   *Reducing Third World debt*
   (b)   *Saving the rainforests*
   (c)   *Cutting out chlorofluorocarbons*
   (d)   *Developing more eco-sensitive household products*
   (e)   *Using catalytic converters in cars*

6. Pick one word or phrase from the list which best describes your feelings
   about random breathalyser testing:

Sensible	*Useless*
Intrusion of privacy	*Safer for everyone*
Good idea	*Should cut down accidents*
Over-officious	*Unnecessary*
Dangerous	*Keeps people on their toes*

OPEN-ENDED QUESTIONS

7. What do you think the government should do about acid rain?

8. Give one word or phrase to describe your attitude towards the
   greenhouse effect.

You also, at this point, need to consider the type of analysis that you're going to have to do, and how it will need to be presented. You must make sure your questions will give you the right kind of information for use in that analysis. Table 5.4 lists a few useful questions you might use to guide stage 2.

Table 5.4   Selecting types of questions

How will you analyse each question?

How subtle or sophisticated does the information each question gives you have to be?

Will you be able to fulfil your aims with category data, or do you need to measure the extent or degree of something?

Do you need open or closed questions?

Will you provide numbers or verbal descriptions in the final analysis?

What form will the written report on your findings take?

Once you know what each question is supposed to be about, and what sort of question styles will be appropriate, you can set about the third stage, which is designing the **questions**. Notice that we talk about 'designing', not just 'writing'. This is because the questions need to be constructed very carefully, and to have exactly the right form and phrasing. During this stage, you need to keep in mind the purpose of each question, as you write it – it's very easy to get sidetracked, or to forget exactly what each question is for. It is best to refer frequently to your list of aims and to your hypotheses at this point: they will help to keep the questions in line. We will look at question writing in a bit more detail later in this chapter.

The fourth stage is that of **piloting** the questionnaire. A pilot test is a test run, which allows you to try out a product or measure that you are designing. In this case, you will need to find out how other people respond to your questionnaire. No matter how much you revise it yourself, there will always be something you haven't thought of – an unexpectedly ambiguous question, or an option that you haven't included. In your pilot test, you try the questionnaire out with a small-ish number of people from your intended sample. Try to be there if you can, so that you can pick up on the verbal queries as well as the written answers that people give. If anyone has to ask you a question while they fill the questionnaire in, that tells you that part of your questionnaire definitely needs to be rewritten!

The fifth stage involves **revising** your questionnaire. This is your chance to go for perfection. Try out your intended analysis on the pilot scores, to make sure that you can do it OK. You don't want to be finding out later that you can't score the answers to the questions because you didn't try the techniques out at this crucial stage! Polish up the phrasing of the questions, make sure you haven't got errors in them, and check the layout. Take account of all of the comments you received during the pilot stage, and adjust the questionnaire appropriately. It's a good idea to keep a list of all of the alterations you have had to make at this stage, and why. That way, when you are looking back or writing up the questionnaire, it will be easier to see and describe how it developed.

Once your questionnaire has been fully revised, you can move to stage six, which is **administering** the questionnaire. There are two sides to this: one is to make sure that your sampling techniques are suitable for the purposes of your questionnaire. We discussed the question of representative samples in Chapter 2, and we will be looking at sampling for questionnaire studies in more detail later in this chapter. The second aspect of administering questionnaires is how you go about it. There are lots of ways of giving questionnaires, and we will be looking at this later in the chapter too. You need to be careful to choose the most suitable technique for the topic that you are researching.

The seventh stage involved in conducting a questionnaire study is **analysing** the data. You need to present your findings clearly in the report. You can use descriptive statistics like bar charts, pie charts and tables, and also measures of central tendency and dispersion (see Chapters 15 and 16). You may want to look at correlations between different questions, or use inferential tests to see if there are significant differences between groups. Or you may have qualitative data to analyse. Whatever you do, make sure the technique you use is appro-

EXERCISE 5.2	Types of questionnaire information

The following list consists of a number of different topics which can be studied using questionnaires. Which of the five types of knowledge listed in Table 5.1 would each of these topics be investigating?

Commuter habits

AIDS-related behaviours

Ozone depletion

Reading habits

Domestic eco-sensitive practices

Holiday plans

Ambitions and careers

Drinking in the street

A new housing development

Sports activities

Reasons for visiting a theme park

CCTV monitoring in parks

Sexual harassment legislation

Reasons for doing a university
  course

Littering

priate for the type of data you have – qualitative, nominal, ordinal, or interval – for each question. If this doesn't make sense to you right at the moment, don't worry. It will all be covered in Part II of this book.

The eighth stage of conducting a questionnaire study is **reporting** your findings. If you are conducting the research project as a psychology student, you will need to write up a formal report containing abstract, introduction, method, results, and discussion – and you will need to include appendices which describe how you carried out the study, and the various stages of development that your questionnaire passed through. A report for publication in a scientific journal is usually more concise, but still contains the same sort of sections.

If the questionnaire study was conducted as part of a professional research project, though, you may need to produce a full professional report of your findings. These reports are usually quite lengthy – much more so than journal articles – and they have more emphasis on discussing the implications of the findings and looking at their professional or commercial implications than on the research design and methods – although you still need to give important details like sampling information. You may even be required to do a verbal presentation of your findings, in which case you will need to have well-presented diagrams to summarise the main points, as well as diagrams illustrating specific aspects of the analysis.

Some common mistakes

These stages show that a researcher conducting a questionnaire study doesn't start writing the actual questions until the third stage – in other words, until it is very clear exactly what the questionnaire is being designed to do, and what is going to happen with the information once it has been obtained. One of the main mistakes which amateurs make when they are constructing questionnaires is to begin by writing out questions, before they have a very clear idea of what they want from the questionnaire. Then they end up with a confused tangle that's almost impossible to analyse. If you know what you want from each question, and exactly why you want it, that's not likely to happen.

Another mistake which amateurs often make is succumbing to the lure of gathering information just for the sake of it. A questionnaire gives lots of scope for information gathering, and it's easy to add additional questions on a 'why not?' basis, just because they might give an extra bit of interesting information. But the greater the number of questions included in a questionnaire, the less thought respondents are likely to give to their answers; the more likely the researcher is to offend people by seeming to intrude into their privacy; and the more likely it is that the respondents won't bother to complete the questionnaire at all.

There is no point including any question unless you know beforehand exactly why you want it there, and how you will use the information it provides. Be ruthless about leaving out the questions that you don't need. Think about the hypotheses you are investigating, and also the length of the final report once you've been through all the answers and connections between questions, and ask yourself whether adding yet another question will be cost-effective, in terms of the time and effort that you will spend analysing it. Including extra questions 'just in case' is not good enough – even one new question can produce a great deal of extra statistical analysis.

Which leads us to the next point, which is how closely analysis and design are linked when it comes to questionnaires. Another common error that amateurs make is not considering how the questionnaire will be analysed until after it has been administered. At that time, when it is too late, they often realise that they have asked a question in the wrong way, or that they really don't know how to use the information they have obtained. So working through the analysis is actually part of the planning stage, which needs to be done when the questionnaire is first piloted. And looking at how different questions link together is also important, because it allows a researcher to work out exactly what will be done with the information from each question, and even how the report will be structured.

Designing questions

A good questionnaire is one which has had careful thought given to the design of the questions. Question design isn't just about the wording and content of the questions; it also encompasses a number of different aspects of questioning, such as the way that the questions are sequenced, the form that they take, and the degree of complexity required in the answer.

Arranging the questions

The sequencing of questions in a questionnaire needs careful thought, because different sequences can produce different results. If a question is asked suddenly, out of the blue, the respondent will answer it as best they can. But what comes to mind is not likely to be as comprehensive as it will be for a question which has been properly 'primed'. The more we think about a topic, the more detail we remember about it – it is a basic principle of memory. So if the questions we are about to answer have already been primed by topics which are relevant, or connected in some way, our answers are likely to be clearer and more accurate.

Priming and cognitive availability

Priming relates to one of the biggest problems of all in questionnaire studies, which is that human beings are many-faceted, and are different in different contexts, or when they are playing different social roles. A young person may have one set of social contexts which encourages them to be acutely aware of social responsibilities – say, being a youth leader – and a different set, such as going dancing with friends at the weekend, which encourages a completely different set of social perceptions. A questionnaire about risky behaviour or some similar topic administered at the youth centre would invoke one set of responses; the same questionnaire administered at the disco might invoke an entirely different set from the same person. And both would be true.

It's not about lying: it's about the fact that we are not always the same all of the time. If you ask people whether they often have sleep problems during a period when their sleep has been troubled, their answer will be affirmative. Six months later, if they have been sleeping well and in a relaxed way, their answer may well be negative. As Bower (1981) showed, when we are feeling good, we tend to recall positive things in our lives and forget negative ones; when things are going badly, we remember more of the negative ones.

All of us have many 'personas' – or different sides to our characters. But when we respond to a questionnaire, we adopt just one of them, and give answers appropriate to that. Priming helps the questionnaire designer to lead the respondent towards an appropriate persona, and so helps to obtain fuller answers. But in a different mood, or in a different context, the same person may give very different responses, even to requests for apparently factual information.

What do these three terms mean?

funnelling

priming

personas

When designing a questionnaire, then, it is important to arrange the questions in order, making sure that each one follows logically on from the other. The technique known as **funnelling** involves moving from general questions to more specific ones – thus allowing the researcher to 'home in' on a specific topic. Sometimes, too, it is appropriate to use **reverse funnelling**, in which a questionnaire, or a section of a questionnaire, begins with very specific questions and then broadens out to more general topics. Both are ways of using priming to prepare respondents for the questions to come.

Writing the questions

Writing the questions for a questionnaire can often seem a very straightforward task. But beware! You may know exactly what you mean, and so to you your questions may seem crystal clear. But unlike you, your respondent will not already know what you are talking about, and may encounter difficulties understanding your question which you had never anticipated. That's why piloting the questionnaire is so vital.

There are some errors which can be anticipated. Table 5.5 lists seven of the most common problems in the phrasing of questions. Leading questions are questions which already imply what the respondent ought to answer (*Do you think it is time the government stopped ignoring the voice of the people?*). Multiple-content questions are those in which the researcher asks for more than one thing in the same question (*Do you think we should have a general pollution tax or should we just fine polluters more?*).

Table 5.5   Some problems of question writing

Leading questions	Over-complex vocabulary
Ambiguous questions	Over-elaborate phrasing
Multiple-content questions	Patronising tone
Implicit questions	

Ambiguous questions are questions which could be interpreted in more than one way. For example, the question *'Do teams need leadership?'* may seem straightforward enough to the person who writes it. But it can actually be read in two ways: either as asking whether a team needs to have a particular person who has been designated the leader, or as asking whether teams can function without anyone taking on a leadership role while they are carrying out their tasks. The two interpretations are very different, but each person who answers it is only likely to perceive one of them. The problem for the researcher is that it is impossible to tell which version the respondent has answered.

Implicit questions assume that the person already knows what the researcher is asking about. For example, asking 'Do you consider conventional footpath erosion strategies to be effective in the national parks?' assumes that the person answering the question will already be familiar with conventional footpath erosion strategies. This type of error is very common indeed, particularly in questionnaires which have been written by specialists or by people who are deeply involved in studying a particular topic.

Some questions use over-complex vocabulary. They use jargon, long words, or over-technical terminology to ask the question, and this can put a considerable strain on the respondent, who has to decode the jargon before they can answer the question. *'What is your evaluation of the efficacy of cognitive strategies in athletic instruction'* is not nearly as clear as '*In your opinion, how useful is mental training for athletes?*' A similar problem is posed by questions which use over-elaborate phrasing, in the form of clumsy or complicated sentence structures instead of clear, simple ones. A question with phrasing like '*In view of the increasing use of metered water systems, and the accordingly greater potential for cholera epidemics, are existing strategies, in your opinion, appropriate?*' requires quite a lot of decoding on the part of the respondent, and is also very open to misinterpretation.

The other problem of question writing which can be found on many questionnaires is that of an excessively patronising tone. Researchers who go to the extreme in trying to avoid the problems we have just been looking at can find themselves assuming that their respondents are stupid or child-like, and phrasing their questions accordingly. Although phrasing questions simply and clearly is important, it is pointless, as well as insulting, to ask questions like '*Do you think advertisers are bad people?*'. It is important to watch the tone and phrasing of your questions, and to choose your vocabulary in a way which is adjusted to the needs of your respondents.

Open or closed questions

<table>
<tr><td>

What do these three terms mean?

leading questions

open questions

closed questions

</td></tr>
</table>

As you can see, then, writing good questionnaire items is a skilled task, and not nearly as easy as it appears on the surface. But there are other decisions which a researcher needs to make when designing the questions which will go on the questionnaire. One of the most important is deciding on the balance of open and closed questions.

Open questions – sometimes called open-ended questions – are questions in which the person is free to answer exactly as they like. They are not confined by a choice of answers from a limited range, and this gives them a number of advantages. They are generally more representative of the respondent's true opinions, less open to the researcher's own personal biases or perceptions, and more true to real life (sometimes expressed as having a higher **ecological validity**). They are often extremely useful for indicating special points of interest, or allowing a researcher to identify aspects of the research topic which they had not previously considered.

On the other hand, open questions do have one main disadvantage, which is that they can be very difficult to analyse. They are most commonly analysed using techniques such as **content analysis**, in which answers are categorised into different types, and the number of each type is counted up. We will be looking at this method in Chapter 15, when we look at descriptive statistics. Sometimes, a researcher may sort the responses, or the themes apparent in the answers to an open question, into 'league tables' of the most popular answers. This, too, is essentially a way of just describing these answers.

The alternative to a descriptive approach in dealing with the answers to open questions is to use a qualitative analysis, which involves making interpretative accounts of the individual responses. We will be looking at qualitative analysis in general in Chapter 10, and at several different kinds of qualitative analysis in Chapters 10–13. But qualitative analysis is time-consuming, and even though the information it gives is much richer than can be provided by closed questions, many researchers prefer to avoid getting into it. After all, some research surveys involve administering a questionnaire to several thousand people, and in that context, the time and labour involved in doing a full qualitative analysis of even one question would become very large.

The alternative is to use **closed questions**. These are questions in which the answers which the respondent can give are prespecified, as boxes to be ticked, points to be marked on a scale, or options to be chosen from a list. Closed questions have some distinct advantages for the researcher, the main one being that they are much easier to score and analyse, because they give predictable outcomes, which are very amenable to statistical illustrations or summaries. As Figure 5.1 shows, they can offer several different types of information, and this information can be analysed using either descriptive statistics (see Chapters 15 and 16) or inferential statistics (see Chapters 17–19).

On the other hand, closed questions have some serious problems, too. These are mainly concerned with **validity** – a concept which we will be looking at in more detail in the next chapter. Because they only have a restricted range of answers available, they are extremely vulnerable to the questionnaire fallacy which we looked at earlier in this chapter; and they are also much more likely to be distorted by the researcher's own personal opinions or bias in some way. In fact, most of the problems of question writing which we have already looked at become most pronounced in closed questions.

What do these three terms mean?
cost–benefit analysis
RDD
response rate

Selecting the question formats, then, involves a series of decisions, which usually take the form of a **cost–benefit analysis** – weighing up the costs, or disadvantages, and comparing them with the benefits, or advantages. The main issues are summarised in Table 5.6. Very tightly specified closed questions are quick and easy to analyse, but only give descriptive information. More flexible closed questions, such as rankings or numerical assessments, give more useful data which are amenable to complex statistical analysis, but they take more time to complete. Fairly constrained open questions, such as those inviting the respondent to provide a single word or phrase, give more valid data but can only be analysed descriptively, whereas fully open questions, in which the respondent can say what they want, are likely to give the most valid data, but are the most expensive and time-consuming to analyse.

Table 5.6 Open or closed questions?

Open questions
More representative of subject's true opinions
Less open to researcher's bias
More realistic / higher ecological validity
Useful to indicate points of interest or weaknesses
Can be difficult to analyse
Usually analysed by:
   content analysis
   interpretive accounts of individual responses
   'league tables' of the most popular themes in responses

Closed questions
Very easy to score and analyse
Give predictable outcomes
Restricted range of answers available
Open to design bias
Useful for statistical illustrations or summaries
Usually analysed by:
   descriptive statistics
   inferential statistics

The only real way of sorting all of this out is to come back to stage one of the questionnaire design – the aims of the questionnaire. The choices of question formats, their analysis, their phrasing and their content will all depend on the aims of the questionnaire, and the context in which the study is being performed. A clear set of aims is the most essential tool of all in questionnaire design.

Administering questionnaires

Once the questionnaire has been designed, it will need to be administered. There are two major aspects to this. The first is the sampling technique which the researcher adopts, and the second is the actual way that questionnaires are given to respondents. We looked at some of the general principles of sampling in Chapter 2, and these are as valid – perhaps even more so – for questionnaires as for any other type of nomothetic research.

Random sampling

Effectively, what we are looking for in any sample is that it should be representative of the population from which it comes. Ideally, a **representative sample** would have all of the important characteristics of its parent population, so that whatever we learn from studying it can also be applied more generally. If we don't take care how we go about it, though, we can end up with a biased sample, which is missing some of the characteristics of the parent population – or, worse still, has some characteristics very strongly, which are irrelevant in the parent population. In that situation, it will not be accurate to generalise any conclusions we draw from our study, so we will lose most of the point of doing a questionnaire study in the first place.

In questionnaire studies, there are four main ways of obtaining our sample. The first, and strongest, is by using a **random sampling** technique. That doesn't mean just choosing the people to participate in the study haphazardly – there's a difference between the meaning of the word 'random' in everyday use and its meaning in statistics and research methods. A random sample is a sample in which every member of the population has an equally likely chance of being selected for the study – and that isn't as easy as it sounds. Most sampling methods will unconsciously favour some people, and not others. Picking names at random out of the telephone directory means that people who are ex-directory are not going to be included. In a psychological study, that could introduce a bias, because those people may be different from others in some important way – for example, by being more suspicious of strangers, or more inclined to anxiety.

A random sample actually has to be obtained very methodically. In practice, truly random samples are quite rare in psychological research. Their main problem is that they have to begin with a list of the entire population, and then select participants from it using some kind of arbitrary system – a bit like pulling names out of a hat. In most cases, that simply isn't possible. If you were interested in studying teenage social representations of recreational drugs, for instance, your population would be teenagers in general – or perhaps the teenagers of a particular country – and that would be an almost impossible list to obtain. You would need to use a different approach to sampling for that study.

If the population is more limited, though, random sampling becomes more practical. For example: if your population is students who attend a particular sixth-form college, and you are worried about whether the college might be developing a 'drug culture', you could select your sample by obtaining a full list of all of the students at the college and selecting names at random from it. You might, for instance, give each student a number, and then select numbers randomly using lottery balls, or some other such system. As we saw in Chapter 2, there is some dispute about whether taking, say, every tenth name on a list is a truly random sampling technique, but for practical purposes that would do too.

Other sampling methods

What do these three terms mean?

quota sampling

representative sample

ecological validity

In practice, most questionnaire studies are performed using a **quota sampling** technique. In quota sampling, the researcher decides on the population characteristics which are important to the study. For marketing research, these are usually age, sex and socio-economic status, because those are believed to be the most salient factors when it comes to purchasing behaviour. For an investigation into sleep disturbance, it might be just age, or perhaps age and sex. If we were looking at reading habits, IQ or educational level might also be important population characteristics.

Once the most important population characteristics have been specified, they are used to identify the subgroups which, taken together, would be representative of the population. Then the sampling procedure is to obtain a certain number – a quota – from each of the subgroups. In this way, it is hoped, the final sample which has been obtained will contain the important characteristics of the parent population, in the right sort of proportions. If you have ever been surveyed by a market researcher who asked you your age group and occupation, and then thanked you and said they didn't need to ask you any more questions, the chances are that person was using quota sampling, and had already obtained their full quota of people in your subgroup.

Another possibility which is sometimes adopted for questionnaires is to use **stratified sampling**, sometimes known as stratified random sampling. This is similar to quota sampling, in that it also involves dividing the population separate subgroups, and selecting the sample from each subgroup. The subgroups are known as strata because, when the method was first discussed, the subgroups tended to be about social class, and the implicit model was of society as 'layered' into upper, middle and lower classes. For modern researchers, the subgroups identified using stratified sampling techniques are still often about income or socio-economic factors, but modern society has some rather different approaches to social class (the disappearance of the term 'lower class' is a good example).

Once the subgroups have been identified, the researcher identifies the proportions of each subgroup in the population as a whole. Then a random sampling technique is applied, to obtain a sample from each subgroup. This is different from quota sampling, where researchers are mainly concerned with obtaining the required quota and have less regard for strict randomisation principles. But, like quota sampling, the final sample has to contain roughly the same proportions of subgroup members as the parent population has.

The fourth main type of sampling used in questionnaire studies is known, loosely, as **opportunity sampling**. Effectively, this consists of asking whichever members of the population are available to complete the survey. If, for example, you are interested in the social representations of recreational drugs held by students at your college, you are most likely to obtain your sample by going to places where the students are likely to be (the canteen or the common room), and asking whoever you see to complete the questionnaire. Opportunity samples are not by any means ideal, and there is a considerable risk that the sample which is obtained by such methods will be biased in some way. It then becomes a matter of judgement whether the bias is such as is likely to affect the conclusions of the study.

Another sampling technique which is sometimes used for questionnaire studies is known as **random digit dialling** (RDD). Using this method, a computer generates random telephone numbers. These numbers are then telephoned, and the researcher asks whoever answers a couple of 'screening' questions, to see whether they have the right characteristics for the study. If they have, the questionnaire is then administered – assuming the individual co-operates. Traditionally, this would have been considered a limited sample because it doesn't take account of those who are not on the phone; but in modern society, this is not considered to be such a small proportion of the population as a whole that it can be ignored. But ethical considerations about intrusion of privacy are more important. We will be looking at these later in this chapter.

Approaching respondents

Effectively, there are four main ways of administering questionnaires – that is, of approaching respondents in order to get them to complete a questionnaire. The first of these is by undertaking **face-to-face interviewing**, in which the researcher speaks directly with the respondent, face to face, and asks them the questions. This offers the opportunity to clarify ambiguities or to explain additional details to the respondent. It also allows for on-the-spot sampling decisions to be taken, and has a reasonably high response rate. On the other hand, it is time-consuming, and expensive if interviewers are to be employed. Interviewers need to be trained, and unless the interviewer has good interpersonal skills, it can come over as artificial.

Handout questionnaires are a cheap and convenient way of administering a questionnaire. They work best with a 'captive', clearly defined population who are all located in one place at a given time, such as students who are participating in a particular course, or sports fans attending a game. But it is not easy to achieve balanced sampling using this technique, nor to clarify problems or misunderstandings which might arise. Layout and presentation are absolutely vital with this type of questionnaire, because they can make a great deal of difference to how the respondent views the issues that the questionnaire deals with. Because of this, handout questionnaires sometimes have quite a low response rate; but in a highly motivated population the response rate increases.

Using **postal questionnaires** makes it easier to get in contact with what is potentially a balanced sample, although the researcher has very little control over who responds. Some studies have shown that for certain topics, postal administration can sometimes produce a slight increase in how openly people respond, but this depends very much on the nature of the questionnaire itself; and again, layout and presentation are really important. The questions need to be extremely clear, and so are not really suitable for populations which, for example, vary widely in their levels of literacy. But the main drawback of postal questionnaires is really their expense. Because they usually have quite a low response rate (generally something between 20 per cent and 30 per cent), a researcher conducting a postal survey needs to send out a great many questionnaires, and printing and postage costs can become very high.

The fourth main method of conducting surveys is by using telephone questionnaires. These are a convenient and easily controlled or supervised way of administering a questionnaire – so much so, that they have become a major tool of marketing research. They do tend to have a high response rate (although as their popularity grows that may change – there is some evidence that frequency of approach affects people's willingness to co-operate). They also attract a freer response because of the anonymity which they provide. However, they are by definition limited to verbal exchanges, so visual aids such as pictures cannot be used. Also, they are expensive to conduct, and at times the invasion of privacy may provoke hostility on the part of potential respondents.

Improving response rates

As we have seen, response rates to questionnaires vary both with the type of sample and with the population concerned. A population which is highly motivated and interested in a topic will obviously produce a higher response rate than one which lacks interest. A highly literate population may respond more freely to any open questions in a written questionnaire; while those with less verbal confidence may leave such questions, or only answer them very briefly – or, if their uncertainties are strong, they may even not complete the questionnaire at all. Questions which induce anxiety, embarrassment or indignation tend to lower response rates, and highly personal or threatening subjects are best investigated using some other method of study – as a general rule, they are not very amenable to being studied by questionnaire.

Response rates also vary according to the technique used to administer the questionnaire. Postal questionnaires generally obtain the lowest response rates, while telephone questionnaires obtain the highest. But it is possible for a researcher to raise response rates by using a number of tactics. One of them is to have some prior contact with the respondents beforehand, so that they are expecting the questionnaire. This can make a great deal of difference. Using follow-up queries, perhaps in the form of letters, postcards or telephone calls, also helps, as does increasing the ease of reply, e.g. providing prepaid envelopes for postal questionnaires. Marketing researchers have also found that providing incentives in the form of small rewards, or having a high-status signatory, or sponsoring organisation, can make a measurable difference to response rates, but these techniques are often considered inappropriate, or too expensive, for psychological research projects.

Ethical aspects of questionnaire studies

The main ethical aspects of questionnaire studies are to do with how they are administered to people, and what is done with the findings once they have been obtained.

The way that people are approached for the study needs to be carefully considered. Like all other forms of psychological research, it is unethical in principle to coerce people into participating in a research project. This means that a researcher needs to avoid situations where respondents are obliged to complete questionnaires because otherwise they will experience some kind of sanction or punishment. It isn't even really acceptable to apply pressure on someone to complete a questionnaire, and sometimes there is a very blurry line between persuasion and pressure.

This also connects with the individual's right to privacy. There is a growing ethical concern about the invasion of personal privacy from telephone marketing, and the use of telephone surveys by psychologists or other social science researchers would come into a similar category. In Britain, those who object to having their address used for 'junk mail' can apply to the Mailing Preference Service to have their name removed from mailing lists, or to the Telephone Preference Service to have their names removed from phone lists, but this does not protect against random dialling techniques, and there is a growing disquiet over the use of telephone sampling by researchers of all kinds. In reality, though, psychological studies which truly use RDD sampling techniques are rare: most psychological research which involves telephoning respondents tends to be restricted to those who have indicated in some way that they are prepared to participate in such a study, which changes the ethical considerations considerably.

The final aspect of ethical considerations when it comes to questionnaire studies is that of confidentiality. As with other forms of research, it is essential that the information provided by respondents is kept unidentifiable. In most types of questionnaire analysis, this isn't a problem, because it is the responses of the sample as a whole which are usually portrayed, using descriptive or inferential statistics. But the analysis of open-ended questions can sometimes provide details which would allow a single respondent to be identified, and the researcher needs to be careful to ensure that this does not happen.

Overall, then, questionnaire studies carry with them relatively few ethical problems, by comparison with other types of research. But then, as we saw at the beginning of this chapter, questionnaire studies are generally a more superficial technique: if we want to probe deeply into a particular aspect of human behaviour, we would generally use a different type of research method. So it is not really surprising that they do not raise such fundamental ethical problems.

Questionnaire studies have their advantages and disadvantages. But they have proved very useful in psychology, for opening up new research topics, and for getting estimates of how widely shared any particular phenomenon or experience seems to be. A well-designed questionnaire can provide the psychologist with access to a large amount of useful data. But a badly designed questionnaire – and many of the questionnaires we encounter in everyday life are designed very badly indeed – gives us problems with the validity of its data, and with the relevance of our conclusions.

In the next chapter, we will be looking at a much more specialised type of questionnaire – the type known as the psychometric test.

 ### Self-assessment questions

1. *What consequences can arise from failing to clarify aims before beginning to design a questionnaire?*

2. *Outline the major problems which can arise when formulating questions for questionnaires.*

3. *Briefly describe the advantages and disadvantages of using open and closed questions in questionnaires.*

4. *In what ways can descriptive statistics be useful for analysing questionnaires?*

5. *What are the four main methods of administering questionnaires?*

Concepts in use

1. *A marketing research company has been asked to find out about the shopping habits of people using town-centre shops. Suggest two different ways that they might administer their questionnaire, pointing out the advantages and disadvantages of each.*

2. *How might you overcome problems of response bias in a questionnaire study of teenage drug-taking behaviour?*

3. *A psychologist wishes to conduct a questionnaire study on the experience of positive emotions. Evaluate three different types of question style in terms of their suitability for this topic.*

4. *What ethical factors might you need to consider if you were conducting a questionnaire study of sleep problems?*

5. *How might you go about obtaining a representative sample for a questionnaire study looking at people's evaluations of bank services?*

6

Psychometrics

Attitude scales
Psychometric tests
Reliability, validity and standardisation
Ethical issues in attitude measurement and psychometrics

In the previous chapter, we looked at the use of questionnaires as a research tool. A questionnaire is a very general method of obtaining information from people, and, as we have seen, it can be quite useful in providing us with largely factual information about people's behaviours or habits. But when it comes to obtaining more subtle information about people, questionnaires are rather more limited.

Part of that limitation comes about because of response bias, in that people are conscious of the way that they are responding to a questionnaire, and generally try to make sure that their answers project the kind of image that they want to give. Another part of the reason is that some information about ourselves is just not open to our own conscious awareness. It can be brought out by the right kind of questioning, or deduced from patterns of responses, but it isn't open to direct self-reporting.

There are ways of obtaining much more detailed, or personal information using questionnaire-type instruments. But these instruments are very different from conventional questionnaires, and constructed in an entirely different way. They can be sorted, loosely, into two groups: attitude scales and psychometric tests. We will look at each of them in this chapter, beginning with attitude scales.

Attitude scales

Attitude measurement is a little more challenging than simply gathering information about someone's likes and dislikes, or their consumer choices. The main reason for this is that many people are not fully aware of their own attitudes, so they find it difficult to report them

What do these three terms mean?

response bias

self-report

lie scale

fully. A simple questionnaire would be a completely inadequate method of measuring attitudes. **Attitude scales** are measuring instruments designed, as their name suggests, to evaluate attitudes. Some of them may appear like questionnaires on the surface, but the process by which they are constructed is more tightly specified and much more rigorous.

Even when people are aware of their attitudes, they still may not like to admit to them. One of the major problems of the development of attitude scales is **response bias** – the tendency that people have to present themselves in the most favourable light. At its worst, this can mean that people simply lie, denying holding attitudes or ideas which they believe will be judged as unacceptable, or claiming to agree with socially acceptable attitudes when really they don't agree at all.

In its milder and more common form, though, response bias has much more to do with conformity than with deliberate deception. There is evidence, for example, that people of all ethnic groups respond differently to attitude surveys about colour prejudice when approached by a black researcher than they do when approached by a white presenter. While response bias may sometimes involve lying, it seems more often to be an unconscious wish to appear socially acceptable, which means that people focus on the more positive aspects of their attitudes, and less on the negative ones. As we saw in the last chapter, very few of us are consistent all of the time, and not many people hold rigidly consistent attitudes which never vary. Indeed, if someone does, there are sometimes grounds for wondering whether they are suffering from some kind of psychological problem – normal human awareness is much more complex, and sensitive to its environment, than that.

One way of getting round the response bias is to introduce a response bias scale – sometimes known as a **lie scale**. This is a set of questions, scattered throughout the attitude scale, designed to show up whether someone is making themselves out to seem better than they really are. They are quite common in psychometric tests, and are sometimes used in attitude scales too; but that depends a great deal on the form of the attitude measure. Sometimes, response bias scales simply aren't practical or appropriate.

Another source of response bias is to do with common patterns of responding. For example, we have a tendency to give consistent answers regardless of the question, and people answer 'yes' much more readily than they answer 'no' – it's another aspect of our tendency to conform to others, and to avoid social confrontation. Because of this tendency, the way that the question is phrased can make quite a lot of difference to the answers. If an attitude scale is organised such that positive attitudes are always indicated by 'yes' answers, its results are likely to become unbalanced. The scale has to be carefully designed, so that 'yes' and 'no' answers are evenly balanced.

Some attitude measures are reasonably straightforward in their design and construction, while others are more indirect. In most cases, it is the straightforward ones where we need to take most precautions against response bias and other types of problem. These are less problematic for the indirect measures since, as we shall see, it is much less obvious how they work or what they are measuring. Nowadays, however, researchers tend to favour direct measures over indirect ones, and perhaps the most popular type of attitude measure of all is the Likert scale.

The Likert scale

A Likert scale is a five-point scale, used to express agreement or disagreement with a particular statement (Figure 6.1). Likert scales have the advantage that they can cope with different strengths of opinion, or even if someone has no opinion at all about a topic. By looking at the combined responses to different items on a Likert scale, it is possible for a researcher to obtain a measure of attitude which is often quite thorough.

Figure 6.1 A Likert scale

I believe that ecological questions are the most important issues facing human beings today.

Strongly agree —— Agree —— Don't know —— Disagree —— Strongly disagree

---

The construction of a Likert scale involves much more than just writing down a sentence and drawing up a five-point scale. Technically, a five-point scale item does not really qualify as a Likert scale unless it gives results which are normally distributed (see Chapter 14). And there is a series of definite steps which need to be carried out to construct a Likert scale properly. They help to ensure that the items which have been selected for the scale are appropriate to the topic, and a good measure of attitudes. The steps are summarised in Table 6.1, but we will look at them in more detail here.

The first step in devising a Likert scale is to decide on the topic of investigation. That might sound obvious, but, as with any other research method, it is very easy to be too vague about what is being investigated. Strictly speaking, the topic of each item in a Likert-style questionnaire should contribute to our theoretical understanding of the phenomenon which is being researched, so it should be possible to explain and produce a full justification of why each item has been included.

The second step is to get several people together, and to generate a broad set of statements about the topic. It's important that more than one person is involved, because it is necessary to have several

Table 6.1 Steps in constructing a Likert scale

1. Decide on the topic of your investigation.

2. Collect a panel of volunteers.

3. Ask them to generate statements about the topic.

4. Collect all the statements and discard those which are repetitive or badly worded.

5. Put the statements into a list.

6. Ask a second panel to evaluate each statement as positive or negative.

7. Discard ambiguous statements, keeping only clear ones.

8. Select an equal number of positive and negative statements and arrange them in random order.

9. Allocate a five-point scale to each statement.

10. Combine your statements into a full Likert-based questionnaire.

different people's points of view. They should generate far more sentences than will be needed in the final attitude scale. Once the statements have been produced, the researcher then discards repetitive or badly worded statements, and collates the rest of them together into a lengthy list. That list is presented to a different group of people, who are asked to judge whether each separate statement is positive or negative, with respect to the topic being investigated. Any statements which are ambiguous are discarded, and only those statements which all raters agree on are included.

The next task is for the researcher to choose an equal number of positive and negative statements which will contribute to the final attitude scale. These are then arranged in random order, so that there is no regular pattern of positive and negative statements which might affect how people respond. The statements are each allocated a five-point scale, which usually goes from 'strongly agree' to 'strongly disagree', but which might be something like 'strongly believe' or 'strongly disbelieve', or some other phrases depending on the actual statement involved. The points on the scale are then assigned score values – usually 5 for an extreme positive response, 4 for a less extreme positive one, and so on – so that the person's responses can be collected to give a general answer.

The semantic differential

The Likert is a fairly direct type of attitude scale: The respondent is asked straightforwardly, about the topics of interest. Some attitude scales, however, approach the question of attitudes much more indirectly. One of the more interesting examples of this is the **semantic differential**, which was developed by Osgood in 1952, as a way of allowing a researcher to develop a much more rounded awareness of an attitude. Instead of seeing attitudes as a purely straightforward matter of cognitive belief, Osgood took advantage of people's ability to think in metaphors, and to express their understanding of concepts by drawing parallels with other aspects of experience.

The semantic differential asks the respondent to express how the target of the attitude measure would rate on a number of dimensions, as indicated in Figure 6.2. It represents an attempt to assess the emotional and associative nuances of an attitude – its connotative meaning – rather than its literal (denotative) meaning. As such, it tries to capture more of the depth in someone's attitude than can be measured by conventional scales.

Figure 6.2 Dimensions of a semantic differential

Father

angular	....	rounded
weak	....	strong
rough	....	smooth
active	....	passive
small	....	large
cold	....	hot
good	....	bad
tense	....	relaxed
wet	....	dry
fresh	....	stale

According to Dawes and Smith (1985), factor analysis of a large number of semantic differential studies, conducted in twenty-six different cultures, indicates that there seem to be three major underlying factors: evaluation (good–bad), potency (strong–weak) and activity (active–passive). In fact, these appear to be so powerful that if it is known how someone rates a particular concept on these three dimensions, it is possible to make a reasonable prediction of how they will respond to the more indirect dimensions of the semantic differential. But there are many advantages of using the full semantic differential rather than just asking someone to rate items on those dimensions, the chief one being that doing so encourages the respondent to think around the topic more deeply, so they are likely to gain a fuller awareness of their personal perceptions of it.

These are just two examples of attitude measurement, but there are many others. Each method of measuring attitudes has its limitations, as well as its advantages. One of the main problems about attitude measurement in general, for example, is that what people say does not always correspond with what they actually do.

Assumptions of attitude scales

There are three basic assumptions made by researchers using attitude scales (see Table 6.2). The first is that attitudes can be expressed in verbal statements – that there is a way of putting the attitude into words. This is fairly tricky, since emotions or feelings are often a major part of an attitude, but it is possible, as we saw with the semantic differential, for words themselves to be used as an indirect expression of feelings.

Table 6.2 Assumptions of attitude scales

1. It is possible to express attitudes using verbal statements.

2. A verbal statement will have the same meaning for all participants.

3. Attitudes expressed as verbal statements can be measured or quantified.

The second assumption is that the same statement has the same meaning for all participants. People often interpret the same words very differently; but for the most part, construction procedures for an attitude measure are designed to minimise this, by using multiple raters for attitude statements and checking on the ways that statements are perceived. But as we will see when we look at repertory grid analysis, everyone makes their own sense of situations, and sometimes people see things very differently from one another.

The third assumption of attitude scales is that attitudes, when expressed in the form of verbal statements, can be measured and quantified. This assumption lies at the heart of attitude measurement, and it applies to psychometric testing too. It also lies at the heart of some objections to attitude measurement and to psychometric testing, since there are some researchers who believe that it is only really possible to look at this aspect of human experience using qualitative approaches, and that attempts to quantify the subtleties of human thinking are misguided. Others disagree, and it is a matter for individual judgement where one stands on the issue. We will be looking at qualitative approaches in Chapters 10–13.

Attitude scales, then, are able to provide us with much more subtle information than can be obtained from a conventional questionnaire, as long as they have been constructed with attention to detail and following appropriate procedures – including the piloting process which is so important in any kind of test or questionnaire development. In a sense, attitude scales are a kind of half-way house between the ordinary questionnaire and that even more rigorous and specialised kind of research tool, the psychometric test.

Psychometric tests

Psychometric tests are tools developed by psychologists in order to gain an insight into aspects of human psychology which are normally hidden, or not immediately apparent. They provide the psychologist, and the person taking the test, with information of which the person was previously unaware. The idea behind most modern psychometric tests is that the information can then be used to help the individual make more informed choices, although in the past they were often used as instruments of social control – see Hayes (2000) or Gould (1981) if you are interested in finding out more about this.

What do these three terms mean?
idiographic tests
nomothetic tests
psychometric tests

Psychometric tests are not all the same, and some work very differently than others. Some psychometric tests, for example, are purely concerned with looking in detail at a particular person, and at how that person sees their world. We call these **idiographic tests**, and they are mainly used to allow a therapist or counsellor to gain an insight into that person's ideas or problems. Other psychometric tests are used to compare people with one another, so they involve measuring each person on a common scale or set of scales. These are known as **nomothetic tests**. Nomothetic tests can be used for all sorts of purposes, including educational and job selection.

Nomothetic tests are the psychometric tests used most commonly in psychological research, although in Chapter 8 we will be looking at how some idiographic tests, too, can be useful research tools for the psychologist. Whether a researcher chooses to use an idiographic test or a nomothetic one really depends on the type of study which is being conducted, and the approach to research which is being adopted.

For example, one issue which will inform the decision is whether the researcher is using an inductive approach or a hypothetico-deductive approach (see Chapter 1 and Table 6.3). Another is whether the researcher is interested in deriving general principles about human functioning from the research, or whether they are concerned with investigating and explaining specific examples of individual human experience. The choice of test will also depend, to a very high degree, on the researcher's own theoretical orientation, and the type of approach to psychology in general which they are adopting. All of these factors will combine to influence the researcher's choice of test.

Table 6.3 Nomothetic or idiographic?

Is the researcher adopting an inductive approach or a hypothetico-deductive one?

Is the immediate goal of the research to identify general principles of human functioning, or to study individual experiences?

Does the theoretical basis of the research emphasise individuality or similarities between human beings?

Test construction

What makes a psychometric test entirely different from an ordinary research questionnaire is the careful process of test construction that it has undergone. In the last chapter, we saw how important it is to pilot a questionnaire, in order to make sure that the questions are manageable and will provide the right type of information. Psychometric tests go through much more rigorous construction procedures, including several pilot stages.

A psychometric test typically consists of a very large number of questions, statements or simple problems, to which the person needs to respond. Sometimes there can be as many as two hundred of them, and there are rarely fewer than forty. They are known as **test items**. During the construction of a psychometric test, each test item is evaluated separately, and then their combined effects are evaluated again. The evaluation procedure is designed to ensure that every test item is reliable, valid and appropriately standardised. The three principles of reliability, validity and standardisation lie at the heart of test construction; so we will begin by looking at each of them.

What do these three terms mean?
reliability
validity
standardisation

Reliability

Reliability is an important principle of psychometric test construction. In essence, it is about making sure that the test gives consistent results in situations where consistency would be expected. For example, if a test is designed to evaluate a person's aptitude for doing a particular kind of work, then we would expect it to produce reasonably consistent results, at least over a short period of time. Our assumption would be that the person's aptitudes wouldn't change much in the short term, and so the test should reflect that consistency. If it gave different results just because the person happened to be in a different mood on another day, we would wonder whether it was really any use.

Effectively, there are three main ways that psychometric tests are evaluated for reliability, summarised in Table 6.4. The simplest way is known as the **test–retest method**, where a test is administered to a

Table 6.4 Ways of testing reliability

The test–retest method	The same test is administered twice to the same participants, on different occasions.
The split-half method	Half of the test is administered on one occasion, the second half on another occasion, to the same participants.
The alternative-forms method	Two equivalent versions of the test are developed. They are administered to the same set of participants on two different occasions.

What do these three terms mean?

test items

reliability coefficient

personality profile

---

group of people on one occasion, and then given to the same group of people on another occasion. Their scores on the complete test, and also on each of the test items, are compared and correlated, which provides a **reliability coefficient** for the test as a whole. We will be looking at correlation in Chapter 15, but a reliability coefficient is a number between −1 and +1 which indicates how similar the two test results are. The closer to +1 the number is, the greater the similarity between them; and in a typical psychometric test, anything less than +.8 would not really be considered reliable.

The test–retest method, though, has some disadvantages. The main one is that the people being tested may remember their original responses to the test when they do it for the second time. If they do, they may simply answer in the same way, without actually considering the test item carefully. That would mean that the reliability coefficient obtained by the test was artificially high, and would distort the test's evaluation.

One alternative to this problem is to evaluate reliability using the **split-half method**. This one is perhaps the oldest method, having been suggested by Spearman in 1907, and it is used for those psychometric tests which consist of a battery of questions. The test is divided into two halves, usually by taking even-numbered test items as one set, and odd-numbered ones as the other. Then a group of participants takes one half-test on one occasion, and the other half at a different time. The split-half reliability coefficient (r_a) is calculated by taking the correlation between the scores obtained from the two halves of the test (r), and applying it to the formula:

$$r_a = \frac{2r}{1 + r}$$

The problem with the split-half method, though, is that the way that the two halves are obtained is somewhat arbitrary. If the test is

Figure 6.3 A personality profile

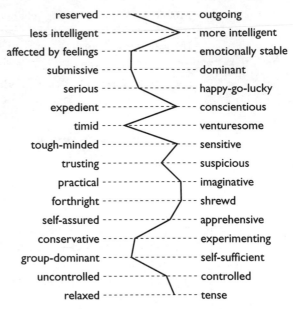

reserved	outgoing
less intelligent	more intelligent
affected by feelings	emotionally stable
submissive	dominant
serious	happy-go-lucky
expedient	conscientious
timid	venturesome
tough-minded	sensitive
trusting	suspicious
practical	imaginative
forthright	shrewd
self-assured	apprehensive
conservative	experimenting
group-dominant	self-sufficient
uncontrolled	controlled
relaxed	tense

Note: Based on Cattell's 16PF factors

What do these three terms mean?

subscales

population norms

standardised administration

divided into two in a different way, it may give slightly different results. Also, many modern tests contain a number of different subscales, and the items for each scale are distributed throughout the questionnaire. Many general personality tests take this form, asking the respondent to answer a large number of questions and then using a complex scoring procedure to organise the answers into a **personality profile**, which shows how the person measures up on several different personality traits (Figure 6.3). With this type of test, we would need to begin by identifying which subscale each item belonged to, and then separate each subscale into two halves – which would be a distinctly cumbersome way of going about things!

The third way of evaluating reliability is known as the **alternate-forms method**. This technique involves the use of two exactly equivalent forms of the same test. During test construction, researchers usually investigate several equivalent but different forms of each test item. Versions which have problems with validity or reliability are discarded, but if the test is being constructed thoroughly, this usually leaves at least two or three items which are precisely equivalent, in that they measure the same subscale and will contribute approximately the same amount of information to the overall result. By matching these items in pairs, and allocating one from each pair to each version of the test, it is possible to develop two precisely equivalent versions of a psychometric test.

Many commercial psychometric tests have two alternative versions, constructed when the test was first developed. Alternate-form reliability

Table 6.5   Types of validity

Face/surface validity	Whether a test seems valid on the surface, or according to 'common sense'.
Criterion validity	Whether the test gives results which agree with other measures of the same thing. Concurrent validity is concerned with comparisons with other measures taken at the same time, while predictive validity is concerned with comparisons with measures taken in the future.
Construct validity	Whether a test truly represents the theoretical construct it was developed to assess.
Ecological validity	Whether a test gives results which are representative of the results which would be obtained from studying that behaviour in the natural environment.

testing involves administering the two versions of the test to the same people, but on different occasions. Since each test item is different in the two tests, there is no problem about people remembering their replies from the last time.

There are still some drawbacks, though. Some psychometric tests require people to solve puzzles or complete tasks under time pressure. The first time someone does this, the time pressure may make an important difference to how they respond: they may rush, or feel under pressure. But a second occasion will feel more familiar. Also, there can be some **transfer of training**: if the test involves solving problems or puzzles, someone can change their scores simply because, having done that particular task before, they know how to go about doing it and so they do it better the second time. Intelligence test scores are particularly vulnerable to this type of improvement.

Validity

Validity is the second major principle of test construction. In its simplest form, validity is the question of whether a test, or a test item, actually measures what it is supposed to measure. Which may sound completely straightforward, but actually making sure that it does is more complex than it might appear at first sight. Table 6.5 lists the main types of validity.

The simplest form of validity is known as **face validity**, or sometimes surface validity. Essentially, it consists of judging that a measure is valid simply because it appears to be so, or it seems likely that it will be. In a questionnaire we might judge face validity according to the contents of the questions: if they seemed to be about the right sort of topic, we might conclude that the measure we were using was valid.

What do these three terms mean?

face validity

criterion validity

construct validity

But we wouldn't use face validity for a psychometric test because it has too many problems.

The main problems have to do with the way that something which seems valid on the surface may actually be nothing of the kind. In the nineteenth century, a number of eminent researchers believed that brain weight would be a good indicator of intelligence, for example. It seemed obvious: intelligence, they argued, depends on the brain, so a larger brain ought to mean higher intelligence. But when researchers actually began to look at the correlation between brain size and intelligence, they found that it was nothing like that straightforward. Some people with very large brains were also mentally retarded, while some geniuses proved to have surprisingly small brains. The idea has high face validity, but turned out to be absolute nonsense.

More recently, in the early part of the twentieth century, researchers believed it was possible to evaluate reading fluency by measuring how quickly people recognised letters and numbers. It seemed obvious that someone who could identify letters quickly would be a fluent reader: the idea had face validity. But later research into reading showed that it wasn't nearly that simple. The context, the person's prior knowledge, and their familiarity with words in general were much more important factors in reading fluency than speed in recognising letters. Face validity always seems logically reasonable at the time; but that can be very deceptive.

An alternative is to evaluate the validity of a measure by comparing it with some other standard which already exists. This is known as **criterion validity**, and it is how physical measures, like weights, lengths and amounts, are evaluated: there are exact measurement 'standards', which are kept in safe places, and used for comparison. The old imperial measures include a standard yard, which is a stick that is exactly a yard long, a standard pint, a standard gallon, and so on. There are also standard metres, litres and kilogrammes, which are physical objects used to make sure that any new measuring device is actually measuring what it is supposed to measure accurately. When we talk of something being used as a 'yardstick', or of something as 'coming up to standard', our words are referring to these measurement standards.

There are two kinds of criterion validity used by psychologists: concurrent validity and predictive validity. **Concurrent validity** is when a psychological test or measure of some kind is compared with a standard that already exists. For example, the results given by new intelligence tests are often evaluated for validity by comparing them with the results obtained by the same people on existing, well-established intelligence tests. Or a test of reading fluency might be compared with the results of a much more lengthy exploration of how fluently people read.

The second type of criterion validity is when the test is compared with some type of criterion which happens in the future, rather than

EXERCISE 6.1   **Test items and construct validity**

One of the main steps in converting a theoretical model into a psychometric test is operationalising the ways that the theoretical concepts can be converted into behavioural questions. Hayes (1997c) argued that one of the important issues in team success was the degree of social identification between members of the team, which could be conceived in terms of the following three dimensions:

Boundaries   establishing a clear distinction between the team and the rest of the organisation;

Cohesiveness   ensuring effective communication with the team and between team members, to ensure a good understanding of one another's roles and contributions;

Pride   identifying achievements and distinctiveness which would enable team members to be proud of, or derive positive self-esteem from, belonging to that team.

Imagine that you are trying to base a psychometric test on this theoretical model. For each theoretical dimension, write three test items which express these ideas in terms of practical behaviour.

How might you go about testing the validity of each of your test items?

being immediately available. This is known as **predictive validity**, because it is really concerned with a test's ability to predict what is likely to happen in the future. For example, a researcher developing a computer aptitude test, designed to indicate whether someone is able to learn about computers relatively easily, might give the test to a set of people who were about to begin working in the computer field. Six months or a year later, the researcher would be in a position to evaluate the predictive validity of the test, by comparing people's scores on the test with how well they had learned about computers.

The third major type of validity is known as **construct validity**. This is concerned with whether a test or measure actually reflects the theoretical constructs on which it is based. Any test will be designed in accordance with a particular theory – for example, a personality test will reflect the particular theory about personality held by those who develop it; or a test used to evaluate teamworking in organisations will reflect what its originators consider important about working in teams. Those theoretical constructions are particularly reflected in how the test is structured – in the number, type and relationship of its subscales. Construct validity is concerned with whether the full set of test items, taken together, will produce outcomes which fit with those theoretical constructions.

To take an example: one of the most well-known personality tests is the EPI, which stands for Eysenck Personality Inventory. This test has three subscales, which aim to measure extraversion, neuroticism and response bias. A construct validation of this test would involve giving the test to a number of participants, and analysing the various correlations between each of their responses. If the test has construct validity, we would expect to find that the neuroticism questions correlated fairly strongly with one another, but less strongly with the extraversion or response bias questions, and that the extraversion questions correlated with other extraversion questions more strongly than they did with those of the other two subscales.

To take another example: the Team Climate Inventory, developed by Anderson and West (1994), looks at the working atmosphere and general conditions for successful teamworking in organisations. It is based on a theoretical model developed by these researchers, which argued that there are four factors required for successful teamworking: support for innovation, participative safety, shared vision, and task orientation. The scales and subscales of the inventory (Table 6.6) reflect that theoretical model, with the addition of a social desirability scale which checks whether the respondents are exaggerating to make everything seem better than it is.

Table 6.6   Scales and subscales of the Team Climate Inventory

Scale	Subscale
Participative safety	Information sharing
	Safety
	Influence
	Frequency of interaction
Support for innovation	Articulated support
	Enacted support
Vision	Clarity
	Perceived value
	Sharedness
	Attainability
Task orientation	Excellence
	Appraisal
	Ideation
Social desirability	Social aspect
	Task aspect

Source: Anderson and West (1994).

A fourth type of validity has become increasingly important in recent years. This is all to do with how much a psychological test, or the measures used in a psychological study, actually reflect their equivalents in real life. It is known as **ecological validity**. Some psychologists, for example, have criticised intelligence tests because they tend to be concerned with pencil and paper problem-solving, and they consider that this is not a realistic description of what intelligence is like in real life, which might include, say, quick thinking at times of emergency, rapid repartee in conversations, and all sorts of other skills.

Several recent approaches to psychometric assessment have attempted to tackle the question of ecological validity by simulating real-life situations. For example, rather than asking people to complete a questionnaire, a test of a manager's decision-making ability to make appropriate decisions might involve giving each manager or potential manager a limited amount of time to make decisions about a number of problems which they might come across in a typical working day. In such situations, the testers hope that the test will be more useful because it is closer to the types of decisions which managers would normally face. In other words, it has higher ecological validity.

Technical discussion: Ecological validity

There have been some frequent misunderstandings about the concept of ecological validity. It is commonly assumed, for instance, that it is all about the environment within which an investigation is set – about how 'realistic' a situation is. There are historical reasons for this, since interest in ecological validity came about as a result of the increasing popularity of ethological observation (see Chapter 4), and the transformation which that made to many areas of psychology. When developmental psychologists such as Rudolph Schaffer were able to throw a completely new light on infant attachments by observing infants in their 'natural environments', psychology began to recognise just how important this type of study could be.

When it comes to the technicalities of the matter, though, ecological validity isn't quite the same as ecological research, even though it may have learned some lessons from it. The generally accepted definition of ecological validity is that given by Breakwell et al. (1995: 221), who described it as 'the degree to which the behaviour of the subjects in the laboratory corresponds to their behaviour in the natural environment'. This definition says nothing at all about whether the environment of the study itself simulates the 'natural environment'. Instead, its focus is on the behaviour of the research participants, and whether their reactions to events and situations are like the reactions they would make in their 'natural environment'.

> **continued**
>
> Cook and Campbell, in 1979, argued that ecological validity is effectively the same as what they referred to as external validity. This is not so much concerned with the 'natural environment' as with how far the findings of the study can be generalised. External validity, they argued, comes from the degree to which the effect can be generalised across different populations, different times and different situations. So in that context, an investigation like Milgram's research into obedience could be construed as ecologically valid, since it has been shown to generalise across populations, times and situations – even though the research itself consists of artificially contrived laboratory situations which are quite unlike the 'natural environment'. But this is a slightly different version of the definition, and not one which is shared by all researchers.

Standardisation

The third principle of psychometric test construction is **standardisation**. There are three different aspects of standardisation as applied to psychometric tests, summarised in Table 6.7. The first is the type of standardisation we encountered in Chapter 3, which involves standardised instructions and procedures. Because psychometric tests are so sensitive, it is important that they are conducted in the appropriate kind of atmosphere; so each test comes with a detailed set of procedures which need to be carried out meticulously by the tester, and also with very specific instructions, which must be read out word-for-word. This is quite unlike a questionnaire study, and it is one reason why the British Psychological Society has established Certificates of Competence in Psychometric Testing, for those who are not psychologists but who are administering psychometric tests.

The second aspect of standardisation is concerned with the test itself. With nomothetic tests, simply knowing how someone has scored on the test tells us very little. We can only interpret test scores when we can see them in the context of what might be expected from people in general. So the construction of a psychometric test also includes

Table 6.7 Types of standardisation

Standardised procedures and instructions.

Population norms providing standard responses from different population groups.

Test standardisation, ensuring that results are compatible with those of other tests in the same area.

---

the development of **population norms** – general tables which describe the typical scores from various groups within the population. The test needs to be administered to large groups of people, so that their scoring profiles can be obtained.

It is at this point that the statistical assumptions underlying psychometric tests become important. Nomothetic psychometric tests are almost all based on the assumption that the scores from a population as a whole would conform to a normal distribution (see Chapter 14). The population norms reflect what type of performance would be expected from different subgroups, and show how they would be placed within an overall normal distribution for the population as a whole. For example, the Team Climate Inventory developed by Anderson and West (1994) has specific population norms for those working in the Health Service, because the concept of teamworking in that context involves individuals from different professional groups, and this is quite different from a production team in, say, a car manufacturing plant.

Population norms are an important aspect of the use of psychometric tests, and using them inappropriately can challenge the validity of the test itself. For example: if a test has been developed and standardised on an American population, the norms for that test will reflect American test responses. If a researcher then takes the test and applies it to a population from a different culture – for example, a British one – they may reach serious misunderstandings about what the test results actually imply. This can mean that the findings obtained from using the test are simply not valid in that context.

The third aspect of standardisation of a psychometric test involves the test as a whole. For a test which is opening up a completely new area, this is not so important. But when a test is in an established field, the outcomes which it gives will need to fit with the criteria which are expected of other such tests. A new form of IQ test, for example, would need to give results which conformed, to some extent, with results from other IQ tests. It would also need to provide results which fitted the normal distribution curve, since that is a major assumption which is made about the distribution of intelligence in the population. Any new IQ test needs to be standardised to conform to these criteria.

There are some problems with this type of test standardisation, as you can see. Some researchers, for example, have questioned whether intelligence really is normally distributed. The assumption derives from an early assertion made by Francis Galton, that since physical characteristics such as weight and height are normally distributed, and since intelligence is presumably dependent on physical characteristics, intelligence too is bound to be normally distributed. But a century of brain research has failed to find any specific physical characteristics on which intelligence depends, and the assertion of normal distribution is as much an article of faith as anything else. The main evidence for it comes from the fact that IQ tests produce normally distributed scores, but this cannot be taken as real evidence since, as we have seen, producing a normal distribution is part of IQ test standardisation.

Reliability, validity and standardisation, then, are important principles of test construction, and they inform just about every step in the development of a psychometric test. It is for this reason that psychometric tests are so very different from ordinary questionnaires. Because they sometimes seem fairly alike on the surface – after all, the respondent just needs to answer a set of questions – it is easy to think that the two are quite similar. But really, they are very different indeed.

Ethical issues of psychometric measurement

Measuring psychological characteristics or attitudes raises a number of ethical problems. Perhaps the main one which is likely to occur with almost every test is the problem of deception. As we saw earlier in this chapter, people's answers to questionnaires, attitude scales and psychometric tests can all be influenced by response bias – the tendency for people to produce what they think are acceptable responses, or the answers they ought to give, rather than answers which truly reflect their behaviours, attitudes or characteristics.

What this means is that an attitude scale, say, which is trying to uncover information about socially undesirable attitudes needs to disguise what it is seeking, because if it is open and transparent, people will be able to see what is being asked and may adjust their responses accordingly. But disguising what the scale is about inevitably means that there is an element of deception – respondents are being deceived about the true focus of the attitude scale.

Deception or technical instrument?

There are several ways of dealing with the problem of response bias – by asking for indirect or hypothetical responses, by disguising the scales, or simply by being open about what is being asked and hoping that response biases cancel themselves out. But dealing with the ethical question is more tricky. As a general rule, researchers take the view that if a participant has given informed consent to participate in an attitude survey, then they have also agreed to be measured. The disguising of the scales is part of the measuring instrument, and contributes directly to its accuracy. So it isn't a question of people being directly deceived: they are aware that their attitudes are being measured, and the technical requirements of a good attitude scale mean that not every aspect of the way that measurement occurs can be instantly open to public view.

The technical instrument argument is even more commonly used when it comes to psychometric testing. Psychometric tests usually deal with the problem of response bias by introducing lie scales, which we met earlier in this chapter. These sometimes consist of specific test items to which only one response is likely to be true – such as 'Have you ever been late for work or college, for any reason?'. Because they are phrased in an exaggerated way, the chances are that the person who answers 'no' isn't telling the whole truth. But just in case they are, a lie scale consists of several of these items, and it is acceptable for someone to score one or two of them. More than that, though, and their answers to the test as a whole are deemed invalid, because of response bias.

Sometimes, lie-detector scales take a different form. In a complex test – and some psychometric tests are very long and demanding – the person may come across the same question more than once. They are not likely to recognise it as being the same, though, because it will have been phrased differently each time. Moreover, that difference will involve a choice of words which leads the response bias in a different direction from the first version of the question. Someone who is answering truthfully will answer these questions consistently, but someone who is lying will give the socially acceptable response to both answers. It won't be apparent in the test itself, or to a casual glance, but the test scoring system will pick it up.

There is, then, inevitably some deception in the actual process of psychometric testing, but again the technical instrument argument applies. It isn't practical to take every element of a psychometric measure and argue that it must be transparent and open to public view. The inner workings of medical scanners or X-ray machines aren't open to public view, either. The details of how they work are available in the technical journals to those who are interested in such things, and the same applies to psychometric tests.

Social uses of psychometric testing

What is of more importance in ethical terms is the use that is made of psychometric test results. Psychology's history is full of wide-scale social consequences from the abuse of intelligence testing in the first half of the twentieth century, which have been documented by Gould (1996) and others. These include, for example, the ideas about inherited intelligence and racial evolution which formed the ideological rationales for racist US immigration policies, in the first half of the twentieth century, and also for the Nazi attempt to annihilate the Jewish people in the concentration camps and gas chambers of World War II.

On a milder scale, in the 1960s there were some rather unpleasant social psychology studies which involved giving students false feedback from psychometric tests, in order to lower self-esteem and see what resulted. Nowadays, of course, that kind of research is totally unacceptable; but any psychometric test requires the person who did it to be given feedback, and that always involves some element of risk.

Ipsative and normative tests

The question of what a test is used for also relates to making sure that a test is used in the right kind of way. Some psychometric tests, for example, are **normative tests** – which means that they give results on standard scales, which are then compared with tables of population norms provided in the test manual, to give the tester an idea of how typical that person's result is. So you can use a normative test to compare one person with another.

However, there is another way of designing a test, which is also commonly used in test design, but is less suitable for comparisons. **Ipsative tests** are used to examine personality structure, in terms of which personality characteristics are stronger or weaker. So an ipsative test assessing a person on, say, the five robust factors of emotional stability, conscience, extraversion, agreeableness and openness to experience would give a result which showed the relative strength of each of these qualities in that person. What it wouldn't show was their absolute strength.

Ipsative tests are useful as the basis for counselling or careers advice. But they are not absolute measures of how strongly a person holds a trait – all they tell us is whether a trait is stronger or weaker than the rest of the set. Someone might score highly on all five, but their Openness score might be slightly weaker than the others. Although the ipsative test would show that as their weakest trait, it still might be stronger than in someone else who had scored it as their strongest one.

A normative test, then, can be used for comparison, but an ipsative test can't. In 1988, Johnson, Wood and Blinkhorn argued that the results from ipsative tests were often used for comparisons when they shouldn't have been, both in research and in job selection. This, they argued, was extremely misleading and amounted to a misuse of the tests.

The way that the test is administered is also important. Psychometric tests may appear easy on the surface, but a good test has been carefully constructed and requires exact conditions for its administration. There are qualifications in psychometric testing run by the British Psychological Society available to non-psychologists, which train people in test administration. No psychometric tests should be administered

EXERCISE 6.2   Which area of psychology?

Psychometric tests are used by psychologists working in many different fields. The main ones are clinical psychology, which deals with people experiencing mental problems or problems in living; occupational psychology, which is concerned with selecting people for jobs or occupations; educational psychology, which is concerned with learning and education; and organisational psychology, which is concerned with the human side of working in organisations.

Listed below are twelve different psychometric tests. Identify the main areas of psychology in which each of these would be most likely to be used.

A computer aptitude test
A diagnostic test for dyslexia
A job satisfaction inventory
A Q sort comparing self concept and ideal-self concept
A repertory grid test identifying someone's personal constructs
A test for visual neglect resulting from head injury
A vocational guidance test for career choice
An IQ test
An organisational commitment questionnaire
A trait-based personality test
A test for specific memory impairment following head injury
The Team Climate Inventory

by anyone who hasn't done this type of training or its equivalent. Most tests are restricted to qualified users, and not available to student research projects, because of the way that psychometric tests can reach sensitive areas, and test results can be badly misused or misunderstood.

For the qualified researcher, though, psychometric tests can be a useful way of obtaining information, as long as the ethical sensitivities of this way of gathering data are respected. There are psychometric tests dealing with personality, intelligence, aptitudes for different types of work, organisational processes such as teamworking, vocational guidance, and many other areas. For the qualified researcher, having this type of instrument available can provide a valuable tool to augment or focus a research study.

In the next chapter, we will be looking at another valuable research tool: the research interview and the several different forms it can take. Interviewing is becoming an increasingly important part of conducting research, as psychologists become more able to deal with the whole person who is participating in their research, and more interested in the way that person experiences the research process. So being able to conduct an appropriate and effective research interview is another important part of the psychologist's research tool-kit.

Self-assessment questions

1. *What are the three main methods for testing the reliability of a psychometric test?*

2. *List two advantages and two disadvantages of the Likert scale approach to measuring attitudes.*

3. *Briefly describe the semantic differential, and explain how it is used to measure attitudes.*

4. *Distinguish between the connotative meaning of a phrase or idea, and its denotative meaning.*

5. *What are the main ethical issues in psychometric testing?*

Concepts in use

1. *Diagnostic psychometric tests are widely used by clinical psychologists and by others working with people who are experiencing emotional or cognitive problems. What issues need to be considered when standardising such tests?*

2. *What are the advantages and disadvantages of using personality tests to select people for managerial jobs?*

3. *How might you go about trying to assess the predictive validity of a computer aptitude test being administered to trainees being taken on by a computer firm?*

4. *What types of problems might arise if the administration of intelligence and aptitude tests to a set of job candidates did not follow the proper standardised procedures?*

5. *How does the principle of the social responsibility of science apply to the practice of psychometric testing?*

7

Interviews

Interviewer effects
Conducting interviews
Stages of interview research
Ethical issues in interview research

Interviews are becoming increasingly popular as a research tool – indeed, when we look at qualitative analysis later in this book, we will find that the research interview is by far the most common way of gathering qualitative data. But in fact, since the earliest days of psychology, psychologists have used interviewing as a useful way of gathering data. The method was disparaged to some extent by the behaviourist school of thought, but even they conceded that 'verbal behaviour' sometimes provides useful research data.

An interview occurs when a participant is asked questions which have been designed to elicit particular types of information. In almost all research cases, those questions will be asked by another person – the person conducting research, or others who have been employed to do the interviewing. Interviews can take many forms: they can vary in time from a couple of brief questions to an in-depth, probing experience which lasts for an hour or more; they can vary in the structure of the answers required, from tightly specified interview schedules which amount to little more than verbally administered questionnaires to schedules designed to obtain open-ended and free-ranging accounts; and they can vary in the amount of interpersonal balance between the person being interviewed and the interviewer.

As an example of the latter, Massarik (1981) discussed how interviews can vary along a number of interpersonal dimensions. These dimensions include how hostile or accepting the participants are of one another; how much trust or distrust exists between participants; how the roles of interviewer and interviewee are played out – for example, whether these roles are extremely unequal or not – and the amount of closeness or 'psychological distance' which exists between the interviewer and the interviewee. Using these dimensions, Massarik identified six different forms of interview, which are listed in Table 7.1.

Table 7.1   Types of interview

1. **The hostile interview**	The interviewer and interviewee have different goals (e.g. a police interrogation interview).
2. **The limited survey**	Little personal involvement on the part of the interviewer, and minimal acquiescence from the interviewee (e.g. a product-based market research interview).
3. **The rapport interview**	Clearly defined but with a high degree of positive interaction and co-operation between interviewer and interviewee (e.g. a research interview about personal experience).
4. **The asymmetrical-trust interview**	One participant is more trustful than the other (e.g. a doctor–patient interview).
5. **The depth interview**	A high level of rapport and trust is established to explore views and motivations of the interviewee (e.g. an anthropological interview).
6. **The phenomenological interview**	This involves a maximum amount of trust and caring between the interviewer and interviewee, with few boundaries or limitations on interview content (e.g. some specialist qualitative research interviews).

Source: Massarik (1981).

Interviewer effects

What do these three terms mean? *non-verbal signals* *interviewer effects* *rapport*

Interviewing is a skilled activity, because of its interpersonal nature. People are extremely good at reading non-verbal signals – the minute changes in behaviour which indicate how information is being received. These are often unconscious on the part of the interviewer, but they can have a profound effect on how people respond. In a face-to-face situation, for example, most people like to be co-operative, and to avoid interpersonal conflict. So an unconscious indication from an interviewer that they disagree with what the person has said, or with a particular option in a question, can lead a respondent to change their answers into something that they feel is more socially acceptable.

Any interpersonal situation also means that people will bring their wider social knowledge and habits to bear on the situation. And this, too, can affect the answers which they produce. It is not uncommon, for example, for people to respond differently to male interviewers than they do to female ones; and studies in America showed respondents reacting differently to black interviewers than to white ones. The age of the interviewer can have an effect too: an older interviewer asking teenagers about their knowledge of drugs, or of youth culture, is likely to elicit quite different responses than a young interviewer would obtain. People adjust their responses according to what they consider is appropriate for the person asking the question.

Interviewer effects of this kind are something which need to be taken account of in any interview study. If the study is concerned with obtaining representative views from a large number of people, then it is likely that more than one interviewer will be needed – perhaps varying gender, age, and ethnicity – to make sure that any interviewer effects are balanced out in the sample as a whole. If the research is an in-depth case study, or some other situation where comparisons between people are less important, it will still be necessary to make sure that the respondent feels able to talk freely and openly with the interviewer. Sometimes people just don't 'hit it off' interpersonally, for reasons which are too subtle to pin down easily; but if that is the case that particular researcher is not going to be the best person to interview that particular respondent.

Interview skills

On the interviewer's side, too, conducting an interview requires a great deal of sensitivity. It involves establishing a **rapport** with the

| EXERCISE 7.1 | Interviewing for the future |

You have been commissioned to conduct an interview study of people's opinions about and use of recreational facilities in your local area. Recreational facilities as far as they are concerned includes sporting venues, theatres and cinemas, parks and allotments. You have free choice in how you will conduct your study, and a reasonable budget; and your report will be used directly to aid the council's future planning.

1. How will you go about finding the respondents for your study? List the characteristics which your pool of respondents will need to have (age range, etc.).

2. Will you conduct structured, semi-structured or open-structure interviews? Give reasons for your choice.

3. What factors will you need to take into account when you are planning your interview schedule?

4. What are the likely sections you might include in your report?

5. What ethical considerations are raised by this type of study?

participants, so that they feel able to talk freely and to give their opinions without being influenced. At the same time, it is an interpersonal affair, so if the interviewer simply acts woodenly, in an attempt to avoid influencing the replies, that in itself is artificial and will affect the way that the interaction proceeds. All of which means that a research interviewer needs to develop both verbal and non-verbal skills.

Verbal skills are involved, because what we actually say in interviews is important. Interviewers need to employ a number of techniques to avoid influencing what the interviewee says, while still encouraging people to talk freely. In some interview studies, particularly those which involve gathering data from large numbers of people, interviewers are given standardised responses they can make. These are similar to the standardised instructions which are sometimes used in experiments, and they are a rather simplistic way of trying to make sure that verbal influences are kept to the minimum.

Standardised responses are problematic for interviews, though, because they tend to make the situation very artificial. Interviewers need to be sensitive to the **speech registers** which are used in social situations; they need to make sure that the way in which they are talking to the other person involves the right kind of register. It can be hard to do this when delivering a pre-established set of responses; but people can be just as sensitive to this type of non-verbal cue as they are to differences between words.

Speech registers are of several kinds, but the five main groups are: frozen, formal, consultative, casual and intimate (see Table 7.2). As a general rule, we use speech registers unconsciously; but one of the differences between a skilled interviewer and an unskilled one is the way that a skilled interviewer will adopt a consultative register; while people who are unskilled at interviewing tend to use frozen or formal

> **What do these three terms mean?**
>
> *standardised responses*
>
> *interview*
>
> *speech registers*

Table 7.2 Types of speech register

Frozen	Speech is ritualised and empty of real meaning (e.g. a shop assistant saying 'Have a nice day').
Formal	Highly structured and very grammatical (e.g. a public lecture or a formal complaint).
Consultative	Friendly but polite (e.g. asking a stranger if the bus is due).
Casual	A relaxed, easy style, not particularly concerned about grammar or vocabulary (e.g. chatting with friends).
Intimate	Well-understood, close conversation with a high degree of shared understanding (e.g. family talk or talk between intimate friends).

EXERCISE 7.2	Choosing the interview type

The list below represents a series of topics for interview research. Which of the three main types of research interview – structured, semi-structured and open-structure – do you feel would be most suitable for each topic?

Absent-mindedness or failing memory
Choices of washing powder and cleansing products
Experiences in hospitals
Holiday plans
Local provision of public transport
Music preferences
Experiences of DIY
Pubs and clubs in the locality
Experiences of management at work
Ecologically sensitive domestic practices
The popularity of different hobbies or leisure activities
Views about ageing

styles, which are often very off-putting for the respondent. Standardised responses make this particularly likely to happen, and a great deal of training is required for an interviewer to be able to overcome that kind of problem. As a general rule, it is better for interviewer training to focus on developing verbal and non-verbal skills so that they can respond flexibly to the different interpersonal issues arising with different respondents.

One of the verbal skills which skilled interviewers acquire is **reflecting**, which is the skill of saying back to the person what they have just said. This isn't mechanical repetition: it generally involves using different words, in order to let the person see that the interviewer has heard and understood what they mean. Another is the skill of **amplifying**, which involves taking what someone has just said and broadening out its relevance or scope, to make the interviewee's meaning clearer. And a third verbal skill involved in interviewing is that of **non-committal agreement** – the ability to encourage another person to continue talking by expressing encouragement, but without actually expressing your own views. By using these skills, interviewers are able to encourage people to speak openly without influencing them unduly, but also without having to pretend to be robots.

Interviewers also need to be sensitive to **non-verbal signalling**. It is very easy to guide people unconsciously by nodding the head, or

What do these three terms mean?

non-committal agreement

verbal behaviour

verbal influences

Figure 7.1 An interview observation schedule

---

1. The amount of time the interviewer looked directly at the interviewee was:

   Far too little   *Not enough*   *About right*   *A bit too much*   *Far too much*

2. Which of these expressions did the interviewer use during the interview?

Smiling	*Sympathetic*	*Interested*
Frowning	*Enquiring*	*Neutral*
Concerned	*Pleased*	*Bored*
Tired	*Questioning*	*Apathetic*

3. Which expression did the interviewer use most often? _____

4. How was the interviewer's tone of voice? Place a mark on the scale in the appropriate position.

Always the same	___ ___ ___ ___	*Very varied*
Suited to topic	___ ___ ___ ___	*Not suited to topic*

5. Was the interviewer's posture:

Alert?	*Yes*	*Mostly*	*Sometimes*	*No*
Positive?	*Yes*	*Mostly*	*Sometimes*	*No*
Neutral?	*Yes*	*Mostly*	*Sometimes*	*No*
Encouraging?	*Yes*	*Mostly*	*Sometimes*	*No*

6. Did the interviewer use appropriate gestures?

   Yes   *Mostly*   *Sometimes*   *No*

7. Did the interviewer employ any noticeable mannerisms (fiddling with hair, pencils, etc.)

   Yes   *Mostly*   *Sometimes*   *No*

8. Did the interviewer show that they were listening by:

Nodding?	*Often*	*Occasionally*	*Hardly ever*	*Never*
Saying 'uh-huh' etc.?	*Often*	*Occasionally*	*Hardly ever*	*Never*
Mirroring expressions?	*Often*	*Occasionally*	*Hardly ever*	*Never*

---

smiling if they say the kind of thing you want them to say, or by frowning if they say something unexpected or unwelcome. But equally well, adopting a rigid posture and refusing to make any movements at all is just as artificial; so again an interviewer needs to be aware of the non-verbal skills involved in interview situations.

A skilled interviewer has a broad knowledge of the kinds of messages which non-verbal signals can convey, and uses these in order to make the other person as relaxed as possible. Details like making eye-contact with the respondent, and using appropriate styles of posture, gestures and tones of voice are important. When they are first learning to conduct interviews, many people find it useful to practise these in front of a video camera or in front of friends. Figure 7.1 gives a sample check-sheet which can be used for observing interviewing style and looking at the different non-verbal dimensions which are involved.

Conducting interviews

One of the first things that a researcher intending to carry out an interview study needs to do is to establish the range of information being sought. Is the purpose of the interview to confirm a series of ideas which have already been established through other research? Is it to begin an investigation of an entirely new area, to see what aspects of it seem to be important? Or is it to look around a topic, to see if there are additional issues apart from the central question which might be relevant? Each of these questions involves a different range of information, and that will have implications for the form of interview that the researcher conducts.

A researcher also needs to consider what type of information they need to obtain. Is it factual information, about what people do or how they organise their time? Is the researcher aiming to collect people's views and opinions on a particular topic? Or is the interview to be concerned with the intimate details of personal experience? These are only examples, of course – there are other types of information which an interviewer can collect. But each of these types also has implications for the form of the interview.

| **What do these three terms mean?**

rapport interview

depth interview

salient quotes |

It is possible to use Massarik's classification, which we looked at in Table 7.1, to organise this information. For example, if the interviewer is collecting people's views or opinions on a particular topic, then a rapport interview would be most appropriate. If, on the other hand, the interview is concerned with something very straightforward, like an investigation of where people find it most convenient to study in college, then a limited survey interview would be more suitable. Or if the interview is to be about something personal, or something which the subject is likely to want to explain in detail, or if the researcher has no clear idea what people might say, then a depth interview might be the most suitable technique to adopt.

Another way of looking at interviews is to consider them in terms of the **interview schedule**. All research interviews, no matter how open or free-ranging they are, will have some kind of schedule, if only one which says how much time the interviewer and interviewee have available and roughly the area they are looking at. That is probably the most unstructured type of interview which takes place in psychological research, and it does have its place. In Chapter 11 we will be looking at phenomenological analysis, which often draws its data from interviews of this kind.

Structured interviews

Most research interviews in psychology, however, have a more structured interview schedule than that. The interview schedule is the way that the researcher makes sure that what is discussed represents the topic of the study. So the range and purpose of the study affect the nature of the interview schedule. In the case of a study where the interviewer requires very specific information, the interview schedule can be extremely tightly specified, stating exactly which questions should be asked, and sometimes even how responses should be coded.

This type of structured interview schedule is extremely similar to a verbally administered questionnaire – indeed, the only difference between the two is that the interviewer is present, and therefore able to explain something more clearly to the respondent if that should be needed. Even then, in this type of study, the interviewer's responses are often standardised, and what they can and can't say is tightly controlled.

We looked briefly at using standardised responses earlier in this chapter. Effectively, what it means is that what the interviewer is able to say has been scripted in advance, and is not left open to the interviewer's judgement. If the answer that the person gives to a question is unclear, and the interviewer needs to ask for further clarification, they use **probe questions**. These are questions which have also been worked out beforehand, in order to encourage the respondent to produce an answer which is more relevant to the researcher's topic of interest. The pre-scripting of questions, though, means that apart from deciding whether or not a probe question is required, there is very little left to the interviewer's judgement or initiative.

There are also issues concerning the way that a structured interview schedule should be drawn up, and these are exactly the same ones as affect the drawing up of a good questionnaire. So if you are planning to conduct a structured interview study, you should look at Chapter 5, and plan the interview schedule following the procedures which we looked at there. A structured interview schedule is suitable for collecting the same type of information as a questionnaire, and may be the best option for getting information from large numbers of people. The fact that they have to be administered personally does make them more expensive and time-consuming than questionnaires, but they do tend to have a better response rate.

On the other hand, this type of interview has its own problems. The rigidly structured approach to interviewing is one of the legacies from behaviourist methodology, with its perpetual quest for 'objective' data

What do these three terms mean?
probe question
consultative register
structured interview schedule

and its insistence that cognitive or motivational aspects of human experience were 'contaminating influences' on psychological research. Unfortunately, though, trying to study people so 'objectively' in itself distorts what happens, because it creates such a peculiar situation. People respond to one another as human beings, and we react completely differently to someone who is unable to act spontaneously than we do to someone who is more relaxed and open. And this kind of difference is one which matters very much in psychological research, because it is concerned with being more open and giving more information to the interviewer.

Semi-structured interviews

Consequently, modern psychologists use interviews very differently. They use them to collect people's ideas, opinions, or accounts of their experiences. This means that modern research interviews rarely conform completely to the structured interview style. Instead, researchers use either semi-structured or open-structure interviews. Semi-structured interviews are not concerned with obtaining coded answers to specific questions. They allow the respondent more freedom to answer the question, and researcher more freedom in the way they ask it.

At the same time, they do collect the responses to a specific set of questions. A semi-structured interview schedule involves a set of questions, which are phrased in such a way as to allow a respondent to answer relatively openly. But the ways that the questions are asked does mean that they have specific answers: it isn't about just allowing the person to talk freely about anything they like.

A semi-structured interview schedule will include a number of 'closed' questions, to which the respondent's answers can be coded or categorised easily; but it will also include a number of questions where the respondent answers in their own words and the interviewer notes down these responses as exactly as possible. The questions are very similar to the open-ended questions in a questionnaire, and the schedule itself often looks a bit like a form with a lot of blank lines for writing in the answers. Figure 7.2 gives an example of a semi-structured interview schedule which was used for collecting data about people's views on environmental issues. As you can see, the questions do have definite answers; but the schedule allows the person to respond in their own words.

Clinical interviews are semi-structured interviews used in a specific setting for research purposes. They are often used as a way of investigating child development, because they allow the researcher to ask very specific questions in a context which seems relatively natural – or at least less formal – to the child. Perhaps the most famous clinical interviews were those conducted by Piaget on children's cognitive

Figure 7.2 A semi-structured interview schedule

Please write answers in the spaces provided, as clearly as you can.

1. What is the Greenhouse Effect, and how is it caused?

2. What are the biggest sources of pollution in this country? What effects is that pollution likely to have?

3. What are the likely consequences of the destruction of the world's rainforests?

4. Why do we need the ozone layer?

5. What causes acid rain? What does acid rain do?

6. Apart from any mentioned here, which environmental issues would you identify as being of primary concern?

development, in which children were set specific problems to solve, and their responses were taken as indicating the level of cognitive development that they had reached.

Other types of clinical interview have been used by researchers in different contexts. Effectively, these interviews are conducted in a setting which is designed to allow them to seem as unintrusive as possible, and which also permits the researcher to observe the way that the person interacts with others or within the setting as the interview is carried out. Clinical interviews may be combined with covert observations, as they are in many family therapy units, for example; or in a therapeutic context such as play therapy for children. They are a bit different from other forms of semi-structured interview because of the context in which they take place, and they are also a bit less structured. But they, too, require good interviewing skills on the part of the person carrying them out.

Open-structure interviews

Another very popular type of interview which is being used increasingly in psychological research is an approach which we might call

open-structure interviewing. These are rapport interviews which do have a structure, but one which is less clearly defined than a semi-structured interview. Rapport interviews which encourage people to give open-ended accounts of their ideas and opinions have become increasingly popular in psychological research. These interviews are much richer in terms of the quality of the information which the interviewer receives, but require the respondent to have the freedom to organise their answers more freely. Often, they come across as if they were just conversations between the interviewer and the respondent.

At the same time, research interviews are usually carried out for a specific reason, and so the research interview does need to be more controlled than an open-ended conversation. Typically, an open-structure interview will have an interview schedule of some kind, but this is very flexible indeed: sometimes it is little more than a list of the main topics which the interview should cover. One such list used in a study of social identification in small companies is shown in Table 7.3. The first question wasn't particularly important to the study, but was used as a **primer** question – one which encourages the respondent to start talking. Once the conversation has started, it becomes easier for people to discuss other issues.

Open-structure interviews are presented to the respondent as a collaborative venture: the purpose of the interview is discussed openly, and if it involves a list of topics, the respondent is shown this from the start, so that they can see what the interview should be covering. The interviewer then conducts the interview in such a way as to make it seem as much like a normal conversation as possible, concentrating on getting the interviewee to feel as relaxed as possible, so that they can talk freely. In this type of interview, the interviewer has freedom

> **What do these three terms mean?**
>
> *primer question*
>
> *emotively loaded words*
>
> *open-structure interviewing*

Table 7.3   An open-structure interview schedule

When did you first join the company, and how did this happen? What did you do before?

How would you describe your role within the company? Who do you answer to mostly?

How do you get to hear about new developments or arrangements within the company?

Do you enjoy working here? Can you give me any examples of events that are typical of working here?

Does the company have any social events outside of working hours?

How would you compare the company with other, similar companies?

How do you think the company is likely to develop in the future?

to phrase the questions how they like, and to make decisions based on their own judgement of how the interview is going and what the person will respond to.

This doesn't mean, though, that they don't have any guidance. The interview schedule defines the topics which must be covered during the course of the interview; but the way in which this is achieved is up to the interviewer. As the period of time allotted to the interview comes to an end (the usual length for this type of interview is about 20 minutes), the researcher and respondent check back over the list of topics to make sure that they have all been covered during the course of the conversation.

Open-structure interviewing, then, requires the interviewer to have good interviewing skills, and to be able to put the interviewee at ease. It also requires the interview to be tape-recorded, since even someone skilled in shorthand would find it hard to note down everything someone says when they are talking openly and freely.

This raises ethical issues, of course. It is essential for the respondent to give their consent to being tape-recorded; and also to give their consent for the content of the interviews to be used for research purposes. Sometimes this doesn't happen. In one case, I was conducting a set of interviews in a small company, which were partly designed to provide information for my own psychological research, but also contributed to a consultancy report, providing anonymous feedback for the managers of that company (this is the study from which Figure 7.2 was drawn). One respondent was happy to be interviewed, but refused to give permission to be tape-recorded. So I was able to take notes and use his opinions for the consultancy report, but the interview couldn't be used for my own research purposes, which required the more detailed record provided by the tape.

Analysing interview data

As you have seen, different types of interview provide different forms of data, and these require different types of analysis. We will be looking at analysis in detail in Part II of this book; but since the analysis needs to be taken into account from the first moment the interview was planned, we will consider some of the main points about it here.

One of the advantages of structured interviews is the way that they provide a limited range of answers, which can be clearly coded and are open to statistical analysis. The answers provided in structured interviews are usually coded by the respondent as they go, and are relatively easy to organise and collect. So the results from this type of study can be clearly presented, with diagrams and numerical summaries of what was found. We will be looking at the statistics available for this type of data in Chapters 15 and 16.

Data from semi-structured interviews can be analysed in several different ways. Any techniques which can be used to analyse open-ended questionnaire data will be suitable for semi-structured interviews as well. The most common one is **content analysis**, which consists of identifying the general themes mentioned in the interviews, and then counting the number of times they are mentioned. We will be looking at this in Chapter 14; but it does allow the researcher to do some statistical analysis, since it provides lists of frequencies for each theme. Again, the most suitable techniques for analysing this type of data are descriptive ones, which will be covered in Chapters 15 and 16. We do need to remember, though, that simply reducing everything to numbers can be misleading, in that how often something is mentioned doesn't automatically show how important the theme is.

Sometimes, it is possible to look at more detailed aspects of the data. If respondents' answers have been collected word for word, it may be possible to go through the material looking for **emotively loaded words**. This is a method proposed by Eiser (1975), and it can often give important clues to the attitudes underlying what people have said in interviews. It is a technique which works best with transcripts of open-structure interviews, but it is also possible to use it with semi-structured data.

Identifying **salient quotes** is also a method which can sometimes be used with data from semi-structured interviews, although it tends to work best with open-structure material, since the answers are generally more spontaneous. This is the most basic form of qualitative analysis, and we will be looking at it in Chapter 10. For semi-structured interviews it is often best to focus on considering the range of answers which were obtained, and looking at some of the direct content which they reveal.

Most of the qualitative analysis techniques which are described in Chapters 10–13 can be used to analyse open-structure interview data. Once the interviews have been transcribed, which is hard work but more or less unavoidable for proper qualitative analysis, then there is a wide range of techniques available to the psychological researcher. If you are conducting a more limited study for coursework, it is sometimes possible to perform a limited analysis which involves listening to the tapes over and over again and identifying salient quotes. That will depend on the topic you have been investigating, and the type of material you have collected.

If you are thinking of using interview studies for coursework, therefore, you need to think very carefully about how you will analyse them, because some of the analytical techniques used by professional psychologists are complex, time-consuming, and require considerable sophistication in the use of computers! However, there are some simpler techniques available for each type of interview, which are more limited but can be used fairly easily, and which can often give interesting results.

Interviewing and everyday life

One of the big advantages of interviews is the way that we can explore people's experiences through the accounts that they give in the interview. For example, Brown and Canter (1985) performed an investigation of how people react in fires, based on interview data, and showed that you could gain a great deal of insight from people's own accounts of their experiences, and what they thought was happening at the time. Interviews have also been used to amplify our understanding of people's experience of common events, as illustrated by the investigation of peaceful crowds conducted by Benewick and Holton (1987), both during and after the Pope's 1982 visit to Britain.

   Interviews can also compensate for the limitations of traditional research procedures. In 1977 Bromley argued that an analysis of the ordinary language that people use to describe things may be richer and more fruitful for psychologists than more traditional research frameworks would be; and that this would more than compensate for the extra trouble which is involved in analysing the data.

Stages of interview research

Interviews, then, are a valuable source of information for the psychologist. Using interviews, we can gain insights into people's behaviour which we simply wouldn't have using other methods. In particular, we can use interviews to find out how respondents understand their experiences and their worlds, and this is something which has become increasingly important throughout modern psychology.

Like any other systematic research technique, conducting a good set of interviews involves a number of stages. These are summarised in Table 7.4, but we will look at them in more detail here. Stage one is defining the aims of the interview. This means examining closely just what the study is for, and whether it is using an inductive or hypothetico-deductive approach. In the latter case, it also means identifying the theory being investigated, and identifying any hypotheses which will be explored as part of the study. The researcher needs to ask why this particular research requires interviews rather than some other kind of research technique.

Table 7.4   Stages of interview research

1. Defining the aims.

2. Deciding the form that the interview will take.

3. Planning the content of the interview.

4. Devising the interview schedule.

5. Conducting the interview.

6. Analysing and summarising the data.

Stage two involves deciding the form that the interview will take. That means deciding whether to use a structured, semi-structured or open-structure interview, and that decision will rest very much on the type of data which is needed, and the way that they are to be ana-lysed. So in order to complete stage two, a researcher really needs to plan the whole study, right up to presenting the final results.

In stage three, the researcher plans the content of the interview. This means deciding what areas are to be covered, and what the focus of the interview is to be. If it is to be a structured or semi-structured interview, then the researcher needs to establish what kind of information is required and what the topics of the questions will be. If it is to be an open-structure interview, the topic areas need to be established, to make sure that the respondents' talk is based around the area of research interest.

Stage four involves devising the interview schedule itself. This is not a simple task: structured and semi-structured interview schedules need to be developed very carefully, following the guidelines for question-naires that we looked at in Chapter 5. In the case of an open-structure interview, the topic areas more or less become the interview schedule, but they need to be phrased carefully, to make sure that the respond-ent understands them properly. And, no matter what type of inter-view is being used, the interview schedule needs **pilot testing**. It has to be tried out on a set of respondents, to make sure that they can understand it easily, and that there are no accidental ambiguities or problems with the phrasing.

Stage five involves conducting the interviews. As we have seen, that means paying attention to non-verbal and verbal interview skills, estab-lishing a good rapport with the respondent, and gaining permission for tape-recording and later use of the data. It is also important to make sure that the data are collected in a clear legible and audible form (the pilot-testing stage should include piloting tape-recordings and transcription: it is amazing how often technical problems produce problems in this type of research.)

Stage six involves analysing and summarising the data that have been obtained, and preparing the final report. This might involve statistical diagrams, of the kind we will look at in Chapter 16; it might involve numerical summaries of the data; or it might involve selecting a series of quotations which illustrate the main findings. Whichever method is the most suitable for the topic, the way that the results will be presented should inform the earlier planning stages, to make sure that the form of the interview and the type of data which have been collected do provide data which can be reported in the type of report which is required.

Ethical concerns with interview studies

Interview studies, like all research methods, raise ethical issues. One of these is the topic of the interview itself, and the competence of the interviewer to explore a particular topic. One of the great strengths of interview methods is that they allow a researcher to investigate personal experience. But in some cases, such as experience of child abuse, or other psychological trauma of another kind, an interviewer can find that their questions have become extremely distressing for the participant, and that the interviewer ends up adopting the role of counsellor.

As a researcher, it is your responsibility to make sure that you do not put yourself in situations which are outside your professional competence. Situations such as these require trained professionals, and it is both irresponsible and unethical to attempt to deal with them in an amateur manner. So although they may seem like interesting areas to explore, it is best to avoid that type of topic unless you are a qualified counsellor or clinical psychologist.

We have already touched on another ethical question, which is the matter of obtaining the respondent's informed consent. Those who participate in interview studies are entitled to say whether or not they will be tape-recorded, and should have the right to refuse, even if this is inconvenient for the researcher. Respondents also need to be asked for their permission if you wish to use the data they provide for research purposes, and it is best to get this permission in writing.

It might not seem necessary to obtain written permissions if you are carrying out an interview study for coursework, in that it might seem obvious what the interview is for; but people are interviewed for all sorts of reasons in modern societies, and obtaining such permission explicitly is a way of making sure that they have given their informed consent. It is also a good idea to obtain their consent for using quotations from their interviews in subsequent publications. Figure 7.3 shows what this type of consent form might look like.

Figure 7.3 A typical consent form for an interview study

I, _____, agree that the interview data which I provide to _____ on this date _____ may be tape-recorded and used for research purposes, provided that my identity is not revealed by the researcher.

I also agree that extracts from the recording can be used in reports relating to that research, providing that confidentiality is respected in all cases.

(signed) _____

You will notice that the consent form includes the proviso that confidentiality must be respected. This is one of the most important ethical issues in interview research. It needs to be routine practice for a researcher to protect the identity of anyone who is interviewed for research purposes, and to make sure that they cannot be identified from the material used in the reports. Most researchers deal with this matter by using identification codes or false names from the time the interview data are first put into written form – that is, when they are first collected or transcribed. By using these pseudonyms from the very start, mistakes are less likely to happen.

Remember, too, that people often speak about others during the course of an interview, and those names, too, will need to be disguised during transcription or reporting. Otherwise it might be possible to identify someone from what they have said about someone else, and that would be breaking confidentiality just as thoroughly as attaching their name to the report. It is always the researcher's responsibility to make sure that their research participants can't be identified by other people.

Interviews, then, are a useful way of collecting data about human beings. One of their great advantages is the way that they offer scope for in-depth explorations of people's experiences. In the next chapter, we will look at how case-study research, too, brings in-depth exploration of human experience within the grasp of the psychological researcher.

Self-assessment questions

1. *Distinguish between structured, semi-structured and open-structure interviews.*

2. *How can a knowledge of speech registers help in training effective interviewers?*

3. *What did the behaviourists mean by the term 'verbal behaviour', and how is this idea different from regarding the information which people give in interviews as 'accounts'?*

4. *List three advantages and three disadvantages of using structured interviews with standardised responses from the interviewer.*

5. *Describe the main verbal skills involved in conducting interview research.*

Concepts in use

1. *What problems might arise if an interviewer with poor non-verbal skills tried to conduct an interview study of child-rearing practices among mothers of toddlers?*

2. *What issues would you need to consider when designing an interview schedule to investigate people's religious beliefs?*

3. *What ethical issues might be raised by an interview study of close family social interactions?*

4. *Describe a typical clinical interview used by Piaget in his research into child cognitive development. What are the advantages and disadvantages of this approach to interviewing?*

5. *What type of interview schedule do you think would work best if you were conducting interviews in a works canteen about equal opportunities within the organisation? Give the reasons for your answer.*

8

Case studies and ethnography

The case-study approach
Case-study research techniques
Ethical aspects of case-study research
Ethnography

Case studies are an approach to psychological research which don't try to gather information from large numbers of research participants. Instead, they focus on single cases and explore them, often using more than one research method. Case studies allow a researcher to investigate a topic in far more detail than might be possible if they were trying to deal with a large number of research participants, and they can often provide the theoretical insights which stimulate other types of research.

Psychology has always used information from case studies. The earliest psychologists recognised their value, as they drew on single cases to develop insights into psychological mechanisms. Many major theoretical perspectives in psychology derived from case studies, such as the Piagetian model of child development. And they form the main part of research into topics such as clinical neuropsychology and other areas of physiological psychology. Since these are the most 'scientific' areas of psychology, it is a little ironic that a culture began to develop in mainstream psychology in the middle and later part of the twentieth century wherein case studies were regarded with slight suspicion, as being 'unscientific'.

These reservations had two sources. The first was a rather narrow perception of the nature of scientific research, which led to the assumption that only nomothetic approaches to research (see Chapter 1) were valid in psychology. That perception originated with the behaviourist school of thought, which asserted that the purpose of psychological research was to identify general laws of behaviour. This, in turn, led to the belief that only research conducted on large numbers of people could be valid, and that belief continued to influence psychological methodology long after psychologists had accepted that identifying psychological mechanisms and processes is just as useful as attempting to identify general laws. Case studies were treated with suspicion because it was impossible to tell whether the individuals being studied were actually representative of the population.

The second reason why many psychologists were uncertain about the value of the case study as a research method has to do with the dangers of anecdotal evidence. Lay knowledge – the commonly accepted knowledge of society – is full of generalisations from single cases, on the basis of personal anecdotes about individual experience. Most of these come to entirely false conclusions about human psychology. Even the most basic study of psychology shows how easily human reasoning is distorted by prejudices, fallacies of reasoning, selective memory, and many other mechanisms. So distinguishing between everyday anecdote and systematic evidence is a major concern of psychological research.

Properly conducted case-study research is very different from the type of anecdotal evidence so prevalent in everyday society. But the fact that case studies draw their evidence from single individuals, for many psychologists, came uncomfortably close to using anecdote to support psychological theorising. It accompanied a wider uncertainty about the value of qualitative research methods, as 'mainstream' psychology held to a belief that only quantitative forms of analysis could be rigorous enough to ensure objective investigation of a topic. This uncertainty has changed over time, as qualitative techniques have developed and addressed the problem of rigour, and as psychology in general has recognised the value of inductive research.

Modern researchers, therefore, are much clearer about the role of the case study in the psychological researcher's tool-kit. Case studies are not used to develop general laws about human behaviour in modern psychology. Instead, they are used to open up and explore aspects of human experience, and to give us insight into how psychological processes may be operating. The fact that case studies allow us to investigate experiences in depth means that we can use them to identify interactions and influences in ways which would not be possible with larger samples. Each of these can then be investigated separately, using different research methodologies.

> **What do these three terms mean?**
>
> *nomothetic research*
>
> *qualitative research*
>
> *inductive research*

Using case studies

Not every topic is suitable for case-study research. In many cases, it is much more appropriate to conduct experiments or large-scale systematic observations. It all depends on the topic being investigated, and what the researcher is actually trying to achieve. Judging whether a research project would benefit from a case-study approach means looking very carefully at what the case-study method has to offer the researcher.

Searle (1999) identified four advantages of case studies, which have been summarised in Table 8.1. The first is that a case study can sometimes highlight extraordinary behaviour, which can stimulate new research. For example, Luria's study of the memory man enabled researchers to begin to investigate cases of unusual memory abilities, and the cognitive mechanisms which made such phenomena possible. Without the case study, it is unlikely that this area of research would have been opened up in the same way.

Table 8.1 Advantages of case studies

Stimulating new research

Contradicting established theory

Giving new insight into phenomena or experience

Permitting investigation of otherwise inaccessible situations

The second advantage is that case studies can sometimes contradict established psychological theories. Searle cites the case study of severely deprived Czechoslovak twins, and the remarkable recovery they showed when placed in a caring social environment, as an example of a case study which challenged the established theory of the early years of life being a critical period for human social development.

Because they are so rich in information, case studies can give us insight into phenomena which we could not gain in any other way. For example, the case of S.B., a blind man given sight in adulthood, gave researchers a particularly detailed insight into the processes and experiences of perception, highlighting aspects of the experience which had not previously been suspected.

The fourth advantage of case studies identified by Searle is that they make it possible for psychological researchers to investigate cases which could not possibly be engineered in the psychological laboratory. For example, the case of the severely deprived child, Genie, enabled researchers to study the effect of extreme social deprivation continued from infancy to puberty. To create such a situation for research purposes would be entirely unacceptable, not to mention deeply unethical; but when Genie was discovered by social workers, the use of case-study methodology permitted much deeper insights into the mechanisms, processes and consequences of her experience and recovery.

Sadly, however, Genie's case – and Genie herself – was a casualty of that suspicion of case-study methodology mentioned earlier. She was discovered during the 1960s, at a time when the influence of behaviourist assumptions about measurement and nomothetic research was at its height. Only quantified data were considered to be truly scientific research evidence, preferably obtained from large groups of people, and the researchers had no way of expressing the extremely rich qualitative evidence they were obtaining, in the kind of quantitative terms which their grant committee would accept. The project's funds were terminated after two years, even though Genie was making good progress, recovering well, and providing psychologists with valuable data about language acquisition and recovery from abuse. The social services department took over her case and placed her with a family where she was abused again and rapidly lost the improvements in language functioning and social skills which she had gained through the psychological research project.

What is a case?

A single case doesn't have to mean just one single person. It might be a family, a social group, or even a single organisation, which might even involve large numbers of people. Table 8.2 lists five different types of case which could be the subject of a case study, ranging from an in-depth study of a single individual to the study of an organisation or an event. So a single case study can involve actually dealing with quite a number of individuals. For example, Hayes and Lemon (1990) described a case study which involved interviewing staff in a small but growing computer company, on the social psychological aspects of managing staff. This information could then be compared with other larger companies, in terms of how they had tackled staff management issues at a similar stage in their history.

Table 8.2   Types of case study

Person	The study of one single individual, generally using several different research methods
Group	The study of a single distinctive set of people, such as a family or small group of friends
Location	The study of a particular place, and the way that it is used or regarded by people
Organisation	The study of a single organisation or company, and the way that people act within it
Event	The study of a particular social or cultural event, and the interpretations of that event by those participating in it

Interviewing is not the only method used by case-study researchers, though. Clinical neuropsychologists who are investigating someone who has suffered a distinctive brain injury will use a number of specific tasks, designed to reveal if there are neurological deficits occurring as a result of the injury. These may range from specific memory tasks, in which the person is asked to listen to something like a news report and then tell the researcher what it was about; to drawing tasks, designed to show whether the person shows any kind of visual neglect; to single-eye and handedness tasks which might indicate whether there are unusual differences in functioning between the two halves of the participant's brain.

In another example, Smith (1997) studied the experience of pregnancy undergone by four women. By seeing each of the women at regular intervals throughout their pregnancy and afterwards, Smith was able to explore detailed aspects of their experiences, and also to see how their memories of the experience changed over time and in retrospect. The women's experiences were explored using a number of different techniques, including repertory grid and diary methods, which we will look at in the next chapter, and depth interviewing, which we looked at in Chapter 7.

Triangulation

What do these three terms mean?

triangulation

systems analysis

psychological field

The advantage of using multiple methods of investigation, as Smith did, as is that doing so gives a researcher a much more rounded picture of whatever it is that we are studying. Using several different research methods to explore the same phenomenon is known as **triangulation** – a metaphor taken from geographical surveying, where taking multiple measurements allows the surveyor to obtain a single result. Those measures may be specific research methods, and we will be looking at some of these later in this chapter. But adopting triangulation as an approach also allows us to take up different perspectives in looking at case studies – perspectives which may help us to systematise our investigations and gain a better all-round understanding of what is going on.

Complex cases, for example, may be seen as social, cultural or psychological systems. In such cases it is often helpful for the research psychologist to adopt a **systems analysis** approach to the study. This involves identifying the four major dimensions of the system: elements, order, processes and functions (Table 8.3). Every system consists of **elements**, which are distinct from each other and undertake different tasks or roles. It also involves some kind of **order**, or coherence between elements, which may take the form of patterned interactions, or may simply be a matter of mutual understandings and expectations. Systems involve **processes** – generally both psychological and physical ones – which may be developmental ones, involving change as a result

Table 8.3 Dimensions of systems analysis

Elements	The separate parts which make up the system
Order	Coherence between the elements, e.g. patterned interactions or mutual expectations
Processes	Changes over time, or transactions or exchanges
Functions	The goals or outcomes of activity within the system

of time and influences, or may involve specific types of transaction or exchange. And systems also involve **functions** and goals: activities occur because they produce certain types of outcome, and the nature of those activities relates to the overall aims or goals of the system.

A case can also be viewed as a **psychological field**. The concept of the psychological field originated with Lewin, in 1952, and was a way of expressing the complexity of social experience by organising it into different dimensions. The dimension of most interest to psychologists, of course, is the **psychological dimension**, which involves aspects of individual experience and identity. But this is not the only dimension worth exploring, even in the case of quite a specialised case study, since the other dimensions of the field will exert an influence on the individual's own experience and identity.

One of those other dimensions, for example, is the **spatial dimension**, relating to the places or locations within which a particular event or experience is set – such as the home, the pre-natal clinic, the psychological laboratory, and so on. As Orne showed in 1962, this is a dimension which can exert a considerable influence over people's behaviour, and also their understanding of what is going on. A psychological case study will also have a **cultural dimension**, relating to the symbols and social rituals involved in its occurrence. Everyday living is full of small social rituals, and studying them and their implications can be very informative for the psychologist (Hayes 1998). There will be a **historical dimension**, too, relating to previous or related events and influencing how this one is perceived and dealt with. And a psychological case will also have a **social dimension**, involving relationships, lifestyles and social networks.

This is not an exhaustive list: there are other possible field dimensions. But the use of this kind of framework for an investigation allows the psychologist to look all around the situation, and to collect contextual information in a systematic manner. No research method, as we saw in Chapter 1, can give absolutely definitive answers. Triangulation allows the psychologist to 'home in' on what is going on, by collecting different types of evidence, and seeing how they converge to influence the experience or behaviour which is being investigated.

Case-study research techniques

One of the most important research techniques used in the case study is interviewing. The fact that the case study involves a relatively small number of participants, rather than large samples, means that the researcher can look into the participant's experience much more deeply. So interview data can be analysed in depth, and are a rich source of material for the case study. We will be looking at some of the approaches to the analysis of interview data in Chapters 10–13.

Vignettes

One technique which is very useful for the case-study researcher is the use of **vignettes**. Vignettes are ways of summarising observations or experiences succinctly, in such a way that they highlight the relevant features of the case, so that they can be identified and will provide important contexts within which more specific information can be viewed. In some ways, vignettes can be seen as a method of analysis of a case study, but they can equally be viewed as ways of organising the information which the researcher is receiving.

Vignettes have been used extensively in clinical settings in the past, but there is increasing interest in the use of vignettes as a general research tool. Miller *et al.* (1997) described how vignettes were used in a series of case studies investigating the problems faced by relatives of drug users. By allowing the researchers to explore the salient features of each case, and also by comparing vignettes of the same case produced by different members of the research team, the researchers were able to produce an insightful and valuable exploration of the topic, with a depth which would not have been practical using other methods.

A vignette actually consists of a short account, rarely more than two hundred words long, which summarises the salient features of a particular case. Some researchers apply a specific structure to a vignette – for example, that it should include a description of setting, of relationships, of salient events, and of reactions to outcomes. Others prefer to leave the structure of the vignette unspecified. In the case of the Miller *et al.* study, for example, at least two researchers would draw up vignettes of the same case, independently; and their styles were often very different. By comparing the two or more vignettes, the researchers were able to identify different aspects of the case, and this helped them to gain a richer insight into what was going on for those individuals or families.

Vignettes usually describe the experiences or behaviour of a single person. But that is not invariable: they can also be used to study

---

EXERCISE 8.1   **Studying the recovery process**

Your friend has broken her wrist in an unfortunate domestic accident. The hospital staff inform her that it is likely to be about three months before she can use her wrist freely again, and you decide to use this opportunity to study some of the psychological dimensions of her recovery. Your friend agrees to participate in the research.

1. What aspects of your friend's experience do you want to find out about?

2. How will you go about collecting the data for your investigation? Will you have just one form of data collection, or more than one?

3. How often will you need to collect your data?

4. What type(s) of analysis will your data require?

5. What ethical considerations will you need to bear in mind as you design and carry out your investigation?

---

families, social groups or even organisations – in fact, anything which lends itself to case-study research. Sometimes, the production of the vignette is considered adequate in itself; but if a vignette is to be compared with others, they are usually analysed using a **thematic qualitative analysis** (see Chapter 10). In effect, it is the increased acceptance of this type of qualitative analysis which has allowed vignettes to be recognised as a valid tool for academic research, even though they have been widely used in applied settings, such as professional education or the management literature.

Prior to the revival of qualitative methodologies in psychology, vignettes were mostly used in psychological research to supplement other methods of investigation – in particular, when researchers wished to highlight distinctive cases which emerged from nomothetic studies. For example, Milgram (1973) used vignettes to describe the two individuals who became distinctive during his research into obedience by flatly refusing to obey the experimenter. His use of vignettes showed how Gretchen Brandt and Jan Rensaleer both had a personal history which had sensitised them to the dangers of unthinking obedience, and which had allowed them to break the social norms of the situation and act according to their own consciences. We will be looking at vignette analysis again, in the context of qualitative analysis, in Chapter 13.

What do these three terms mean?
repertory grid
diary methods
vignettes

Repertory grids

Some of the methods used by case-study researchers are **idiographic** measures – psychometric measures which are not concerned with comparing people with each other, or with gathering information about large numbers of people, but which are concerned with identifying and exploring the distinctive individual qualities of a single person. The repertory grid is one of the most useful of these idiographic approaches, and is used in a great deal of case-study research.

Repertory grids are based on the theory of **personal constructs**, which was developed by the clinical psychologist, George Kelly. Kelly was interested in the distinctive ways that people interpret their individual worlds. From his clinical work, Kelly came to the conclusion that people do so using their own distinctive set of personal theories about how the world works and what people are like, which come into play whenever the person has to interpret a social situation. He referred to these as personal constructs, because they are what we use to construe, or make sense of, social situations.

Everyone interprets the world in their own way, so the set of personal constructs each person has is distinctive and special. A case study using this approach will be aiming to identify the individual set of personal constructs which the research participant uses. There are two common ways that this is done: using repertory grids, and using laddering.

The repertory grid technique is a method which Kelly developed to allow a psychologist to explore a client's personal constructs. We will be looking at the specific construction of a repertory grid in Chapter 13; but what it does is to allow the researcher to identify a set of personal constructs used by a particular individual, and to see how relevant each of those personal constructs is to how the person goes abut their day-to-day life. The technique can highlight a range of personal constructs, and it also allows a researcher to distinguish between more relevant 'core' constructs and relatively superficial 'subordinate' ones.

Laddering

Laddering is another technique based on personal construct theory which is quite often used in case-study research. It's actually a style of interviewing, which encourages the person who is being interviewed to reveal more of the constructs that they are using. During any conversation, people reveal personal constructs that they are using; but these are often relatively superficial ones. By careful questioning, an interviewer can ask for more information about these constructs, and these questions will often result in the person revealing more detail about the more fundamental constructs which they are using.

Laddering, however, doesn't involve interrogating participants in an assertive or aggressive manner. That's just likely to mean that they close up and become defensive. Part of the skill of using laddering in case-study research is making sure that the tone of the interview remains light, almost like a casual conversation. In that way, the person feels secure and able to reveal more personal information.

There are ethical implications to this, of course, in that it can be used as a rather manipulative technique. Used in the wrong way, it could involve people being 'tricked' into revealing more personal information than they would otherwise have wished to do. So it is important that research which involves laddering, or repertory grids for that matter, also involves the participant giving informed consent to the researcher, and being fully debriefed afterwards. The usual way that researchers do this is by sharing their research observations openly with the participant once the interview is over, and before the material has been used for other purposes.

What do these three terms mean?

idiographic techniques

psychometrics

laddering

What is particularly useful about these idiographic techniques, in terms of case-study research, is that they allow the researcher to gain an insight into the person's own distinctive way of seeing the world, so that investigations can explore issues and experiences in more depth than might otherwise be possible. Effectively, they provide a window into the unique experience of the individual or the case being studied. They also, which is equally important, provide the researcher with a way that a case study can be structured so as to provide systematic, but also richly meaningful, data.

Disadvantages of case-study research

Case studies are a valuable way of gaining insights into some of the more detailed or personal aspects of human experiences. For the psychological researcher, they offer opportunities for in-depth exploration of issues which are simply not possible in nomothetic studies involving large numbers of people and aiming to identify regularities of behaviour. But case studies, like all research methods, are at their strongest when used in conjunction with other techniques.

Searle (1999) identified a number of disadvantages to case-study research. The first one is that of uniqueness – no two cases are the same. While this is a strength in some forms of research, it is a weakness for others, because it means that findings cannot be replicated, and so some types of reliability measures are very low.

Another criticism raised by Searle is that the researcher's own subjective feelings may influence the case study. This is particularly true of many of the famous case studies in psychology's history, especially the case histories reported by Freud and several others. In unstructured or clinical case studies the researcher's own interpretations can influence the way that the data are collected. This criticism also ties in closely with the third criticism, which has to do with selectivity of reporting. Case studies are complex and involve very large amounts of data, so any attempt to summarise them involves leaving out some material – an open opportunity for subjective bias to distort the findings.

Similarly, some case studies are based on retrospective material, in which information about past experiences and events is gathered as part of the study. Memories are notoriously subject to distortion, and very few people have full documentation of all various aspects of their lives. In addition, there is always a tendency for someone looking back over the past to 'home in' on the factors they believe to be important, while remaining entirely unaware of other possible influences. We will come across this point again in the next chapter when we look at diary research; but the inaccuracies of data collection make retrospective case studies a very questionable form of research.

The most common criticism of case studies is that it is impossible to generalise from the results, since the person or situation being studied may be atypical. This criticism, though, is less significant than others, since case-study methods are deliberately idiographic rather than nomothetic. The purpose of nomothetic research, as we saw in Chapter 1, is to identify general laws and principles of human behaviour, and for this type of research, generalisation is all-important. Case studies are only used in this type of research to supplement or illustrate other research methods. But idiographic research is directly interested in charting uniqueness, and not in looking for typicalities. What makes a human being distinctive is just as important as what makes a human being like everyone else, but looking at it involves different research methods.

Ethical aspects of case-study research

Like all research methods, case studies present their share of ethical problems to the researcher. The most important one of all is that of **confidentiality**. In a case study, a researcher is often obtaining deeply personal information, which is not usually shared widely with other people. But the nature of the study means that some of this information will be published, or at least written up as a research report. It is therefore essential that anyone conducting a case study is very protective of their research participant's identity. That means obscuring small details which could lead to their identity being deduced, as well as hiding or changing all names.

Case studies, especially in clinical research, can also raise problems of labelling and attribution. Highlighting a particular problem, or a distinctive way of looking at the world, or the effects of an illness, can lead to individual or idiosyncratic behaviours from that person all being attributed to the problem or distinctiveness. As a result, the person becomes labelled by others, and faces an uphill struggle to be recognised as an individual in their own right.

Issues like this underlie the reasons why students undertaking case-study research need to make sure that they are not taking on something outside their professional competence. As we saw in the last chapter when we looked at the ethical issues related to interviewing, it may seem interesting to want to explore anorexia or child abuse or some other such issue, but when you are dealing with individual people it is very easy to get completely out of your depth, and to find that the case study or interview has brought up issues which really need to be dealt with by a trained professional. Similarly, psychologists looking at head injury, or dyslexia, have to be careful about issues of labelling and attribution.

That doesn't mean that you should avoid case studies. They can be both useful and informative, and it is a good idea to get experience of ways of dealing with that type of richness of data. But if you are doing research as part of your psychology coursework, you do need to choose your topic with some care. Assuming you do that, however, you will find that the case-study method is a valuable tool for learning about people and psychology.

Ethnography

What do these three terms mean?

data collection

retrospective studies

ethnography

Ethnography is an approach to data collection with a very long history – one which pre-dates the systematic organisation of psychology and sociology. Its main purpose is cultural description, which means that it is concerned with life as it is lived from day to day. Ethnographers document and observe salient aspects of everyday living, and use these to gain insight into the experience. Ethnography has its roots in anthropology and sociology, although there has been a long-standing psychological tradition of enquiry using this method as well, particularly in cross-cultural psychology. As the importance of cultural contexts and social awareness to psychology became more apparent, so increasing numbers of psychologists began to use ethnographic techniques to explore some of the complexities of modern society.

Taylor (1994) lists four key aspects of ethnographic research (Table 8.4). The first of these is that it is characterised by gathering data from a **range of sources**, rather than just one single source.

Football and ethnographers
Marsh, Rosser and Harré, in 1978 conducted a psychological ethnographic study on the experience of football hooliganism. They studied a particular set of football supporters, participating in their supporter-relevant activities, observing their behaviour and talking with them. By joining in with the crowd, they were able to gain an acceptance of their presence which enabled them to observe directly how these 'hooligans' actually conducted themselves.

One of the most interesting findings to emerge from the study was that the supporters' behaviour was much less random and uncontrolled than was generally supposed. Much of the 'aggression' which so alarmed the media and the police actually took the form of explicitly patterned activity, which had more to do with ritualised verbal insult and face-saving exchanges than direct hostility. A later ethnographic study conducted with West Ham supporters, and reported by Taylor (1994), found similar findings, implying that the perceptions of the police and the media were perhaps less accurate than was widely believed.

Ethnographers use interviews with people in the culture that they are studying, but they also examine relevant documents, talk with others who may come into contact with the main participants of the culture, and observe behaviour directly, often in a participative manner. The interviews conducted by ethnographers are rarely formal, since, as we saw in Chapter 7, formal interviews may contain content which is structured and organised to fit the demand characteristics of the interview itself. Instead, they are more likely to take the form of everyday conversations, documented later by the ethnographer.

The second distinctive aspect of ethnographic study is that behaviour is studied in its **everyday contexts**, rather than under experimental conditions. Since it is the culture which is the focus of interest, rather

Table 8.4   Key aspects of ethnographic research

1. Data are obtained from a range of sources, not just one.

2. Behaviour is studied in everyday contexts, not artificial laboratory conditions.

3. Early stages of data gathering are unstructured by the researcher, and determined by the situation and context.

4. The exploration is conducted in depth, and not superficially.

Source: Taylor (1994).

EXERCISE 8.2   Case studies or not?

Some research topics are more suitable for case-study research than others. The list below identifies a number of different research topics. Some would be highly appropriate for case-study research while others would be inappropriate. Decide which category each research topic falls into.

The shared characteristics of popular teachers
Management practices in a highly creative design company
Memories of a specific Millennium event
Driving behaviour of Volvo owners
Personality traits in military personnel
Recovery from skin cancer
Types of road accident involving pre-school-age children
Sport and exercise habits in middle-aged people
The experience of pregnancy
Memory impairment following brain surgery
The pre-schooler's growth in social competence
Visitors' reactions to hands-on exhibits in a science centre

than the individual's behaviour, it is important that the culture itself is what is studied; so explorations of how individuals might act in a different context are not seen as particularly relevant. The researcher, too, is not aiming to provide an externalised, objective account, but to explore the experience of belonging to that culture, from the point of view of the participant. As Uzzell (1995) described it: 'the view is not the outsider looking in, but the insider looking around.'

The third key feature of ethnographic research identified by Taylor (1994) is that it uses an **unstructured** approach to data gathering in its early stages. This enables the researcher to approach the topic in an open manner, without preset hypotheses. Inevitably, hypotheses will develop during the course of the study, as people respond to the situations and relationships in which they find themselves. As the researcher explores these hypotheses as they arise, key issues gradually become apparent, until by the end of the study it is possible to identify some theoretical perspectives. But the initial data-gathering period needs to be open and unstructured.

The fourth key feature of ethnographic research is that of **depth**. It is not possible to use ethnography to conduct a rapid, superficial survey of a group or culture. Because of the complexity of the subject matter, and the need to ensure that the information which is being received is actually an appropriate reflection of the culture itself, ethnographic research takes time to conduct. It takes time to explore a culture, and even more time for the explorer to become accepted enough by members of that culture for an analysis to be worth conducting. An ethnographic analysis, therefore, will almost always consist of an in-depth study of just one or two situations – it is more closely linked with the case-study method in psychology than any other, and in some ways can be viewed as a case study whose target is a culture, rather than an individual or group.

Ethnographic research is a method of collecting information, rather than an analytical technique. Sorting out the data does involve a certain amount of 'telling a story', in the sense that ethnographers are concerned with making sense of, and also illustrating, the social situations which they have been experiencing. But it also involves more detailed analysis, which often draws on qualitative research methods such as those outlined in Chapters 10–13.

In the next chapter, we will be looking at the type of research which involves collecting information from other documents. Diary methods are a useful way of gathering data while people are going about their day-to-day lives; and other forms of documentation can also be useful for the research psychologist. In that chapter, too, we will be looking at meta-analysis, which is an increasingly important technique for bringing together and summarising large numbers of research projects dealing with a similar topic.

Self-assessment questions

1. *Distinguish between core constructs and subordinate constructs in personal construct theory.*

2. *Outline the main types of cases which might be studied by psychologists in case-study research.*

3. *Describe the use of laddering in personal construct interviewing.*

4. *What are the main problems associated with case-study research?*

5. *What are the key features of ethnographic research?*

Concepts in use

1. *A researcher has decided to use in-depth case-study methods to investigate the psychological effects of retirement. What are the advantages of this decision?*

2. *How might you apply the concept of triangulation in an investigation of the relationship between social aggression and violence on TV?*

3. *Explain how an investigation of children's classroom behaviour might have a spatial dimension, a cultural dimension, a historical dimension and a social dimension.*

4. *What ethical considerations might be raised by an ethnographic exploration of football 'hooliganism'?*

5. *How might the four concepts of elements, order, processes and functions manifest themselves in a systems analysis of a residential care home for the elderly?*

9

Analysing documents

Diary studies
Document research
Meta-analysis

Not every form of psychological research involves direct interaction with research participants. Sometimes psychologists use the evidence provided from documents to learn about human experience, or to analyse what other psychologists have learned so far. In this chapter, we will look at two major ways of obtaining psychological evidence from documents: diary methods of investigation, and the research method known as meta-analysis.

The diary method

The diary method is an approach to collecting data in which respondents are required to keep notes about a particular type of experience or event, at appropriate intervals over a period of time. The notes provide the basic data for the research, which can be analysed using a variety of different methods, both quantitative and qualitative. Diaries can vary in form, ranging from a tightly structured questionnaire, which needs to be completed on a regular basis, to open-ended reports, in which the person notes down their experiences from time to time. But whatever form they take, diary methods always involve the participant making repeated recordings over time, and this allows the researcher to explore issues of development, change or recurrent experience in a way which is very difficult using other research techniques.

> **What do these three terms mean?**
>
> *structured questionnaire*
>
> *open-ended format*
>
> *diary record*

Advantages and disadvantages of diary methods

There are several advantages to using a diary approach for the researcher. Breakwell and Wood (1995) identified seven in all, which are listed in Table 9.1. But perhaps the most important advantage of all is

Table 9.1 Advantages of diary methods

Familiarity	The person understands the task the researcher is asking them to do.
Cost-effective	A diary is an economical and practical way of gathering data over long periods of time.
Data sequencing	The information is sequenced, so the order in which things happened is clear.
Intimacy	A diary is a personal and reasonably private way of collecting data, which may encourage honesty on the part of the respondent and allows a researcher to collect very personal information.
Exploration	A diary allows a researcher to explore new issues or approaches to understanding a topic.
Spontaneity	Using diaries which people have kept for their own purposes gives the researcher spontaneous data which have not been generated specially for research purposes. There are many advantages to this, although there are disadvantages too.
Historicity	The analysis of themes in private diaries over time can allow a researcher to perceive historical developments.

Source: Breakwell and Wood (1995).

that diary studies bring the task of data collection into the person's own everyday world. As researchers have repeatedly shown, context exerts a huge effect on what we remember, what we feel and how open we are to suggestions. The human mind is complex, and different aspects of it come to the fore in different circumstances. So a method which provides a researcher with data that have been recorded in the everyday context of their research participants' lives is extremely valuable.

Another advantage of diaries is that they offer the opportunity to study change over time. Many forms of psychological research ignore the time dimension, and simply provide the researcher with a 'snapshot' of what is happening at a particular moment. But this can be misleading, because so much of what we do is part of a whole sequence of activity, not an action in itself. For example, in the past psychologists have studied people's actions while they stand at bus stops, and their patterns of conversation. But for the person who is actually engaging in that behaviour, standing at a bus stop is a relatively minor part of a much more important event. Their journey will be being made with some kind of purpose in mind. It is likely to have been preceded by other such journeys, and to be followed by consequences of some kind.

Table 9.2 Disadvantages of diary methods

Control of content	The researcher does not have total control over what the diary includes.
Dropout	Some people may fail to complete their diaries over the full period of time.
Poor recruitment	Diary studies can be easily affected by volunteer effects or other artefacts.
Veracity and verification	It is rarely possible to check diary entries for accuracy or truthfulness.
Reactance	People may change their behaviours as a result of completing the diary.

Source: Breakwell and Wood (1995).

The bus-stop waiting activity may be of interest, but if we really want to understand something of someone's experience, we need to look at their actions in a time context. Diary methods allow us to do that.

In the case of the open-ended, phenomenological type of diary study, the diary also allows a researcher to gain insight, in a very direct manner into a person's actual experience and how they perceive it. The person records their ideas, experiences and impressions in the diary, and when this is analysed, it allows the researcher to see how these have developed or changed. Diaries can give the researcher access to someone's personal way of looking at the world, and reveal what that particular person thinks of as important. For example, the diary entries made by women during the course of their pregnancy gave Smith (1997) some interesting insights into the ways that their perceptions of themselves, the pregnancy and their future baby changed over time.

Diary studies have some disadvantages, too. Breakwell and Wood (1995) identified five of these, listed in Table 9.2. One of the ones they identify is having control over the content of the diary. An open-ended diary leaves the respondent free to write whatever and how much they like, and they may focus on different aspects of the experience. Once the diary study is under way, the researcher has very little control over the content, and if the respondent is noting down information which is of no value to the study, it may not be discovered until the end of the data-collection part of the project.

Another disadvantage for some researchers is the problem of **reactance**. Reactance occurs when the process of participating in the study actually changes the participant in some way. For example, a diary study aimed at investigating the extent to which someone engages

What do these three terms mean?

reactance

priming

document analysis

in ecologically sensitive household practices may sensitise the person who is completing the diary into acting in a more ecologically conscientious manner. If the study is being conducted within an action research paradigm (see Chapter 11), this is not much of a problem, since that approach to research assumes that the process of studying people will have consequences for those people's behaviour. But most psychological research is conducted within a more positivistic paradigm, in which researchers try not to influence their research participants. Reactance presents real problems for that type of research; and it occurs in many other types of research method, not just diary studies.

Perhaps the most important disadvantage of diary studies, though, is that the researcher has no actual reality check on the data. If the respondent chooses to put information in the diary which doesn't actually correspond with their experience, the researcher is stuck with it – and may not even know that it has happened. By far the majority of people participating in a diary study will try to be truthful, and to report the right kind of information to the researcher. But if the study is badly designed, it may lead people into providing inaccurate information, much as badly designed questionnaires do. It is for this reason that researchers need to take great care when conducting a diary study – they are not necessarily the easy option that they may appear on the surface.

What do these three terms mean?

primacy effects

action research paradigm

positivistic paradigm

Designing diary studies

There are several things which a researcher needs to be careful about when designing a diary study. One of them is the form that the diary will take. Most diaries are written documents, but sometimes it is a good idea to allow the research participant the opportunity to record or note them down in some other way. Obviously, if the researcher is dealing with people who do not find writing easy, as a result of handicap or some other factor, then using a method such as a tape-recording or video is an advantage. Or if the researcher is studying busy executives, it may be more useful to have the diary take the form of an electronic record on their computers, than for it to be a paper document.

For the most part, though, a diary will be kept by the research participant writing on paper. But the actual layout of the diary can be very influential. It may, for example, contain questions that the person needs to answer (time of day, nature of occasion, etc.), as well as a space for their own personal statement. Many of the decisions which researchers have to make in questionnaire studies are relevant here, in that the more structure the researcher provides, the easier it will be to compare data from different respondents, but the less likely it will be that the data will fully reflect what the person experiences.

Unlike questionnaire studies, however, it is more common for diary researchers to use an open-ended format – partly because a diary study doesn't usually involve as many people as a questionnaire study, so there is more opportunity to look at the results in depth, and partly because diary methods are usually used in **idiographic** rather than **nomothetic** research. Diary researchers tend to be more interested in gathering detailed individual accounts of experience, and less interested in comparing one respondent with another. Questionnaire researchers, however, operate using a nomothetic approach – they are less interested in individual experience, and more in the general experiences of people as a whole.

Nomothetic or idiographic?

Diary methods can be used either as nomothetic research or in a more idiographic manner. For example, Reason (1979) used diary methods to study errors of memory. People were asked to note down any memory lapses or other errors that they made, as soon as they noticed that they had made them; and this data allowed Reason to identify a number of factors in everyday errors, which could then be used to structure further research. This was an example of nomothetic research using a diary approach: the results from several research participants were aggregated together to identify general trends and mechanisms.

Linton (1975), on the other hand, kept a diary in which she noted down two significant events a day over a five-year period. Every few months, she selected two items randomly, read the description, and tried to recall the date on which it had happened. If she had no recollection at all of the event, it was dropped from later samples. The pattern of forgetting and memory loss which Linton experienced over the five-year period illustrated a number of different principles of memory such as primacy effects and the importance of rehearsal. But it also gave some surprising results – for example, that highly emotional events did not turn out to be any more memorable than others, when she tried to recall them. This idiographic study had only one research participant, and used a very different approach to methodology than the one Reason had used. But the data it gave to cognitive psychology were just as useful.

It is important, too, that the instructions which the person receives should be clear and unambiguous. Breakwell and Wood (1995) suggest that it is often a very good idea to provide a respondent with a completed example, so that they can see the types of entry which the researcher expects, and model their responses on that. In a purely phenomenological study (see Chapter 11) this would be unacceptable. It would be considered that 'priming' the research participants like this was contaminating the data, since the research participants would shape their responses in ways that they would not have done otherwise. But for most forms of psychological research, providing examples and encouraging the research participants to respond in certain ways is the most practical way of ensuring that the data arrive in a form which the psychologist can use.

Reminders

One of the disadvantages of diary method research can be that people drop out of the study – they become bored with filling the diary in, or they forget for a while and do not resume it when they remember because they think there is 'no point'. Researchers can reduce the amount of drop-out by keeping in contact with their research participants. This is usually done by an occasional telephone call or postcard, or more recently an e-mail; and it can make quite a lot of

---

EXERCISE 9.1   Using documents in research

List A describes various types of documentation which might be used in a psychological research project. List B describes a number of different research projects. Match the items in list A with the items in list B.

List A	*List B*
hospital accident records	localisation of cortical function
a politician's published diaries	safety behaviours in the home
diary records of everyday errors	reflections of the self-image in art
printouts of statistical calculations	strategies of excuse and justification
old psychology textbooks	gender role perceptions
newspaper cuttings	diagnostic strategies for mental disorders
autopsy records of brain lesions	absent-mindedness
magazine advertisements	development of psychological epistemology
photographs from an art gallery	fraudulent evidence in the IQ debate
psychiatric records	discursive frames and football supporters

difference. Some researchers have adopted some of the techniques of questionnaire administration – using incentives, lotteries and the like – but for many, there is little need to resort to such tactics, unless it is a very large-scale study. Personal contact with the researcher, and the opportunity to express their individual experiences, can sometimes be enough to maintain motivation in smaller studies, and the judicious use of reminders can back this up very effectively.

The data which the diary provides can be analysed using either quantitative or qualitative forms of analysis. We will be looking at these in the next few chapters; but the decision as to which form of analysis to use will have been partly taken when the diary study was first designed. Open-ended diary entries require qualitative forms of analysis. A researcher may begin with a quantitative approach – usually by conducting a content analysis, counting up how many times different topics are referred to – but that is not likely to be the sum total of the analysis.

Information obtained from open-ended diary formats is usually very rich, and needs to be analysed using the types of qualitative technique that we will be looking at in Chapters 10–13. More structured diaries lend themselves readily to quantitative analyses, and we will be looking at these in Chapters 14–19. But at the very least, the time dimension available in the diary makes it likely that the researcher will attempt to develop a profile of how events or categories of experience have varied over time.

> **What do these three terms mean?**
>
> *idiographic*
>
> *nomothetic*
>
> *replication*

Diaries and documents

The previous discussion has dealt with the type of diary study in which the diary is specifically generated for research purposes – without the research, there would be no diary. But there is another kind of diary study, which involves looking at diaries which have been written for a different purpose – memoirs, personal diaries which have become available after someone's death, and so on. Diary studies of this kind are connected with other types of **document analysis** – research which involves analysing these existing documents for what they reveal about underlying or recurrent psychological processes and mechanisms.

Document analysis doesn't only deal with diaries. For example, Wood (1981) analysed a series of interviews and biographical writings compiled by Ghiselin, in 1952, which aimed to capture the creative experience of eminent artists, musicians and scientists. The data provided by this material enabled Wood to identify four 'themes' which seemed to be recurrent in the process of creativity: the idea of an 'inner dialogue' between the conscious and unconscious mind; the perception of self as a kind of spectator to the creative process, rather than as agent; a strong distrust of words; and the vital importance of practice in establishing the prior skills and expertise without which true creativity is not possible.

Documents, in the context of document research, are recorded media. Most of the time, this refers to records which have been made on pieces of paper of one form or another. But this isn't always the case. In 1981, for example, Manstead and McCulloch reported a study of 170 British television commercials – the total set of advertisements portraying adults, broadcast by one TV channel during the evenings of a single week. The researchers were interested in sex-role stereo-typing, and conducted a content analysis of these advertisements, look-ing at aspects such as mode of presentation, credibility, role, location, argument, reward type and product type. Their documents, in this context, were the recordings the researchers had made of the advertise-ments, rather than documents on paper.

Problems of pre-existing material

There are some problems with using published memoirs or other pre-existing diaries as the material for diary research. The most important of these is that they may not provide the full information which a researcher needs. Since they have been written for different purposes, they may omit information which researchers consider important, and include information which the diarist thought significant, but which is irrelevant in terms of understanding the psychological dimensions of their experience.

Another problem, particularly with published diaries, is that the material has almost always been re-worked, either by the diarist or by the person who is submitting the diaries for publication. This re-working will be aiming to enhance the readability and coherence of the diary, but in the process it can lead to distortions of the original meaning, or even to changes designed to cover up material which might be embarrassing or lead to social condemnation.

Sometimes it may be possible for a researcher to obtain private diaries which were never intended for publication. These can be immensely valuable as a direct glimpse into the individual's personal experience; and they suffer from very few of the social bias problems of published diaries. The most famous diary of this type, of course, is the diary of Anne Frank, a young Dutch Jewish girl whose whole family hid from the Nazis for two years, before being discovered and sent to concentration camps. Anne's diaries, which she had used to express all her private thoughts and emotions, were saved by family friends, and give a direct insight into her experience.

That particular diary, however, was distinctive, in that Anne wrote in a particularly clear and articulate way, treating her diary as if it were a real person to whom she was writing letters. Many other personal diaries involve personal codes or shorthand, or other idiosyncratic ways of referring to events; and this can make it difficult for the researcher to understand what was actually going on at any one moment. Nonetheless, spontaneously generated diaries, whether published or not, can often provide a psychological researcher with insights which they would not otherwise have obtained, and in a time context which is particularly valuable.

Meta-analysis

The research technique known as **meta-analysis** is another, more specialised form of document analysis. This time, though, the documents consist of published research findings. Meta-analysis is becoming increasingly popular in psychological research, as a way of making sense of the findings of many different studies. Replication, as we saw in Chapter 1, is an important part of nomothetic research. But the need for researchers to replicate studies, and the need for that replication to occur in a wide variety of contexts, means that any one topic can result in hundreds, or even thousands of studies, each with slightly different outcomes. As a result, it can be very difficult to identify exactly what is going on, or even to summarise the implications of all that research.

> **What do these three terms mean?**
>
> *meta-analysis*
>
> *narrative review*
>
> *file-drawer problem*

Science very rarely involves certainty or agreement – or at least not when a phenomenon is first being investigated. As research evidence mounts in a particular field, it is almost always equivocal. Some studies may seem to provide evidence that a phenomenon exists; others may imply that it doesn't; and different researchers dispute with one another about the implications of findings. All of this is a normal and even a desirable part of scientific research, but there are times when it is helpful to be able to take a more general perspective, and summarise the overall implications of research findings to date. And this is where meta-analysis comes in.

In some ways, any examination of relevant literature is a kind of meta-analysis, particularly if it leads to new theoretical insights. And every research report and major study involves some kind of examination of the relevant literature. But for the most part, these take the form of **narrative reviews** – accounts of studies, linked together by contrasts or highlighting points drawn out by the person compiling the review. The huge amount of information available to modern researchers means that some selection of the material is

Table 9.3 Levels of analysis in research

1. **Primary analysis**	The original data analysis of a study.
2. **Secondary analysis**	Reworking of the research data using different statistical techniques.
3. **Meta-analysis**	Analysing the data from a large number of individual studies statistically.

Source: Glass (1976).

always necessary; and this, together with the need to interpret the material and draw conclusions from it, makes the process very open to subjective bias.

In 1976, Glass suggested a way that explorations of the relevant literature for a research topic could become more systematic and scientific. Glass identified three levels of analysis in research topics (see Table 9.3). The first and second relate to individual studies; but the third, meta-analysis, treats the findings of many such studies as a complex data-set – much like the set of different results obtained from different research participants in one single study. This data-set is open to statistical analysis which can draw together and summarise the various research findings. This approach is quite different from the narrative review, for a number of reasons which are summarised in Table 9.4.

Table 9.4 Narrative reviews and meta-analysis

Narrative reviews	*Meta-analysis*
Narrative reviews are often selective, not comprehensive	Incorporates every known study of the topic
Tend to focus only on statistical significance of studies	Can take into account effect size as well as significance
Have difficulty dealing with conflicting results	Deals with conflicting results by identifying sources of error and artefact
Conclusions reflect aims and concerns of individual researcher, and so are difficult to replicate	Conclusions are readily replicated by other researchers
Can be valuable in developing new theoretical insights	Used only for summarising existing research findings

Meta-analysis and parapsychology

The difference between meta-analysis and narrative analysis, and in particular the increased objectivity of meta-analysis, has meant that it is a very useful research tool for highly controversial topics. Parapsychology is one such area, where some sceptics feel very strongly that research findings are simply the result of artefacts, and the use of narrative reviews has simply led to accusations of partisanship and bias. In recent years, many parapsychologists have begun conducting meta-analyses of particular research topics. Radin (1997) showed how these meta-analyses often reveal remarkably consistent findings, even though the effect sizes may be quite small. For example, a meta-analysis of 832 micro-PK studies showed a small but consistent effect which was extremely unlikely to be simply a matter of chance. Moreover, there would have had to be roughly 54 000 failed studies to cancel out the effects of the studies analysed in the meta-analysis.

While sceptics still argue about the methodology of the research, and the way in which studies have been incorporated into the analysis, the use of meta-analysis has provided parapsychological researchers with a much more objective way of summarising and evaluating the many different studies conducted in this area. And not every meta-analysis is positive – parapsychology journals are very aware of the problems of publication bias, and of the need to address the sort of methodological criticisms levelled at them; so their editorial policies are such that they take care to publish negative findings and replications, as well as just positive results.

Conducting a meta-analysis

There are several different ways of approaching meta-analysis. One of the more straightforward was developed by Glass *et al.* (1981). It has six steps, which are summarised in Table 9.5, but which are worth exploring in a little more detail here. The first step involves selecting the dependent and independent variables which you are interested in – see Chapter 3 for a reminder of what they are. A meta-analysis may be concerned with more than one pair of independent and dependent variables – for example, a researcher might want to explore text length and reading fluency as one pair in a meta-analysis of reading studies, and teaching method and task completion as another.

The second step may seem straightforward – identifying and obtaining all of the relevant studies – but this can involve some intensive searching, using different keywords in electronic databases, to make sure that all of the relevant studies really have been identified. Once

Table 9.5   Steps of meta-analysis

1. Select the relevant independent and dependent variables.

2. Identify and obtain all relevant studies.

3. Identify characteristics which may be pertinent to the outcome of the study (e.g. gender, age, type of learning method) and code each study according to these characteristics.

4. Calculate effect-size estimates for the relevant independent/dependent variables.

5. Calculate mean and standard deviation of the effect size across all the studies.

6. Compare the effect-size summaries with the characteristics identified in step 3, to identify connections or correlations.

Source: Glass *et al.* (1981).

they have been identified, the person doing the meta-analysis needs to obtain full reports, which provide relevant data for the analysis. All of this is quite a lengthy and time-consuming process.

The third step is all about identifying possible factors which could have influenced the outcomes of studies. For example, in a meta-analysis of studies of methods of teaching children to read, there will be several differences between studies. The ages of the children in the different studies, or their socio-economic backgrounds may vary. The length of time they received the training may also vary, or the degree to which parents were involved. The researcher needs to identify as many of these factors as possible, and to code each of the studies with respect to each factor – so it is easy to see, for example, which studies provided the children with most training time, and which provided the least. Some forms of meta-analysis leave this stage until later in the process, but Glass *et al.* (1981) considered that it was more objective to do it at an early stage in the proceedings.

Effect size and statistical significance

The fourth step involves calculating estimates of the **effect size** for each study. The effect size is all about how extreme the differences between samples are. Most statistical analysis used in psychology is concerned with **statistical significance**. This, as we will see in the next chapter, is concerned with how likely it is that the results of the study have happened purely by chance. Even quite a large finding, which seems to be very convincing, can sometimes happen just because of random factors or sampling errors.

But statistical significance isn't the whole story, because it also makes a difference whether the results show a very big effect or an almost unnoticeable one. In a study of learning to read, for example, one teaching method may give results which are significantly different from another, but those differences may be really quite small. Another teaching method may give dramatically different results, most of the time, but not consistently enough to be statistically significant.

Glass *et al.* (1981) developed a formula for calculating effect sizes, which they referred to as *d.* The formula is as follows:

$$d = \frac{\text{Mean of experimental group} - \text{Mean of control group}}{\text{Standard deviation of control group}}$$

We will be looking at **means** and **standard deviations** more closely in Chapter 15. But using the Glass procedure, *d* needs to be calculated for each of the studies, for each pair of independent and dependent variables that the researcher is interested in.

The fifth step of the meta-analysis involves taking a good look at the effect sizes which have been obtained. There should be one *d* statistic for each study in the analysis, and they will not all be the same – in fact, each study will probably show a different effect size. So the researcher needs to calculate the mean effect size for the studies as a whole, and also the standard deviation, to see how much effect sizes vary. It is this calculation which will allow the researcher to draw some general, overall conclusions about the topic which is being researched.

This leads into the final step of the meta-analysis, which is to look back at the characteristics which were identified and coded in step 3, and to see whether they seem to show any particular **correlation** with the effect sizes which have been obtained. It may be, for example, that studies of reading which involve parents show larger effect sizes than those which don't. That's something that we would expect to find, and which might easily be picked up in a narrative review. But equally, it might be that this isn't the case – that the studies as a whole don't indicate larger effect sizes, even though one or two do. By analysing the studies using a meta-analysis of this kind, we can obtain objective evidence about whether parental involvement and learning to read do show a connection – or at least, evidence which is much less open to accusations of subjective bias from other researchers.

This is not the only way of conducting a meta-analysis. Hunter *et al.* (1982), for example, produced a model for meta-analysis which is similar to the one we have just discussed, but includes some corrections to deal with sampling errors or other artefacts in the various studies. They took the view that studies with larger sample sizes would be less likely to show **sampling errors** (we will be looking at these more closely in Chapter 14), and so introduced a correction into the analysis which takes into account the sample size when calculating the effect size. A fuller account of their method can be found in Wood (1995).

Problems of meta-analysis

Meta-analysis is a useful technique for researchers, but like all research methods it has its drawbacks. One of them is the problem of defining just what we mean by all of the studies in an area. It might sound straightforward, but in many cases the boundaries of a research topic are not clear. For example, there may be some studies which have been mainly concerned with something else, but which have looked at the topic of the meta-analysis just incidentally. Should these be included? Then there may be studies conducted by researchers from other disciplines, looking at the same problem. Their research will be conducted in slightly different ways from the psychological research, reflecting the different approaches to knowledge in their discipline. Should these studies be included in a meta-analysis? As you can see, it can be tricky knowing just where to draw the line, and to some extent it comes down to the researcher's judgement, just as it does with narrative reviews.

Another major problem in meta-analysis is the question of studies which are badly designed, or methodologically flawed in some other way. In a narrative review, the researcher will simply omit those studies, because their design problems mean that they can't be taken as good evidence in the relevant research area. But the principle of including all studies is a very important one in meta-analysis, and the method leaves no way of distinguishing a well-designed study from a badly designed one.

What do these three terms mean?
artefacts
GIGO
mean effect size

Researchers have not come to any agreement about this matter: some, such as Hunter *et al.* (1982), argue that even badly designed studies should generally be included, on the grounds that the design problems may not actually have biased the findings. Others, such as Eysenck (1978), adopt the computer acronym GIGO – which stands for 'Garbage In, Garbage Out' – and argue that it is impossible to draw meaningful conclusions from an analysis which includes badly designed studies.

The third major problem for meta-analysis is known as the **file-drawer problem**. This is the argument that, as a general rule, only positive findings are submitted to journals for publication; and even if a researcher replicates a finding successfully, editors rarely accept it for publication because it is not saying anything new. So successful replications or studies with negative findings are not sent for

EXERCISE 9.2   **Studying studies of risk-taking**

You have been asked to conduct a document analysis on studies of risk-taking behaviours in teenagers. This will involve making a number of decisions. Answer the questions below, which will provide you with some basic information which may be helpful in carrying out your study.

1. What characteristics do you think might be relevant to the outcome of your study (age-range, education, etc.)? List the important ones.

2. Decide on the types of behaviours you include as risk-taking. Ask yourself whether you will include long-term risk-taking such as smoking, as well as short-term risk-taking such as mountain-climbing.

3. Develop a list of behaviours which you consider to be risk-taking. Discuss the list with others, asking them to rate the list from most risky to least risky, and to add any other behaviours which they believe to be left out.

4. If you have access to a library database such as PsycLit, use that to search for all of the studies which mention the behaviours on your list. Check the abstracts to make sure that they relate to young people, and then compile a list of these studies. This will give you a set of data which you could use as the basis for a meta-analysis.

5. If you don't have access to PsycLit, go to your local reference library and search the science magazines, using indexes such as the *New Scientist Index*, which the library will have available. Make a list of the number of times each of the behaviours on your list has been mentioned during the past five years. This set of data would not be full enough for a meta-analysis, but would allow you to do an interesting narrative review.

publication, but instead are filed away in a drawer, with nobody knowing about them except the people who carried out the study.

Some researchers, such as Hunter *et al.* (1982), argue that this is not really a problem since it is the methodological quality of a paper which determines whether it will be published or not. Other researchers, though, see this as a bit idealistic, and have attempted to address the file-drawer problem in a different way. Rosenthal (1979) developed a formula which examines effect sizes and other aspects of the meta-analysis data, and calculates just how many failed studies would need to have been relegated to file drawers in order to cancel out the effect. This approach has been put to good use by many researchers.

Meta-analysis, then, is a useful technique for researchers, and it is particularly valuable for dealing with the vast amounts of information generated by researchers in modern times. But not many would suggest that it can completely replace narrative reviews. What it does is to augment them, and to provide some objective data on which a reviewer can base opinions. But the task of theoretical synthesis – of exploring past research for suggestions about future theories, or patterns which may indicate unsuspected relationships, is still something which requires a combination of meta-analysis and narrative review.

This chapter concludes our exploration of specific ways of gathering data for research. Now, we will move on to Part II, where we look at ways of analysing data – although we have already looked at some methods, such as ethnography, where the two are seen as inextricably linked. It has been useful in this book to separate the two, but, as we've already seen several times, research design needs to consider the possible analysis from the very beginning, to make sure that the data have been collected in the most appropriate way. So an understanding of a broad range of analytical techniques is as important a part of the psychologist's research tool-kit as an understanding of a broad range of methods of data collection.

Self-assessment questions

1. *What are the main disadvantages of diary methods?*

2. *Distinguish between idiographic and nomothetic approaches to diary research.*

3. *List three types of document, other than diaries, which might be studied by psychologists, identifying an advantage and a disadvantage for each one.*

4. *In what ways is a meta-analysis different from a narrative review?*

5. *What is the file-drawer problem, and how have psychologists attempted to deal with it?*

Concepts in use

1. *List some of the main problems which might emerge when using a video diary approach to study students' leisure activities.*

2. *From your knowledge of existing psychological research, describe a published psychological study which has used the diary approach.*

3. *How might reactance become an issue in a diary study of the practising habits of young musicians?*

4. *Imagine that you are conducting a major research project to explore the issue of child safety in the home. How would a document-based study help your investigation of this topic?*

5. *Meta-analysis has become a popular technique in controversial research areas such as parapsychology. What are the advantages and disadvantages of using meta-analysis in these areas?*

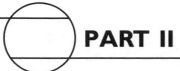

PART II

Making sense of data

In this part of the book, we go on to look at different forms of analysis. Analysis is all about making sense of the data which have been collected, and there are different types of analysis depending on what it is that we are interested in and want to find out. If we want to look at people's descriptions of events that have happened in their lives, or their personal experiences, there would be very little point in trying to do so by converting the information into numbers, and conducting a quantitative analysis. We would lose so much information that what remained would really tell us very little.

But if we wanted to examine the acquisition of a specific skill, such as reading fluency, then adopting a research method which allowed us to convert the information into numbers and conducting a quantitative analysis would be much more useful. The analysis would allow us to look at our information objectively, and to see patterns in it which might not be apparent if we adopted a more qualitative approach.

A research psychologist, therefore, needs to have a good knowledge of analytical techniques, as well as a good knowledge of research methods. In the next few chapters, we will look at both quantitative and qualitative analysis. Familiarity with both quantitative and qualitative methods provides a psychologist with a versatile and wideranging psychological 'tool-kit'. Knowing when these techniques are appropriate and when they are not will allow a researcher to choose the best way of analysing the research data, no matter what sort of research project is involved.

10

Introducing qualitative analysis

About qualitative research
Thematic qualitative analysis
Theory-led thematic analysis

Our exploration of different research methods is now complete, and we are moving on to the other part of the research process: analysing the data. In many ways, the research method we use to collect information about something and the analytical method we use to make sense of that information are inextricably linked together: each one influences the other. There are as many ways of analysing data as there are of collecting it, and each one has its own requirements.

There are also, as we saw in Chapter 1, different philosophical approaches to the research process. Sometimes, the research we are undertaking is very specifically hypothetico-deductive in nature. We conduct our research to refute or confirm specific hypotheses, in order to verify or refute a specific theory. As a result, the data we collect will also be very specific in nature, and the way that we analyse them will reflect the exact question we are asking.

On other occasions, we may want to conduct research in areas where specific theories have not yet been developed, or in a context where we have reason to doubt the theories which exist and want to begin again from scratch. At such times, we are more likely to adopt an inductive approach, collecting data which are not constrained by specific hypotheses, but instead are open to new ideas or possible explanations. That type of data requires a different type of analysis: one which will be open to alternative possibilities.

About qualitative research

In the first part of this book, we looked at ways of collecting data, and many of those approaches involved the collection of qualitative

EXERCISE 10.1   **Topics for qualitative methods**

List A gives a number of different approaches to qualitative analysis. List B gives a set of brief statements, each of which might be considered to describe one of the approaches, or at least some aspect of it. Match up the two lists.

List A	*List B*
action research	identifying recurrent ideas or themes within the data
conversation analysis	applying ideas or themes to the data to see if they fit
protocol analysis	exploring the data for theoretical insights
grounded theory	using the data to explore the respondent's own world
vignette analysis	producing change as part of the research process
inductive qualitative analysis	exploring the structures and mechanisms of social exchanges
phenomenological analysis	
discourse analysis	exploring how experience is socially constructed
repertory grid analysis	exploring the personal constructs used by the individual
thematic qualitative analysis	recording what people say about how they carry out a task
	summarising experiences in small descriptive accounts

data. Interviews and diary methods, for example, are ways of collecting qualitative information, as are some types of observation. The researcher who has collected this type of information then has a choice. The data can be converted somehow into numbers, and analysed using the kind of statistical techniques that we will be looking at in later chapters; or they can be kept as they are, and analysed using qualitative analysis.

Each of these options has its advantages and disadvantages. Converting the information into numerical form has the advantage that it helps the researcher to make comparisons between different people, and to identify general trends more reliably. But it also means that a lot of the information is lost in the process, and a great deal of its human meaning. Using qualitative analysis on this type of data allows the researcher to focus on the human meanings in the information, and to understand the nuances of what participants are communicating more fully; but it also makes it more difficult to draw comparisons between people, and to be sure of how reliable the information is.

For many psychologists, deciding between quantitative and qualitative methods involves making a trade-off between reliability and validity. We looked at these concepts in Chapter 6, in the context of psychometric testing, and we saw then that they can be broadly summarised as reliability being whether a measure gives consistent results over time, while validity is concerned with whether the measure truly addresses what it purports to be measuring. Some researchers see quantitative research techniques as emphasising the importance of reliability: rigidly controlled experimental or observational techniques are used to collect numerical data, with their emphasis being on research procedures which can be replicated and will produce the same or similar results whenever they are carried out, but which mean that the information that is collected loses validity in the process.

Qualitative research methods, by contrast, emphasise validity. The main goal of the researcher is not to produce results which can be replicated, but to develop a true understanding of what is going on. As a result, the emphasis is on the communications which come from research participants and the social processes which are taking place. The researcher acknowledges that the uniqueness of human beings means that the research findings are unlikely to be replicated very easily. They have validity, but not reliability.

As we've seen many times in this book, almost any kind of research involves making decisions and trade-offs of one sort or another. For many researchers, the decision to use either qualitative or quantitative techniques is one which takes in the aims of the research, the nature of the topic which is being studied, and the way that the research information will be used when the project is completed. Some research projects lend themselves more readily to quantitative research methods, some to qualitative ones. Increasingly, though, researchers are using combinations of the two.

Qualitative research and objectivity

Qualitative analysis is not new in psychology. It has been used by psychologists continuously, ever since psychology first began. But the advent of behaviourism, and its long-lasting influence, meant that for some years in the middle part of the twentieth century qualitative research was regarded as 'unscientific', and not the kind of thing that a serious researcher should do. This attitude was a little odd, since it is exactly those parts of psychology normally regarded as the most 'scientific' – brain research and clinical neuropsychology – which

---

What do these three terms mean?

reliability

validity

transcription

have continued to use qualitative methodology throughout the whole century. But this contradiction passed unnoticed by the psychological community as a whole.

The opposition to qualitative analysis may have been a little irrational, and was certainly carried further than was good for psychology; but it wasn't totally without foundation. Many psychologists, such as Orne and Rosenthal, had demonstrated how psychological research could be seriously distorted by assumptions and expectations; and other psychological research had shown how human thinking is not always strictly logical, and can often be over-influenced by language and specific examples. This research produced a great deal of concern about the way that psychological research could be distorted by the assumptions and beliefs of the researcher.

This concern expressed itself in anxieties about qualitative research, since most forms of qualitative analysis involve the researcher interacting very strongly with the material. It is the researcher who decides on themes for analysis, who identifies what is important in the data and what isn't, and who selects the form of analysis in the first place. For many psychologists, this seemed to be open to problems such as self-fulfilling prophecies, bias and distortion. As a result, there has been a considerable amount of attention given to addressing the problems of rigour in qualitative analysis.

Many of these concerns actually stemmed from a misperception of qualitative analysis. It was viewed as being largely unstructured, with the researcher simply picking out information that they were interested in, regardless of what was contained in the rest of the data. But in reality, qualitative analysis doesn't operate in that way at all. There are many very explicit approaches to qualitative analysis – we will be looking at some of them in this and the next few chapters – and absolutely none of them involves just picking out the bits of information you are interested in regardless of the rest. In fact, as we will be seeing, qualitative analysis involves a number of very explicit and distinctly rigorous steps; and the selection of the appropriate method is as important in this field as it is in quantitative analysis.

In many ways, qualitative analysis is much harder to carry out than quantitative analysis. Qualitative analysis involves much more work for the researcher, and doesn't give simple, easy answers at the end. Moreover, psychologists using qualitative analysis need to be extremely vigilant about the problems of bias and distortion, and this means that even the simplest analysis can involve a great deal of re-analysis and reappraisal. But the rewards are high. What qualitative analysis can do is provide us with much richer information about the topic we are investigating. It allows us to avoid regarding a human activity as a simplistic, robotic action without motives or thought, and

---

What do these three terms mean?

rigour

bias

reappraisal

enables us to identify some of its complexity. As a result, we can gain a much deeper understanding of our topic, and one which reflects the complexities of human experience much more accurately.

Frameworks for qualitative analysis

The chapters in this book illustrate a number of different approaches to qualitative analysis. They have been deliberately selected to give an idea of the range of approaches and ideas in this area. It is quite common to hear psychologists talk of qualitative analysis as if it was just one method, but in fact there are almost as many ways of doing qualitative analysis as there are ways of doing quantitative analysis.

Unlike quantitative approaches, however, there are some major philosophical differences between different approaches. The first approach we will be looking at is the basic form of qualitative analysis which is still the most popular among researchers. This is known as thematic qualitative analysis, and is a useful way of exploring the richness of qualitative data. But as we will see, conducting a thematic qualitative analysis properly is a rigorous and demanding process.

Thematic analysis, as its name suggests, involves identifying particular themes which occur in the material which is being studied. Those themes may emerge from the data as they are analysed, taking the form of recurrent statements, attributions or assumptions which people make. Alternatively, the themes may have been determined before the analysis began, and the analysis may consist of identifying statements which relate to them. This type of thematic analysis is theory-driven, and allows the researcher to use this kind of qualitative analysis to test specific hypotheses and ideas.

Chapter 11 deals with some very different approaches to qualitative analysis, beginning with grounded theory. This is a way of using qualitative methods to build up a theoretical understanding of an area or topic. It can be a lengthy process, since the researcher has to return to the material again and again in order to check and revalidate their original understanding, and to draw out more of the subtleties in the material. But the idea is that the end process will result in a theoretical overview which is a reasonably thorough reflection of the data which have been collected, and which can serve as the basis for future research into the area.

The phenomenological approach to qualitative analysis isn't particularly concerned with understanding objective reality – indeed, phenomenologists challenge whether such a reality exists. Instead, phenomenological qualitative research aims to understand the internal world of the research participant, and how they perceive events and experiences in that world. It is a more individualistic approach than the social constructionism applied by discourse analysts, and involves a deep penetration into the individual's mental world.

We will conclude Chapter 11 by looking at action research, which isn't always a strictly qualitative technique but has been very closely linked with the challenge to conventional methodology presented by the qualitative approach. Action research also emphasises the importance of approaching psychological research from the participant's point of view. Action research challenges the conventional assumptions of objectivity in psychological research, and argues that it is often more effective for researchers to be consciously aware of the effect that they are having, and to build such effects into their research designs.

Chapter 12 deals with forms of qualitative analysis which specifically deal with conversations or discourse. The first part of the chapter describes conversation analysis, which is an approach to understanding conversations which looks particularly closely at structures and mechanisms in the conversational process. Conversational analysis draws on research from several different disciplines, and combines these to provide the researcher with a far more complete picture of what is going on than could be obtained from a single mode of analysis.

The other approach we will be looking at in this chapter – **discourse analysis** – involves a rather different set of assumptions. Like phenomenological analysis, discourse analysis is not particularly concerned with external objective reality. Most discourse analysis is conducted on text or verbal interactions between people, and we will begin by looking at this. But in this chapter we will also be looking at how psychologists can use this, and other qualitative techniques, to analyse artwork or other visual material.

Discourse analysis operates from the principle that our experience is constructed by and through our interactions with other people – the sense we make of our experience is socially constructed, so effectively our understanding of the world is socially constructed too. The way in which this social construction happens is through conversational strategies, shared symbols and meanings, and frames of understanding, and so this is the focus of this type of qualitative analysis. But discourse analysis recognises that the researcher is also part of the social construction process, and so are the meanings which the researcher puts on the material being studied.

In Chapter 13, we will be looking at some more specific approaches to qualitative analysis. As we will be seeing later in this chapter, theory-led thematic analysis is one of the approaches to qualitative analysis which can be used within the positivistic hypothetico-deductive research paradigm that most quantitative researchers use. The other one in common use is known as **protocol analysis**. This is

> **What do these three terms mean?**
>
> *qualitative research*
>
> *quantitative research*
>
> *behaviourist*

a qualitative approach which is becoming increasingly popular in cognitive psychology, as researchers study how people interpret their own actions. It involves asking research participants to describe their thoughts and ideas as they carry out specific actions, collecting information about how they see what they are doing. Sometimes that information may reflect what is going on, but often it reflects something rather different – the person's own theory of what they are doing, which may not be the same thing at all.

We will continue Chapter 13 by looking at repertory grid analysis, a specific idiographic technique which enables researchers to explore the internal world of their research participants in a manner which combines insights from both qualitative and quantitative research. In that chapter we will also look at vignette analysis, which is an approach to qualitative analysis used productively by several research teams dealing with real-world problems, and one which allows the researchers to combine more than one person's perspective in a coherent manner. Vignette analysis combines phenomenological insights with theory-driven evaluations, and as such is able to develop insights into problems which might be more elusive using just one or other of these approaches.

These techniques fall loosely under the category of qualitative analysis, but in many ways they challenge conventional assumptions about the qualitative–quantitative divide. So we conclude Chapter 13 by looking explicitly at that distinction, and some of the issues which it raises.

There are, of course, many other approaches to qualitative research. This book aims to give a sample, not a comprehensive coverage, and there are many good books on the market which go into specific detail on particular techniques. If you plan to do a detailed research project using these techniques, you should consult these. What is provided here should be enough for a general understanding of the approach, and provide a 'taster' for the way that the method works. But qualitative analysis is complex, and undertaking a full-scale qualitative study can be a very lengthy and tedious process. If you're looking for an easy option on the analytical front, stick to the numbers!

Thematic qualitative analysis

Thematic qualitative analysis is, as its name suggests, qualitative analysis which involves sorting information into themes. Themes, in this context, are recurrent ideas or topics which can be detected in the material which is being analysed, and which come up on more than one occasion in a particular set of data. Because the data are qualitative, often taking the form of interview data from research participants (but sometimes being other data, such as descriptions of events), the information can vary a great deal. The same theme may be described using different words, may emerge in different contexts, or may be raised by different people. Often, it is all of these. So thematic qualitative analysis involves the researcher searching diligently through the data in order to identify these themes.

As a result, thematic qualitative analysis is almost always a long and tedious process. There are one or two computer programmes which can be used to help researchers conducting qualitative analysis, but using them still involves the researcher going through transcripts or tapes over and over again. Each time a new theme is identified, the researcher needs to go back through the previous transcripts to see if it was there before and wasn't noticed. Since a qualitative analysis can involve more than twenty different themes, this is quite a lot of work.

Stages of thematic analysis

The process involved in thematic qualitative analysis, then, begins with the preparation of the data. This has to be done in such a way that the researcher can return to them over and over again. In the case of interviews, that almost always means transcribing them so that the researcher can use a typescript of the results. In the case of observational data, the information obtained by the observers also needs to be put into written form, and those notes need to be as

---

EXERCISE 10.2   **A trial thematic analysis**

Try carrying out a small thematic analysis on the passage below. Use Table 10.2, and carry out the steps from step 3 onwards. Do it as if you were going to use it for a research report. You might find it interesting to compare the outcome of your analysis with that of a friend, to see if you came up with similar themes.

An unexpected encounter

The train stopped. She jumped out, and hurtled towards the spaceport. She felt a sudden urgency to get clear of this planet. Quickly, in case another of those storms blew up and grounded her for another week. She moved quickly through the walkways, striding from one to another, single-minded in her intent. She cannoned into the girl in the exitway.

'What the . . .' Char stopped. For an instant, she had caught sight of an unmistakable expression on the girl's face as she gazed outwards. An expressing of longing. And something else – of being trapped? As

the girl stammered apologies, Char glanced from her to the shuttle, and hastily bit back the angry remark on the tip of her tongue. She knew that feeling. She'd felt it often enough herself over the past few weeks, hadn't she?

She looked at the girl again. Adult, but young. Duffle, travelling clothes. Not the cleanest in the world, but you could see they'd been clean not so very long ago. Neat. Obviously on the move. Equally obviously, no clear destination. Well the rest of her journey might have been wasted, but she could do something about this.
'Sorry about that. Looking at the shuttle? That's OK.'
'Thanks.'
'What's your name, kid? I'm Char.'
'Jani.' Just like that. No flicker, no sign of recognition of her name. Were on-world visits from spacers so common, then? No, she knew they weren't. Well, she'd ask later. Meanwhile, she wanted to get off-planet. And so, from the looks of her, did Jani.
'Like to come aboard?' she asked.
'Huh?' uncomprehending.
'Aboard. You. On my ship. The shuttle there. This is an invite.'
'The shuttle? It's yours? Me? But I thought . . .'
'It doesn't matter what you thought.' Char was in no mood for explanations. 'It's mine. My property, my invite. I say again: like to come aboard?'

The girl nodded dumbly. She accompanied Char up the ramp and into the little shuttle, Looked round, stowed her duffle into the clip. Settled herself in the seat that Char indicated. No hesitation. Good. Char checked the girl's webbing, strapped herself in, and radioed for take-off clearance. It came quickly: they must have been expecting it. No matter. As the earth fell away, she looked at her passenger. Bright cheeked, bright-eyed, obviously thrilled to bits. She'd do.
'Want to radio your folks?,' Char asked, 'tell someone where you are?'
'Huh? Oh, no, thanks. No one to tell, anyway, really.'
A shrug. Elaborately casual. Too casual. But understandable, perhaps. None of Char's business.
'When do we get to the ship?'
'Fifteen minutes, maybe twenty. We're in a close orbit, this time.'
The dam broke: 'What's the ship like? Are all the crew on board? What's she called? How's she fuelled? Do you go interstellar?'
'Easy, Jani,' Char said, laughing. 'you'll see it all in time. The ship's the Astra. You can see all round her, if you like. This your first trip up?'
Jani shot her a strange look. 'Of course.'

complete as possible so that details don't get lost. It is for this reason that it is so important to sort out the method of analysis you are going to use in the first planning of a research project. Otherwise, you might find that the way that the data were collected doesn't provide the right type of information for the analysis.

Once the data have been prepared, you can begin to identify themes. There are two ways of going about this. One is to use themes which have been established beforehand, as the likely outcomes of a particular psychological theory. This is known as **theory-led thematic analysis**, and we will look at it more closely later in this chapter. The more common approach is known as **inductive thematic analysis**, and often just referred to as thematic analysis. In this approach, the themes emerge from the data collected.

 In an inductive thematic analysis, the second stage of the research (after the data-preparation stage) consists of reading carefully through all of the data, and noting down any items of interest or other bits of information which seem to be relevant to the research topic. This has to be done separately for each transcript or observational record. Those topics might be noted using a computer package like Nudist+, or in the old-fashioned way, by noting them down separately on index cards or slips of paper. At this point, the themes haven't yet emerged: what the researcher is dealing with are specific items of information which seem to have some relevance to the topic which is being investigated.

The third stage involves sorting out these various bits of data, and it is here that the themes begin to emerge. Items which appear to be dealing with similar topics are placed together – literally, if the researcher is using paper records, or electronically in a computer system. (The old way of conducting thematic analyses generally involves the researcher spending quite a lot of time sitting on the floor surrounded by small pieces of paper!) The piles which develop as a result of this sorting process represent the themes which will form the basis of the analysis.

At this stage, though, they are not the themes in their final form. Each pile represents the beginning of a theme – a kind of 'proto-theme', which will develop and change as the analysis proceeds. The researcher now has to take each pile separately, and examine it to see exactly what this theme is. The theme will have to be given a provisional name, and at this point a researcher may also attempt the first draft of a written definition.

Once this has taken place, the researcher then needs to take the themes, one at a time, and go back through each of the transcripts again. Each one must be carefully re-read, to see if it contains anything which is relevant to the theme which the researcher is currently exploring. It's an important part of the analytical process, because of the way that human perception is selective and it is so easy to overlook information if we are not actually looking for it. But it takes quite a long time, because each interview or other chunk of data has to be examined again for each theme. That means that if the data have thrown up ten themes, each interview transcript will be systematically examined at least eleven times – once for the first analysis, and then separately for each of the ten themes.

When this second 'trawling' of the data has been completed, the researcher is in a position to take each theme and construct its final analytical form. This has three parts. The first is a name, or label for the theme. It will have had some kind of label earlier in the analysis, but themes have a habit of changing their focus as they become clarified, so early labels are sometimes inappropriate by the end. Table 10.1 shows some labels for themes which emerged from a study of environmental concerns, in response to questions about the main consequences of pollution. The second is a definition of the theme, which again may have adjusted itself as the analysis progressed. And the third part is the data which are relevant to the theme. In the case of interview data, this will consist of quotations; in the case of observational data, of relevant observations.

What do these three terms mean?

inductive approach

themes

inter-rater reliability

Table 10.1   Themes from an environmental analysis

bad air quality	global warming
ill health and disease	death of marine life
destruction of environment	damage to life in general
water pollution	contamination of land
loss of ozone layer	damage to children
acid rain	disruption of climate
poisoning of food chain	damage to monuments and buildings

In reporting a qualitative analysis, it is often impractical for the researcher to report every single quotation which is relevant to every theme. To do so would make the research so unwieldy that it could never be reported. So a researcher reporting a qualitative analysis will tend to select a couple of quotations or observations which reflect the theme most clearly.

It is for this reason that some researchers who are not familiar with qualitative analysis view it as selective and biased. But what they often don't realise is that the analytical process involves a much more com-prehensive approach – *all* of the quotations relevant to the topic have to be identified, and the full qualitative analysis which the researcher carries out has to deal with each one.

There are, then, several distinct stages to carrying out a thematic qualitative analysis. They have been listed in Table 10.2 for quick reference. They show us that conducting a full qualitative analysis can be a lengthy process. There is really no way of reducing it and still retaining the scientific rigour which is needed for research. Students often think that qualitative research is an easy option, because on the surface it looks as though it only involves picking out a few interesting quotations. But that is anecdote, not qualitative analysis, and the real research process which goes into producing the illustrative quotations seen in qualitative reports is actually much more thorough.

Table 10.2   Stages of thematic analysis

1. Prepare data for analysis – transcribe interviews or notes.

2. Read through each interview, noting items of interest.

3. Sort items of interest into proto-themes.

4. Examine proto-themes and attempt an initial definition.

5. Take each theme separately and re-examine each transcript carefully for relevant material for that theme.

6. Using all of the material relating to each theme, construct each theme's final form: name, definition and supporting data.

7. Select the relevant illustrative data for the reporting of the theme.

Content analysis

You may occasionally come across a reference to **content analysis** as a form of qualitative analysis. This is an extremely contentious classification, since content analysis is really a type of numerical coding. In the days before the richness of qualitative analysis was widely recognised in psychology, though, content analysis was the main technique researchers used for dealing with complex meanings.

Effectively, the method consists of establishing a number of different content categories, and counting up the number of times items relevant to each of them occurs in a particular set of data. It might be used, for example, to analyse common themes in television advertisements, or in written material. One particularly influential content analysis conducted in the 1970s analysed a popular set of children's books, and showed how very different, and stereotypical, the roles played by boys and girls were. The analysis was useful because it highlighted issues which had been overlooked; but the process of reducing the information down to numbers meant that it lacked much of the subtlety and richness of modern forms of qualitative analysis. We will be looking at it in more detail in Chapter 15 when we look at quantitative techniques.

Thematic qualitative analysis is the original, and probably the most straightforward method of all the different qualitative techniques. There are, however, a great many more approaches to qualitative analysis, and they vary from those which see it as an additional tool which enhances conventional scientific research, to approaches which challenge the fundamental assumptions of the research process itself.

Theory-led qualitative analysis

Some qualitative research operates within the hypothetico-deductive research paradigm (see Chapter 1). This is a framework in which theories are explored by generating specific testable hypotheses. These hypotheses are predictions which are tested by setting up experimental or observational situations which will show whether they hold true in reality, or not. The purpose of the qualitative analysis in this type of research is the same as it is for quantitative analysis: to provide information which will allow the researcher to come to a conclusion about whether the hypotheses seem to have been supported or not.

Thematic qualitative analysis can be used in this way. The version of thematic qualitative analysis which we have just looked at involves allowing the themes to emerge from the analysis as it is carried out. There is, however, an alternative to this, which is to have the themes pre-established as a result of the application of a particular psychological theory. Ordinary thematic qualitative analysis adopts an **inductive** approach to research, in which theoretical insights emerge from the data as opposed to being imposed beforehand. Theory-led qualitative analysis, however, adopts a **hypothetico-deductive** approach in which the theory comes first and generates predictions which the research is set up to test.

Hypothetico-deductive research lends itself to quantitative data analysis, mainly because it is usually testing very specific predictions which can be measured precisely and numerically. Sometimes, though, predictions made within a hypothetico-deductive research framework are tested more effectively using qualitative methods. If the research consists of interview data dealing with human thoughts, feelings or emotions, for example, it may not be appropriate to reduce the information to numbers. We would lose too much detail that way, and might end up failing to grasp any of the real meaning of the data. We need a way of looking at what people have actually said, and exploring how that fits with what we might have expected them to say.

The process of conducting a theory-led thematic analysis begins rather differently than a conventional thematic analysis. The first stage is to identify the theoretical themes being applied in the analysis. This doesn't involve the data in any way: rather, it involves analysing the

> **What do these three terms mean?**
>
> *theory-driven analysis*
>
> *inductive thematic analysis*
>
> *hypothetico-deductive research*

theory which is being investigated, and identifying specific predictions about what the data are likely to contain. These predictions form the basis of the themes of the analysis.

The themes themselves are a little more general than the predictions themselves. They are the types of topic likely to be generated by answers connected with those predictions. For example: if we were conducting an investigation of the psychology of food beliefs, and the relationship between emotive information and consumer behaviour, we might make a prediction that information about battery farming will make omnivorous research participants more likely to purchase free-range meat. But we might conclude that we were interested in at least two themes which related to that prediction: one theme to do with 'animal welfare', and a second theme to do with 'meat purchasing habits'. Both of those themes would be likely to contribute to the investigation of our prediction.

Once the themes have been identified, the second stage is the same as a more conventional thematic analysis: preparing the data. The information has to be converted into a form in which it can be used again and again. It's an almost inescapable part of conducting qualitative analysis – no matter which technique you adopt, you will almost always find yourself transcribing tapes of recorded data at some point. It is the only way we can be sure that the analysis is really focused on the information that has been collected, and not on our own erratic memories of it.

The third stage in the analysis consists of taking each theme separately, searching through the data, and identifying all of the items of information which relate to that theme. It's a lengthy process, and generally needs to be done at least twice for each theme, since the definitions of what should and shouldn't be included in a given thematic category can change a bit in the first run-through. Sometimes, too, we find that the same chunk of information seems to fit into two themes. It isn't really a problem: it gets included twice, but with a cross-reference between the two.

Once all the items have been collected, the researcher takes one theme at a time, and sorts through the data looking at the meanings and implications of what people actually seem to be saying with regard to that particular theme. The difference in this stage, though, is that there is already a prediction about what is likely, so part of this sorting process is looking to see how well what has been said concurs with what was predicted. It is this stage which indicates how far the research outcomes support or challenge the predictions.

The use of predetermined themes to structure the analysis means that a researcher can deal with quite large amounts of data. Interviews, particularly if they are open-ended, can generate huge amounts of information, and reducing these to manageable proportions is quite a task. This method makes it possible for a researcher to use this kind of

---

What do these three terms mean?

proto-themes

content analysis

attributions

Theory-driven themes and theory-driven data
Sometimes, it is useful to specify not just the topic, but also the form of the items making up a particular thematic analysis. For example, Hayes (1997a) described a study of social identification in small companies, in which the material subjected to the thematic qualitative analysis wasn't just any verbal data, but attributions. Attributions are statements indicating causality, or causal beliefs, and the study was specifically focused on social identity processes. Attribution theory indicated that looking at causal attributions was a useful way of bringing hidden assumptions to the surface, so the analysis took the form of looking at different aspects of social identification, as indicated in the causal attributions made by employees.

The study, then, was theory-led in two different respects. Psychological theory had dictated the choice of themes for the analysis, but it had also determined the type of material which was included in the analysis.

data to investigate a single issue or prediction. The search through the data, rather than being an open-ended and iterative process, is much more straightforward, since it is focused on just one theme at a time.

This type of analysis also allows the researcher to compare different research participants' views on the same topic. If two people have both searched the same interviews for statements related to animal welfare, it is possible to see how closely their decisions connect. It is even possible to carry out a correlation test (see Chapter 18) and obtain an **inter-rater reliability coefficient**, to show how closely the two researchers have been in their judgements.

The third advantage of this approach to qualitative analysis, of course, is that it can be used to investigate existing psychological theory. Because of this, it can be used as a supplement to other forms of research, to provide enriching qualitative material that will 'flesh out' the numbers. Or it can be used as a method of analysis in its own right.

It does have some disadvantages, though. The main one is that this particular way of going about thematic analysis doesn't allow the researcher to identify new or unexpected bits of information, unless they relate directly to one of the pre-established themes. It isn't a substitute for an inductive thematic analysis, because that serves an entirely different research purpose. What theory-led thematic analysis allows a researcher to do is to use qualitative analysis to support and enrich a specific investigation of an established theory. In areas where theory is less well established – where the researcher is investigating a completely new area, for example, then a researcher would need to conduct a full naïve thematic analysis, or use another inductive technique such as discourse analysis or grounded theory.

Theory-led thematic analysis, then, is a form of qualitative analysis which can be used in conjunction with existing psychological theory to provide qualitative insights into the ways that particular predictions may have meaning for human beings. Other forms of qualitative analysis are also used in conjunction with existing psychological theory, and one of the most popular of these is protocol analysis, which we will be looking at in Chapter 13.

In the next chapter, we will be looking at the data-driven approaches to qualitative analysis known as grounded theory and phenomenological analysis, and we will also look at another approach to research which similarly challenges assumptions of objectivity and detachment: action research.

Self-assessment questions

1. *What is the qualitative–quantitative decision?*

2. *Outline the stages involved in carrying out a thematic qualitative analysis.*

3. *Why has the idea of content analysis as a form of qualitative analysis been challenged by some psychologists?*

4. *State two advantages and two disadvantages of carrying out qualitative analysis using interview transcripts.*

5. *What is the difference between an inductive approach to thematic qualitative analysis, and a hypothetico-deductive one?*

Concepts in use

1. *How would the reliability–validity trade-off apply to a study of old people's gardening habits using qualitative methods?*

2. *Drawing from your knowledge of existing psychological research, describe a specific example of qualitative analysis in a psychological study.*

3. *Explain how a psychologist might use qualitative analysis to enrich a quantitative study of mathematical skill acquisition.*

4. *Taking the particular topic of anxiety disorders, describe how a qualitative approach to studying it would be different from a quantitative approach.*

5. *Imagine that you are conducting a major research project investigating young people's religious beliefs. What would be the benefits of a thematic qualitative analysis of your data, and what would be its limitations?*

Grounded approaches to qualitative research

Grounded theory
Phenomenological analysis
Action research

The last chapter ended with a theory-led approach to qualitative research – that is, an approach which is used to test or evaluate existing theories. In this chapter, we will be looking at forms of qualitative research in which the theory emerges from the data and isn't imposed beforehand. We will be looking at two main examples of this approach: the development of **grounded theory**, in which qualitative data are used to develop a theoretical base which can then be used for future explorations; and **phenomenological analysis**, in which the research data are collected to provide an insight into the participant's own subjective world.

Following that, we will go on to look explicitly at an approach to psychological research which, while not explicitly qualitative, takes as its starting point the idea that it is important to deal with the way that the research participant is an active individual, making their own sense out of what is going on, and acting accordingly. Action research has existed in psychology for a long time, but the growth of qualitative perspectives has meant that it is becoming increasingly recognised as a valuable research technique for psychologists.

What do these three terms mean?
grounded theory
taxonomy
objectivity

Grounded theory

The term 'grounded theory' was introduced by the sociologists Barney Glaser and Anselm Strauss, in 1967, in response to several debates which had been taking place about the value of qualitative as opposed to quantitative analysis. Grounded theory, in Glaser and Strauss's view, was theory developed in an inductive manner, from a close inspection of qualitative sources such as unstructured interviews or participant observational data. The concept was taken up by a number of psychologists as well as sociologists, and over time the term 'grounded theory' was extended to include the methodology involved in developing the theory, as well as the theory itself.

The process of conducting grounded theory research isn't just a matter of looking at the data and developing a theory from it. Instead, it involves what researchers call an **iterative** process – that is, a cyclical process in which theoretical insights emerge or are discovered in the data, those insights are then tested to see how they can make sense of other parts of the data, which in turn produce their own theoretical insights, which are then tested again against the data, and so on. These reiterations (or, literally, re-iterations) mean that there is what Pidgeon and Henwood (1997) call a continual 'flip-flop' between the theory which is being developed and the data which are producing it. So although it is an inductive method of analysing data (see Chapter 1 for a clarification of the difference between inductive and deductive research), a lot of the process involves deduction as well.

The important thing about grounded theory, though, is that what is produced in the end is exactly what the name suggests. It is theory which has been firmly grounded in observation of reality – not theory which has been developed because it seems to be logical, or because it mirrors someone's hypothesising about the likely mechanisms involved in something or other. The theory which is produced using a grounded theory analysis may sometimes be very context-specific, applying only in a relatively small number of situations; but because it is always grounded in data collected from the real world, it can serve as a very strong basis for further investigations, as well as being a research finding in its own right.

What do these three terms mean?
inductive
deductive
iterative

Preparing the data

The first step in conducting a grounded theory analysis involves getting the data into a form which means that they can be explored in detail, over and over again. If it is interview data, this means that the interviews need to be transcribed fully and carefully. If it is participant observational data, the source material is likely to be notebooks and diaries, and again these need to be transcribed so that they can be read through and explored easily.

Transcriptions almost always include both page and line numbering, because this allows a researcher to find a specific part of the text quickly and easily. It's important, because the next step of the analysis involves inspecting the data very closely. The aim of this inspection is to develop a set of concepts and codes, which will eventually be capable of describing the data.

The coding always involves a certain amount of judgement. Qualitative data are very rich, and the aims of the study, the interpretations of the participants, and the viewpoints of the researcher will all affect which facets of the data are highlighted by the coding system. Nonetheless, these categories are different from thematic analysis or traditional content analysis, because they are not pre-established. Instead, they emerge from the data, and are developed by the researcher in the process of reading through the material.

Indexing

The categories are noted using an open-ended indexing system. The initial entry in the index is the first indicator for a concept, which is developed and refined as the analysis proceeds. Pidgeon and Henwood (1997) describe the first step in constructing an indexing system as looking at the first paragraph of the transcript, and asking 'What categories, concepts or labels do we need in order to account for what is of importance to us in this paragraph?'. The concept is given a label which doesn't need to be short or snappy, but does need to reflect the meaning which the researcher is perceiving.

From there, the researcher works through the data systematically, adding and adjusting categories and concepts. The label for any particular concept is likely to change in response to the data, and the way that the data are perceived can in turn be affected by the labelling system. In Pidgeon and Henwood's terms, there is a continual 'flip-flop' between the data and the indexing categories. So the construction of the indexing system is a creative process, not a mechanistic one. It develops as the ideas for the categories and codings emerge in response to the data.

One of the important differences between a grounded theory analysis and other types of coding is that the researcher is not particularly interested in establishing how many examples of each concept occur in the data. Instead, the emphasis is on the range and diversity of how each concept is used. So the researcher needs to be alert to the similarities and differences between different occurrences of the same concept; and each index card describing that concept ends up containing a lot of different indicators, which each illustrate a different facet of that particular idea.

The core analysis

The need for creativity continues as the researcher moves on to the **core analysis**. In this stage, the indexing system becomes more refined, categories are linked together, and the researcher writes a number of memos which describe meaningful aspects of the categorisation and coding system. But this process doesn't just happen once. It goes through several iterations, or cycles, as the categories are explored and new concepts are introduced. The researcher needs to find categories which will interpret the data to the researcher's personal satisfaction, but will also fit the data, in the sense of providing a recognisable description of them. The idea is that what begins as a set of unstructured material becomes a coherent set of theoretical concepts, codes and instructions, and this can be a lengthy process.

Eventually, a concept becomes saturated, in the sense that the analysis of the material is no longer throwing up new facets or suggesting new connections. At this point, the researcher needs to begin to summarise the concept, usually by writing a fairly comprehensive definition of it. This can be demanding, since the definition needs to incorporate all of the different facets of the concept which are reflected on the card; but it does help the researcher to articulate and refine the meaning of the concept which has emerged from the data.

The grounded theory itself develops as a synthesis of these definitions, the memos the researcher wrote during the core analysis, and the relationships between concepts which the researcher has perceived and noted during the course of the analysis. It is the integration of all of these that produces a way of understanding the topic under study. That understanding is as full and reasonably comprehensive as possible; but it also gives insights into how the topic is actually perceived by the participants. So it provides a theoretical viewpoint which is often very different from a perspective obtained using more quantitative approaches.

Outcomes of grounded theory research

Some criteria for the evaluation of grounded theory projects are listed in Table 11.1. Pidgeon and Henwood list three types of outcome from grounded theory work. The first is **taxonomy development** – the use of a grounded theory analysis to identify a practical set of concepts which can form the basis for further research. This is particularly useful when beginning to explore an entirely new research area, because it gives researchers an idea of what type of questions to ask, and what avenues to explore.

The second type of outcome is **local theoretical reflection**. This is using the analysis to explore issues relating to a particular event or circumstances. It might involve comparing the insights from the analysis with established theories to see how well the two match up (or don't), or it might involve taking one or two core aspects of the analysis and seeing what they mean in that particular context. It is possible, too, for the 'local' part of this type of outcome to refer to theoretical implications, rather than the specific context; but this can

Table 11.1   Evaluating grounded theory projects

1. **Keeping close to the data**	The building blocks of the theory should fit the data well.
2. **Rich and integrated theory**	The theory produced should be rich, complex, and such as can provide connections between different levels of analysis or abstraction.
3. **Reflexivity**	Research activity shapes the object of enquiry in social research, and the theory should reflect this interdependency.
4. **Documentation**	The research process itself needs to be documented, as well as its final outcome. This allows the development of the theory to be open to academic scrutiny.
5. **Negative case analysis**	Exploring cases which do not fit the emerging theory is helpful in evaluating the theory and developing it more fully.
6. **Sensitivity to participant realities**	The theory should be generally recognisable to participants in the study, although it needs to be borne in mind that people are not always fully aware of reasons for their actions.
7. **Transferability**	While grounded theory is, by definition, firmly located in its context, a rich theory will tend to suggest other areas of relevance and application.
8. **Persuasiveness**	A rich theory which fits the data well should be challenging, stimulating, and yet highly plausible, and therefore likely to be persuasive.

Source: Pidgeon and Henwood (1997).

get rather technical. If you're interested in this way of using grounded theory, you would need to look at the method in much more detail than is included here.

The third type of outcome identified by Pidgeon and Henwood (1997) is fully-fledged **grounded theory**. This is the attempt to develop a full account of the topic being investigated, which generalises far beyond the specific context. It incorporates so much depth and detail that it can be treated as a full explanation and used as the basis of future research. This is an ambitious goal, and one which would require a very lengthy and detailed set of grounded theory analyses.

Nonetheless, this type of qualitative analysis does have this potential, and when that potential is realised, it gives us a rich source for the advancement of knowledge.

What do these three terms mean?

context-specific

core analysis

saturation

In general, however, grounded theory analysis is most suited for identifying general themes and issues arising from qualitative data. In a student project, or a small research project, the identification of these themes can be an end in itself. The themes provide insights which arise from the data themselves, and are not imposed by prior theory. As such they can be regarded as a much fuller reflection of the meaning of the data than other, more limited approaches to analysis. And, of course, it is always possible to use these insights to direct and structure other forms of research.

Phenomenological analysis

In the previous chapter, we looked at a type of qualitative analysis which psychologists often use alongside, or to supplement, quantitative research, and we will be looking at some others in Chapter 13. Both thematic qualitative analysis and protocol analysis are easily used with positivistic research methods – those approaches to research which focus on measurement and attempt to describe an objective or independent reality. But the next form of research we will be exploring is very different. It does not concern itself with external reality, and indeed comes from a philosophical tradition which questions whether such a thing actually exists.

Phenomenological research comes from the phenomenological tradition, which argues that meaning occurs through subjective experiences or phenomena. If we are to understand human experience, therefore, we need to explore the personal experience – the phenomena – that each individual experiences. The task of the researcher, therefore, is to try to penetrate as deeply as possible into the research participant's internal, personal world, and to try to understand their experience as completely as possible.

Phenomenological research, almost inevitably, requires a rather different relationship between the researcher and the research participant than is usual in most psychological research. We looked at the phenomenological interview briefly in Chapter 7, as one of several different approaches to interviewing; and this was the one which involved the building up of a trusting relationship between the researcher and the participants, so that they can feel free to talk openly about their own inner experiences. Analysing the data once they have been obtained involves four basic steps: bracketing, analysing, intuiting and describing (Table 11.2). We will look at each of these in turn.

Table 11.2   Steps of phenomenological analysis

Bracketing	Bringing prior knowledge to the surface so that it can be separated from the analysis
Analysing	Looking at the whole experience and selecting the focus and scope of the study
Intuiting	Exploring the data as open-mindedly as possible
Describing	Pulling together insights obtained from earlier steps into a coherent whole

Source: Lemon and Taylor (1997).

Bracketing

Nobody comes to a research project with an empty mind, and our own ideas, preconceptions and assumptions can sometimes interfere with our attempt to enter into the participant's phenomenological world. So bracketing is an important first stage. It involves the researcher making a continuous attempt to suspend their prior knowledge about the phenomenon, not through denial, but by attempting to bring that knowledge to the surface. Once it has become apparent, it can be recognised and separated out so that it doesn't interfere. It's not possible to be totally free of bias, but as long as we know what our bias is, we can try to control its influence.

The first step for the phenomenological researcher, then, is to engage in a period of self-reflection, which is used to identify presuppositions and biases. This process can also suggest research questions which might be helpful in clarifying different aspects of the experience which is being investigated. The researcher explores their own ideas about the topic being investigated, their personal meanings for the terms which they are using, and the ways that these terms may be reinterpreted by others. Quite often, this process leads to the focus of the research being reformulated, and it often helps the researcher to clarify their own perceptions in a helpful way.

Analysing

The second step in phenomenological analysis is known as analysing. It is about bringing the whole experience together, and making decisions about which parts of the experience should be included in the study, and which should not. Some phenomenological projects are **introspective**, with one person being both the researcher and the person being researched. In these cases, the analysing stage involves a combination of personal memory and self-reflection. Most of the phenomenological projects conducted by psychologists tend to involve other people, though, and for these the analysing stage consists of a series of choices about the form of the experience which is being explored.

Those choices, in turn, involve other choices. The researcher needs to make decisions about whose experiences should be collected and included; and which are the best methods to use for structuring those experiences and recording them. The insights and understanding which the researcher has obtained during the first stage of bracketing are directly involved in guiding these decisions, and helping to structure the research. For example, a researcher may choose to focus on a particular aspect of the experience as a result of finding out, during the bracketing stage, that it was this particular part of the experience which was their main topic of interest.

Intuiting

The third stage of phenomenological analysis, intuiting, is all about adopting a particular frame of mind or mental approach to the data. The previous assumptions and beliefs which have been identified during the bracketing stage are consciously set aside, and the researcher attempts to explore the phenomenon in as open-minded a way as they possibly can. The idea is to be as open as possible to what the research participant has to say, and to make sure that this is not interfered with by prior assumptions and beliefs. The researcher needs to be able to feel what it would be like to be that person, or rather, to live in that person's world.

> **What do these three terms mean?**
>
> *bracketing*
>
> *introspective*
>
> *presuppositions*

Many researchers brought up in the orthodox scientific tradition find it difficult to accept intuiting as a valid research process. The whole procedure is very personal, and involves the researcher in a manner which is nothing like the idealised detached observer of orthodox science. But this is not a side-effect of the method: the phenomenological approach is a conscious rejection of the goal of 'objectivity' and detachment, since phenomenological researchers believe that it is not possible to get a true picture of someone's life experiences by objective means. What is important is the person's subjective experience, they argue, and that can't be comprehended from the outside. It can really only be comprehended by the researcher sharing that experience as far as possible, using a combination of intuition, empathy, imagination and open-mindedness.

Describing

In the fourth and final stage, the researcher tries to pull together the insights which have been obtained from the research. This stage is similar to the ethnographic process of developing the story – the

---

EXERCISE 11.1   **Bracketing**

Imagine that you are about to conduct a phenomenological analysis of exam stress. The data will be collected in the form of six in-depth interviews with your research participants, who have experienced a variety of examinations. However, before you begin interviewing, you need to carry out the first stage of your analysis, which is the bracketing of your own beliefs, assumptions and presuppositions.

This is likely to take some time, and it is worthwhile exploring the ideas that you already have on the subject. Begin by writing a few headings, such as 'knowledge', 'thoughts', 'ideas' and 'opinions', and jot your ideas down under those headings. Soon you will probably introduce some more headings, for things which don't quite fit, and as you get into the swing of it you may find you can dispense with the headings altogether.

When nothing more occurs to you on the subject, take a look at what yours notes reflect. Can you think of some better ways to organise them? Did any of your ideas, feelings or opinions surprise you?

---

researcher is trying to link together the different experiences gathered through the research project, so that they can make intuitive sense to other people. In doing so, the researcher uses the participants' descriptions of their experiences as evidence, and also, partly, as a way of testing whether the researcher's insights really are appropriate.

The other test, of course, is the way that the researcher's 'story' is received by the research participants themselves. If they feel that the account is a valid, if somewhat condensed, account of their own experience, the phenomenological researcher can feel confident that the process has been reasonably successful as a research process. If there is no resonance between the researcher's account and the research participants' own experience, it has not.

There are, then, two types of validity testing for phenomenological research. The first is a test of **internal validity**, in which the researcher's own account is matched with what the participants themselves have reported during interviews. The second is an **external validity** test, in which the researcher's final product is evaluated, subjectively, by the participants to see whether they find it an accurate rendering of their experience. In many forms of research, such a subjective evaluation would be unacceptable, but since the whole goal of phenomenological research is to reflect subjective experience, this is the most appropriate form of validity test the material could receive.

Table 11.3 How to do phenomenological analysis

1. Prior to any data-gathering operation, 'bracket' your presuppositions about what the nature of the research question is, so as to identify biases and presuppositions, as well as to suggest questions which may clarify the experience to be investigated.

2. Make decisions based on this about what types of data are to be gathered and from whom.

3. Adopt an 'intuitive' approach to this experience, which will enable you to approach your informants' accounts of the experience by seeing it through their eyes.

4. Describe your findings through:
   (a) Gaining familiarity with the transcripts by reading and rereading in order to acquire a feeling for them and to make sense of them.
   (b) On the basis of this extract significant statements that describe the phenomena, for analysis.
   (c) Formulate meanings by reflecting on the meanings of the significant statements for each transcript.

5. Group these into themes of related meaning. Internal validation of these themes can then be achieved by referring back to the original statements to judge their adequacy.

6. Formulate these themes into a description of the phenomenon as perceived by the participants.

Source: Lemon and Taylor (1997).

The process I have described here is the full one for carrying out a phenomenological study. Sometimes, however, we want to apply a phenomenological analysis to interview data that have already been collected. (This can only apply to open-ended data, of course – it would be completely meaningless to attempt to apply these methods to structured interview data, since those data would only reflect the beliefs and presuppositions of the person who developed the interview schedule.) Lemon and Taylor (1997) identified five steps in carrying out a phenomenological analysis of interview data. They also identified six stages in a full phenomenological analysis, which are listed in Table 11.3; but we will look at the steps for interview analysis separately, here and in Table 11.4.

Assuming that the interviews have already been transcribed, the first step involves reading and re-reading the transcripts until they are completely familiar, and the researcher begins to develop a sense of understanding the person's point of view. It's an inductive process, which involves being open-minded and empathic, and really trying to see the world using the mental framework of the person giving the interview.

Table 11.4 Analysing phenomenological interviews

1. Read and reread the transcripts.

2. Put significant statements on to file cards.

3. Analyse the statements in terms of their subjective meanings.

4. Group the statements into themes.

5. Examine and elaborate the themes.

The second step involves getting significant statements on to file cards. The researcher needs to identify meaningful statements or phrases which occur in the transcripts. There are usually quite a lot of these in a given interview, and each of them needs to be put on to a card, together with information such as whereabouts the comment appeared in the interview transcript, and which interview it was. The position of the statement is usually given in terms of page and line numbers – most word processors have a facility for numbering the lines on a page – and the interview is usually identified by a code number, to protect confidentiality.

The third step is analysing the statements in terms of their subjective meanings. The researcher reads the cards through over and over again, and writes down the meanings of each one. (The re-readings are necessary, because they often bring out new meanings which weren't noticed before. A single statement can often have several different meanings.) It is also useful at this stage to replay the original tape of the interview, since tones of voice and timings can sometimes help in the process of gaining subjective insight into what the person is saying.

In the fourth step, the researcher groups the statements into themes. The process here is similar to that in the thematic analysis which we looked at in Chapter 10, and the use of index cards means that the process can often take the form of a physical sorting process. It is reasonable to assume that themes which come up often during the course of the interviews are those of particular concern in the subjective world of the participant – although it isn't as simple as a mechanical counting process. The frequency of a theme is a guide to its significance, but not an infallible indicator.

The fifth step involves examining the themes, elaborating them – that is, spelling them out where they seem to be a bit obscure or personal – and grouping together in ways that appear appropriate. At this stage, the researcher may also bring in wider theoretical issues, which may help to provide insight or clarify some of the themes. By the end of this process, the themes have been structured and organised into an account which forms as complete an account of the phenomenon being studied as the researcher feels able to manage.

What do these three terms mean?

phenomenological

empathy

ethnographic

Conducting a phenomenological analysis, then, is very far from just listening in an open-minded way and trying to write down one's understanding of what one has heard. Listening is involved, certainly, and so is producing an account; but on their own those are little more than anecdote – open to presuppositions, assumptions and distortions. The complex and demanding procedures of phenomenological analysis aim to reduce these personal distortions, and enable the researcher to produce as valid an account as possible.

This approach has some limitations, as all research techniques do. Its main problem is the way that the research method has little means for dealing with an account being challenged or questioned. Since it is, by definition, a subjective account, there is no way to fall back on objective measures of reliability or representativeness; and it is for this reason that it is so very important for phenomenological researchers to follow, and document, their research procedures rigorously.

Having said that, there are many aspects of human experience which are enriched and strengthened if we understand them from the inside. Smith (1997), for example, conducted a detailed study of four women who were going through pregnancy for the first time. Smith used a variety of methods of collecting data, including phenomenological interviews, repertory grids (see Chapters 8 and 13) and diaries (see Chapter 9). The in-depth phenomenological analysis which he conducted produced a number of insights into the way that the experience of pregnancy proceeded and changed over the nine months, and also into how that experience was reconstructed by the mother, after the baby had been born. By allowing this detailed exploration of the person's world, the phenomenological analysis was able to operate at a very different level of analysis from traditional positivistic research.

Action research

One of the greatest advantages of qualitative analysis is that it allows us to recognise that the research participant we are dealing with isn't just a passive provider of data, but a living person, with ideas and opinions of their own. As a living human being, they will be making their own sense of the situation, and acting according to their understanding of what is going on. Moreover, their actions and understandings will be directly affected by their relationship with the researcher. This takes us into the idea of **action research** – the idea of the social research process as a dynamic, interacting process, not an external objective observation. Not all qualitative research involves action research, but the two are often found together.

One of the paradoxes of research with human beings is that human beings are both the subject of the research, and the researcher.

EXERCISE 11.2   **Choosing a research method**

Six different research topics are listed below. Although some of them could be studied by more than one method, each is particularly suitable for one of the three methods described in this chapter. Taking each one separately, state whether you think it would be best studied using a grounded theory approach, a phenomenological analysis or action research by circling the method of your choice. Note down a brief explanation for your choice.

People's relationships with their pets
Grounded theory   Phenomenological analysis   Action research
Explanation _____

_____

Gardening among old-age pensioners
Grounded theory   Phenomenological analysis   Action research
Explanation _____

_____

How weather affects people's emotions
Grounded theory   Phenomenological analysis   Action research
Explanation _____

_____

The effect of a yoga exercise programme on older people
Grounded theory   Phenomenological analysis   Action research
Explanation _____

_____

Twins' relationships with one another
Grounded theory   Phenomenological analysis   Action research
Explanation _____

_____

Ways of reducing conflicts between two groups of teenagers
Grounded theory   Phenomenological analysis   Action research
Explanation _____

_____

Moreover, human beings influence one another in all sorts of subtle ways. Action research acknowledges those influences. It takes the view that the researcher, far from being a dispassionate and uninvolved observer, is an active participant in the research process, producing change as a direct outcome of the research. And the participant, far from being a passive 'subject', is actively making sense of their experience and acting in ways they believe to be appropriate to the situation. All of which makes the research process a much more dynamic social process than is often recognised.

Where other approaches to research try to minimise the effect of the researcher's presence, action research aims to take advantage of it – studying how the researcher's intervention has its effects, and the processes which become apparent as a result. The social interactions of the research process are built into the research design – behaviour is expected to change as a result of the researcher's intervention, and the researcher takes that into account when collecting and analysing the findings.

Many action researchers regard their approach as a much more honest way of going about research. They see the idea of the objective, detached and neutral research as a myth. People respond to the researcher, and may act differently than they would if they were not participating in research. Silverman (1977) showed how even operant

---

Action research and ethnomethodology

Sometimes the best way to understand a system may be to disturb it. The sociologist Garfinkel in 1967 discussed the process known as **ethnomethodology**, whereby previously invisible or implicit social assumptions and habits are made visible through the researcher's challenging actions. By acting in ways that were considered socially unacceptable, and sometimes outrageous, ethnomethodological researchers were able to demonstrate the implicit rules and assumptions of social life. As a general rule, psychological examples tend to be rather less dramatic, but the principle of disturbing a system in order to identify its elements and processes has been used very effectively by family researchers and a number of others.

Action research isn't quite the same as ethnomethodology, however, since action research relies very strongly on the idea of the research participant consciously collaborating with the researcher in a joint research process. The 'subject' of ethnomethodology, by contrast, is likely to be unaware of the research process which is actually going on (which raises some interesting ethical questions). There are several similarities between the two approaches, but this is one very fundamental difference between them.

conditioning experiments – usually considered to be examples of direct learning which don't involve any cognitive input at all – are influenced by the participants behaving in the way that they believe the researcher wants them to behave. Since this social influence between researcher and participant is going on all the time, action researchers argue, why not make it explicit, and recognise it as part of the research process?

Action research as a principle is not new: it began with the work of Kurt Lewin in the 1930s and 40s (e.g. Lewin 1946), and became widely used in organisational and occupational research. Mainstream psychology, however, remained relatively uncertain about the method. This uncertainty mainly arose because the psychology of the time based its ideas about 'scientific' research on examples from physics, which has a somewhat more passive subject matter than psychology. However, like qualitative research in general, action research came back into popularity in the 1980s, as researchers looked for more meaningful ways of studying people.

Most psychologists who use action research see it as another research method – part of the tool-box which can be adopted when required by the circumstances. But some researchers regard it as something more than that. Reason and Rowan (1981) argued that recognising that research is never fully 'objective' or 'neutral' leads almost inevitably to a new paradigm in social research techniques. Their 'New Paradigm Research Manifesto' is a series of statements about the nature of research which imply a greater awareness of values, more respect for research participants as active, enquiring human beings, and a fuller examination of the implicit assumptions being made by the researcher than happens in more conventional research. (The manifesto is summarised in Table 11.5.)

These different approaches to action research also affect the way that researchers go about collecting data. Some researchers adopt a relatively conventional attitude to data collection, combining orthodox measurement techniques with the conscious and active involvement of the participants. Others, however, take a social constructionist position (we will hear more about this in the next chapter), and reject the conventional 'objective' forms of data collection as being dehumanising and inappropriate.

Involving participants

Action research as a method of studying human beings has been popular in applied psychology, and also in evaluation studies of one kind or another. But in the past, its slightly ambiguous status in mainstream psychology as a whole meant that the findings from action research projects were sometimes ignored by other researchers. For example, Sommer (1983) compared the influence of five different lines of research

Table 11.5   The New Paradigm Research Manifesto: a summary

1. Research can never be neutral. It has effects and side-effects which can benefit or harm people.
2. Even the most static research exposes patterns which are enabled to change in the process, whether the change is intended or not.
3. New paradigm research involves a closer relationship between the researcher and the researched.
4. It is the shared language and assumptions of the researcher and participants which creates the 'world' which is being studied.
5. New paradigm research aims to produce active knowing and self-awareness, which will facilitate autonomous, self-directed action and self-determination.
6. New paradigm research seeks knowledge which can be used in living, not just as an abstract process in itself.
7. New paradigm research aims to develop a tight and rigorous synthesis of subjectivity and objectivity – a new rigour of 'softness'.
8. Studying people will show up tacit understandings, contradictions, imprecisions and other potentially painful sources of insight and change – which means that emotional support also needs to be built into the research process.
9. The purpose of generalisation is to learn about the power, possibilities and limits of people acting as agents, not for deterministic predictions.
10. Studying the person-in-context as a whole leads to the use of multi-level, multi-disciplinary understandings.
11. Truth and verification are important, but should not be used in such a way as to deny human values. People should be treated as people, not as 'things'.
12. The outcome of research is knowledge, which is also power. The nature of that power depends on the nature of the research, which is never neutral.

Source: adapted from Reason and Rowan (1981).

in the same psychiatric hospital over a five-year period. The 'orthodox' studies of perception and psychopathology influenced research but not practice; whereas action research studies of staff reorganisation influenced practice, but vanished very quickly from the literature. In another study by the same researcher (Sommer 1987), companies which were actively involved in the research process had disseminated and used the findings of the intervention, and also regarded it more positively, than companies which had simply received the intervention in a more passive, conventional manner (Sommer 1987).

Involving participants and providing recommendations during the course of the research is a challenge to the conventional notion of detached study of the research 'subjects'. But the active involvement of research participants has three advantages. The first, as we have already seen, is recognising the fact that people are not that passive, and that some effect will always be produced by the mere presence of a researcher. Active involvement and participation in the research, far from contaminating it, actually serves to reduce such extraneous variables, since the presence of the researcher is accounted for.

The second advantage is mainly relevant to applied psychological research, and this relates to the need for people to 'own' changes which affect them. Organisational psychologists and others have repeatedly found that change operates much more effectively, and is much more lasting, if the people affected have had some involvement in the process of developing and implementing those changes. The third advantage is that action research gives the researcher the freedom to develop and refine the research process as it happens, and to respond to new circumstances, instead of needing to get everything cut and dried beforehand. Often, some new event, such as a food scare or transport disaster, can change people's responses overnight. That can cause difficulties for a conventional research project, but is much more readily accommodated within an action research framework.

The action research cycle

Lewin (1947) developed the idea of the **action research cycle** (Figure 11.1). The action research process begins with a diagnostic stage, which draws on scientific laws and theory as well as on direct observations. The diagnostic stage then leads to the development of a change strategy, in which the intervention is planned. This stage is then followed by the action stage, in which the intervention is carried out; and that in turn is followed by the evaluative stage, in which researchers and participants analyse what has happened and what more needs to be done. The identification of what more needs to be done leads on to another diagnostic stage, and so the whole cycle begins again.

Action research illustrates a number of issues for psychologists. There is the question of whether it is just another research method, or whether it represents a whole research philosophy; and this is reflected

> **What do these three terms mean?**
>
> *New Paradigm Research*
>
> *the action research cycle*
>
> *change strategy*

Figure 11.1 The action research cycle

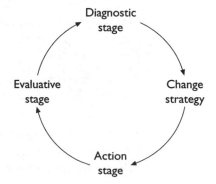

in the debates about qualitative research which we will look at in Chapter 13. There is the question about the influence of the researcher on the outcome, and how this is recognised and acknowledged. And there is the question of the degree of separation between the researcher, the participants and the research process itself.

We will begin the next chapter by looking at ways of analysing how people use language and other forms of symbolic expression. The first part of the chapter deals with Conversation Analysis, which is a technique for exploring the nature and structure of conversations. The second part deals with the social constructionist approach known as discourse analysis, in which researchers explore the ways that meanings are constructed and developed as a social process.

Self-assessment questions

1. *What are the main characteristics of an indexing system for grounded theory research?*

2. *Describe the three types of outcome from grounded theory research.*

3. *Outline and discuss the concept of intuiting in phenomenological analysis*

4. *Distinguish between internal validity and external validity.*

5. *What are the main differences between the role of the researcher in conventional experimental research, and the role of the researcher in action research?*

Concepts in use

1. *What problems might you encounter if you were trying to conduct a grounded theory investigation of illiteracy among adults?*

2. *Taking the particular topic of motivation at work, describe how a grounded theory approach to studying it would be likely to differ from a phenomenological approach.*

3. *How might a phenomenological analysis of the experiences of casualty nurses be of practical use to a management consultant working for a health care trust?*

4. *You are about to conduct an action research study of the relationship between diet and subjective energy levels. Describe what the four stages of your action research cycle would involve in practice.*

5. *Give a specific example of an action research project. If you like, you can describe one which you are aware of from your existing knowledge of psychological research.*

12

Conversations, discourse and images

Conversation analysis
Discourse analysis
Analysing visual material

In this chapter, we will be looking at ways of analysing how people communicate with one another. We will begin by looking at the approach known as **conversation analysis**, which explores some of the observable processes occurring during conversations, seeing them as an example of social behaviour with its own patterns and rules for conveying meaning. There are several different perspectives which researchers can adopt while they are analysing conversational data, ranging from an objective description of the timings and speech behaviours shown by individuals, to an exploration of how social meanings and consensual interpretations of acts are constructed during the course of a conversation.

Discourse analysis – the other approach we will look at in this chapter – deals with communication in a slightly broader sense. Although discourse analysts do study conversations, they also study other ways that human beings convey information – through written text, through explanations or formal interviews, and even through visual material. Discourse analysts see meaning as a co-operative process, not an individual one, and conversation as one of the ways that meaning is developed. The conversation is studied as a social event worthy of analysis in itself – as one of the ways social meanings are constructed.

Conversation analysis

Conversation analysts are also interested in the construction of shared meanings, and many of them work quite closely with discourse analysts – indeed, conversation analysis is sometimes described as a kind of discourse analysis. But not everyone who uses conversation analysis shares the methodological viewpoint which is associated with discourse analysis, so it is best studied as a separate system. The focus of conversation analysis is mainly on describing the conversation in terms of its structure, strategies, and what it can reveal about the mechanisms of this type of human communication.

Conversation analysis as a technique didn't come out of nowhere. Psychologists have studied the way that conversations happen between people for many years, and so have researchers in other disciplines. In fact, the historical origins of conversation analysis lie in anthropology and sociology rather than in psychology, although several modern psychologists are finding it to be a useful way of looking at qualitative data. The technique developed as social researchers began to recognise that conversations often reflect much deeper levels of meaning than appear on the surface. By exploring the conversation itself in depth, researchers found that it is possible to highlight patterns of interaction which reveal a great deal more about what is going on than can be identified using straightforward quantitative analyses.

These patterns are of interest in their own right, but they are also important because of their deeper meanings. Heath and Luff (1993) described the purpose of conversation analysis as identifying the **social organisation** underlying the way that everyday social actions and activities are produced. Because of this, it is important that the initial approach used in conversation analysis is as 'theory-free' as possible. The researcher needs to avoid imposing prior understandings and knowledge on the conversational material as it is analysed. This is one of the key differences between conversation analysis and discourse analysis.

What do these three terms mean?
conversation
discourse
visual representations

Transcribing data

The first stage in conversation analysis, as with all qualitative techniques, consists of preparing the data for analysis. The data can take several forms, but are most likely to consist of tape-recordings of one or more conversations. Collecting these tape-recordings can be complex, since it is important that the conversation is as 'natural' as possible. Interviews conducted for research purposes are not the best possible material, since the conversation in a research interview is usually quite artificially structured – unless, of course, you are interested in conducting a conversation analysis of the nature of conversational interaction in research interviews!

To do conversation analysis, therefore, it is better to have tape-recordings of conversations which would take place even if they were not being recorded. But it is unethical to tape people without their knowledge, and people sometimes talk differently if they know they are being taped. There are three main ways that researchers deal with this problem. One of them – the one used by 'fly-on-the-wall' documentary makers – is to do so much taping that the participants become completely used to it. Another is to get participants to give their consent to clandestine taping for research purposes. And the third is to be completely open about the taping and simply hope that it is not going to distort the conversation too much.

Once the tape-recordings have been made, they have to be transcribed. Conversation analysts don't see the transcript as their primary data – it is the conversation which provides the data, and the transcript is simply one of the ways of recording the conversation for analysis. The other is the tape of the conversation itself. Some aspects of a conversation are not apparent on the first listening, but only become clear after several repetitions, so doing conversation analysis also involves a great deal of referring back to the tape, and listening to segments of the conversation over and over again.

Transcription for conversation analysis is a much more complex procedure than the sort of transcription which is usually used for research interviews. The reason for this is that the researcher is going to be paying much more attention to the precise detail of the conversational interaction. Where a transcript of an ordinary research interview can focus purely on what the respondent has said, the conversation analyst needs to know the inflections that the person used, the ways that they have pronounced words (sometimes a conversation may include a correction of pronunciation, in which case using conventional spelling wouldn't be helpful), the precise timing of gaps between utterances, and many other features.

Ten Have (1999) lists eight different 'elements' which a transcript made for the purposes of conversation analysis needs to include. These are listed in Table 12.1, but we will look at them in a little more detail here. The first is that the transcript should begin with the time, date

Table 12.1 Elements of a conversation analysis transcript

1. Time, date and place of the original recording

2. Identification of the participants

3. Words as spoken

4. Sounds as uttered

5. Inaudible or incomprehensible sounds or words

6. Spaces/silences

7. Overlapped speech and sounds

8. Pace, stretches, stresses, volume, etc.

Source: Ten Have (1999).

and place of the original recording, which is pretty straightforward but also very important. The second is a means of identifying the participants. This is less straightforward, because the researcher has an ethical responsibility to respect the confidentiality of the respondent, so it often consists of some kind of coded identification.

The third element is capturing the actual words as spoken. This may seem straightforward, but there is a great tendency for people who are transcribing spoken material to ignore incompleteness, or to 'fill in' words which haven't actually been said. It is important that the transcript only contains the actual words that were said. For similar reasons, conversation analysts often use phonetic spelling so that the transcript does represent the word as it was said, rather than some ideal form.

The transcript also needs to include the various sounds that people often utter as part of a conversation. This includes partial words, grunts, 'umm-hmm' noises and others. Sometimes, the tape will also include sounds or words that are incomprehensible. These too need to be included in the transcript, because they may contribute to the overall pattern of speech – to its rhythms, or overall sound.

Spaces and silences are important too, and these need to be timed very carefully. There are culturally established conventions regarding the length of time people leave between utterances, and the meanings of periods of silence. A long silence will convey very different meanings than a short pause between two utterances, so the conversation analyst needs to have information about the length of pauses and silences to hand when conducting the analysis.

People often overlap speech and sounds during conversations. These, too, may have cultural significance and are certainly important for understanding the patterns of information in the conversation itself, so they, too, need to be recorded. The same applies to variations in the ways that things are said – changes in pace or timing, changes in volume, or a particular emphasis on a word or phrase.

We can see, then, that the development of a transcript for conversation analysis is a complex process, mainly because it needs to include so much information. What this also means is that a transcript produced for the purpose of conducting a conversation analysis can sometimes look rather odd. The important thing is that the transcript should capture the conversation, in the form in which it takes place. The conventions and notes aren't important in themselves – they are important because they reflect something about the conversation which took place.

Formatting transcriptions

Transcriptions made for the purposes of conversation analysis, therefore, tend to adopt a distinctive format. This isn't just a matter of preference: it has implications for the analysis and how it will be

---

What do these three terms mean?

consensual interpretations

social organisation

transcription conventions

carried out; so it is worth looking at it explicitly. The first point to note is that each separate line of the transcript is numbered. That isn't unique to conversation analysis – indeed, it is usual to do this for interview transcripts as well, since it makes referring to different parts of the transcript so much easier. Most word-processing packages have a facility for numbering lines automatically.

The second point is that the lines of a transcript are usually quite short. This isn't absolutely necessary, but it does make the analysis a bit more straightforward, and it also allows you to make additional marginal notes as you work through the analysis. Again, you can achieve this very easily in a word-processing package, simply by moving the right-hand margin.

EXERCISE 12.1   **Developing a CA transcript**

Make a short tape-recording of a conversation between two of your friends. Choose a subject for the conversation beforehand – for example, the latest film that you have seen – and don't worry if it seems a little artificial at first.

Listen to the tape, and choose a small section of the conversation, with between six and ten exchanges or 'turns'. The task is to try transcribing that section of conversation as if you were going to use it for a conversation analysis.

The best way is probably to follow the 'rounds' described by Ten Have. In this way you will be able to build up your transcription one step at a time, instead of having to include everything at once. Begin by simply transcribing the conversation, and keep a spare copy of this transcription. Then go through it four more times, adding in:

- phonetic spellings to represent the words exactly as they were spoken;
- grunts, 'ums', coughs, and any other additional sounds;
- timings for all of the pauses;
- any other bits of information which you can hear on the tape, and so should be represented somehow on the paper.

Use the conventions summarised in Table 12.2 to describe the material.

When you have finished, look at the final version of the transcript you have prepared, and compare it with your first version, where you simply wrote down the words.

What were the main differences between the two transcripts? And how would these differences be important to a researcher?

What is a little more challenging is the way that the lines are arranged relative to one another. The most usual convention is that a new utterance by any speaker begins on a new line; pauses have a line of their own which contains the time they took in brackets; and any overlap between speakers – where one person speaks at the same time as someone else – is indicated horizontally. The last part means that overlap in speech is indicated by overlap in lines. First, you identify the point in the previous utterance where the new person begins speaking, then you begin the record of their 'utterance' (what they say) exactly below that point on the transcript. This is more tricky to do on a word-processor, since changing the size of the font will affect spacings along a line; so you will need to decide beforehand which font and size you are going to use, and stick to it.

Ten Have (1999) suggests that the best way to make a transcript is to do it in 'rounds'. The first 'round' consists of a standard record of what has been said. In the second 'round', you listen to the tape again and adjust the spellings so they represent the sound of what has been said more exactly. The third 'round' might consist of listening to the tape again, adding in grunts or other extra sounds. A fourth 'round' could time the pauses; and so on. Table 12.2 lists some of the

> **What do these three terms mean?**
>
> *phonetic spelling*
>
> *sequence organisation*
>
> *repair organisation*

Table 12.2 Some conventions used in conversation analysis (CA) transcripts

underlining or *italic*	stress on that particular word or part of word
CAPITALS	particularly loud compared with the rest of the utterance
↑	rising inflection
↓	falling inflection
:	prolonged sound from the previous word
•hhhh	an intake of breath
hhhh	an outbreath
(h)	a breathy section inside a word, such as a sob, or laughter
° . . . °	the part between the degree signs was quieter than the rest of the utterance
< . . . >	the part between the symbols was said faster than the rest of the utterance
[. . .	beginning of overlapped speech
]	end of overlapped speech
=	no gap between this and utterance on the next line
(2.0)	pauses, timed in seconds and tenths of seconds
(.)	a small gap between utterances
( )	the transcriber couldn't hear what occurred here
(( ))	this is the transcriber's description

conventions that a typical transcript for conversation analysis might use to indicate some of these features. In this way, the transcript gradually builds up until it contains all the appropriate information. By far the best way to do this is to hire or borrow a transcription machine, because this will allow you to go back over the same bits of tape as many times as you like.

Analysing the data

Once the transcript has been made, it is time to analyse the data. The essence of conversation analysis is that the information emerges from the conversation itself, and isn't imposed by the researcher. It isn't about looking to see whether the conversation reveals a particular thing, but about looking to see how the conversation has taken place in order to see what it reveals.

Patterns or sequences in the structure of the conversation can often help the researcher to understand something of the basic underlying social organisation which it reveals. Different researchers have identified different ways of going about this, although there are many similarities between them. Table 12.3 describes the five steps proposed by Pomerantz and Fehr in 1997. Ten Have (1999) suggests a four-step strategy, which involves taking a selected sequence of conversation, and looking through it for examples of turn-taking organisation, sequence organisation, repair organisation, and the organisation of turn construction or design.

Turn-taking organisation includes exchanges of conversation between people, pauses, overlappings of statements, and so on. It's also particularly useful to note down any cases where the turn-taking seems

Table 12.3 Analysing CA sequences

---

1. Select a sequence of interest, bearing in mind that sequences often overlap and don't have clearly defined endings.

2. Characterise the actions in the sequence, and identify any of their distinctive features.

3. Look at the way that speakers have 'packaged' their actions (e.g. by choice of words or images) and how these affect the recipient's options.

4. Look at how timings, turn-takings, pauses and interruptions affect how matters will be understood.

5. Look at the implications in the conversation for identities, roles and relationships (e.g. using 'local' relationships such as questioner–answerer, and also 'wider' relationships such as doctor–patient).

Source: Pomerantz and Fehr (1997).

to be unusual, or interrupted in some way. Sequence organisation involves looking at sections of the conversation which seem to belong together – and to note down the pattern they seem to follow. Repair organisation includes cases where one or more of the participants has adjusted or corrected an utterance, or taken the conversation in a different direction as a result of not receiving an expected response; and the organisation of turn construction or design is all about who chooses to speak when, who initiates and who responds, and any regular patterns that can be detected of this kind.

The outcomes of these four steps can then be brought together as general rules or principles which describe what is going on in the conversation. That will give a basic structure for the analysis, which can be amplified and developed further by the addition of unusual or distinctive features of the conversation which the researcher has noticed. 'Noticing' is very important in conversation analysis, since it is one of the ways that important information comes to the researcher's attention. So one early step is to look through the transcript and listen to the tape as open-mindedly as possible, and to note down impressions or unusual patterns of exchange, which can be explored more deeply as the analysis proceeds.

Conversation analysis, then, places a strong emphasis on the structure and organisation of the conversation. The idea is that analysing these will give a researcher a deeper insight into the underlying social processes and structures which form the basis of the conversation in the first place. It is a data-driven technique, in which the researcher consciously avoids imposing prior knowledge on the material, but instead looks to see what the data themselves can reveal. In that respect, it is very different from the next form of qualitative analysis we will be exploring. Discourse analysis is a technique in which the researcher consciously applies prior knowledge of social meanings and implications to the data.

What do these three terms mean?

data-driven technique

theory-led investigation

validity

Discourse analysis

As we have seen, approaches to qualitative analysis differ in their fundamental assumptions. When we look at protocol analysis, in the next chapter, we will see how it assumes that the speech acts which people produce reflect inner cognitive processes, and that interpreting these speech acts allows the researcher to 'look inside' the human mind to see something of the processes which are going on. Phenomenological analysis takes a somewhat different stance when it comes to the idea of objectivity, but it too sees the speech acts which people perform as reflecting some kind of inner state. In this case, it sees the speech acts as reflecting personal experience and meaning – as an insight into the individual world of the speaker. Conversation analysis studies the forms and structures revealed in conversations, in order to get a picture of the underlying social organisation which it reveals.

Discourse analysis, however, does not make these assumptions. Like conversation analysis, discourse analysis often uses material from conversations; and it is possible to use conversation analysis within the same kind of framework as discourse analysis. But conversation analysis can also be used as a quantitative technique, and even in the context of positivistic, hypothetico-deductive research (see Chapter 1), whereas discourse analysis directly rejects that kind of approach to methodology.

Most of the research methods that we have examined in this book have tended to emphasise the study of either observable behaviour or human cognitions. But Edwards (1997) argued that this is both limited and impractical – that it doesn't take into account that human actions are flexible, and the way we shape and reshape our experiences through discourse. If we are to achieve any kind of realistic understanding of human social interaction, he argued, we have to adopt ways of exploring the social discourses within which human experiences are shaped.

Validity and reliability

Discourse analysis takes a very different approach to validity and reliability. These are not seen as arising from any 'objective' evaluation of the data, and are not really separated from one another in the way that they are in positivistic research. Potter (1996) identified four important considerations relating to reliability and validity in discourse analysis, which are very different from those we looked at when we were considering reliability and validity in Chapter 6.

| What do these three terms mean?

deviant case analysis

reflexivity

immersion |

The first of these is **deviant-case analysis**. Discourse analysts often make claims about patterns or regularities – things which often or usually happen in discourse. The validity of these claims is sometimes highlighted by looking at cases where the pattern has been broken – where there is deviation from what is expected. The example which Potter gives comes from studies of political interviews, in which the convention or pattern is that the politician does not treat the interviewer's questions as if they represented the interview's own views, but instead treats them in a more detached, 'professional' manner. So exploring the occasional instances where a politician does treat a question as if it represented the personal views of the interviewer, and how this disrupts the whole tone of the interview, is a way of exploring reliability and validity.

EXERCISE 12.2   **Conducting a discourse analysis**

Use the four themes described in Table 12.5 to conduct a discourse analysis of the material below. You might find it interesting to compare your analysis with one carried out by a friend. Were there points of similarity, or major differences? Can you combine your approaches to enrich each other's analysis?

INTRODUCING . . . *THE SUNDAY PSYCHO*!!!

Following the success of the blockbuster film *Four Psychologists and a Computer*, it's high time for psychology to reach into the realms of popular journalism! Accordingly, we are pleased to announce the birth of the *Sunday Psychologist*, or *Sunday Psycho* for short!

Following the highly successful template developed by the *Sunday Sport*, the *News of the World*, etc., we will ensure that the *Sunday Psycho* provides full coverage of all major topics of interest! Our unique psychological perspective will introduce a new dimension to these stories: investigations of the life of Elvis, for instance, will draw from psychological research on obesity, drug abuse, teenage marriages and, of course, psycho-biological and socio-cognitive insights into reincarnation!

Our psycho-journalists will find plenty of material in their investigations of the Royal Family. Maternal deprivation theory, non-verbal implications of dress style and gesture, and family dynamics will all contribute to our penetrating appraisals of events! Sports psychology, too, has a great deal to offer, and our ethogenic and even ethological discussions (inter-tribal conflicts, courtship rituals and the like) will form fascinating reading, as will our detailed analyses of the personality problems of certain football team managers! Our approach will make a major and distinctive contribution to the popular sports page!

IN THIS WEEK'S ISSUE!!
- Elvis is alive and working as a Chartered Psychologist somewhere in Epsom!
- Was Cyril Burt really an Alien? We ask the questions no one else dares to ask!
- 'I was just working through my Oedipal Conflict' – a football hooligan speaks!

PLUS SEXY PSYCHOS!!!

Our readers' poll: you tell us your votes for the handsomest hunks in psychology, including:

- Dishiest TV psychologist
- Most cuddlesome columnist
- Sexiest book cover photograph

special feature – THE SECRET PSYCHOLOGISTS!!!

Our intrepid reporters reveal the closet psychologists who dare not reveal their true profession! Learn the truth about:

- Benny from *Crossroads*
- Frank Spencer
- The Incredible Hulk
- Eddy Edwards
        and many more . . .

PLUS!!

Psychological jargon – our step-by-step guide reveals the hidden nuances. You'll never be lost for words again!

ALL THIS AND MORE . . . COMING SOON!!!

Discourse analysis is also concerned with participants' own understandings of a particular statement or event, rather than imposing an external interpretation on them. A remark which may appear as a compliment to an 'objective' observer may not be taken as such by the recipient. If that is the case then it is the recipient's understanding which must be taken as the more valid in exploring the social construction of knowledge which is taking place. How the person has interpreted the remark affects the whole nature of the communication.

Reliability and validity also emerge through the **coherence** of a body of work. As researchers continue to explore issues and topics, each new piece of work may provide additional confirmation of the previous studies, or may challenge the work of previous researchers. Rather than looking for independent 'tests' of validity or reliability in a single project or measure, discourse analysts explore these issues in terms of cumulative bodies of knowledge, seeing it always in its social and epistemological context.

The fourth important consideration relating to reliability and validity is to do with how the readers evaluate the study. This highlights one of the most important aspect of discourse analysis, which is **reflexivity**. Discourse analysis is not about applying some external measuring device to an existing social phenomenon. Instead, it is a reflexive process, which means that there is a dynamic interaction between what is being studied and the way that it is being studied:

each changes the other. Social meaning is both reflected in, but also constructed by, the analysis. So the sense that readers make of the study, and the way that they assess the interpretations which the analyst brings to bear on the materials, contribute to the validity of the piece of work.

Transcription and immersion

As with most types of research method, there are different ways of approaching discourse analysis and different styles of conducting the analysis itself. But always, one of the first things a researcher needs to do is to prepare the data. If the data consist of taped interviews or conversations, the researcher will use both the original tape and a transcript, so the transcript needs to be carefully prepared. It needs to be a little more than simply a record of the words which were spoken. Discourse transcripts are not usually as complicated as ones prepared for conversation analysis, but they do need to include some symbols which will give information about the ways that things were said, because these can give important information about subtleties of meaning. The most common ones are described in Table 12.4.

Table 12.4 Common transcription symbols for discourse analysis

bu-	sharp cut-off of the word
underline	emphasis on the word
(.)	small but noticeable pause
(1.2)	pause lasting 1.2 seconds
:	extension of the previous sound
,	continuing sound at the end of a word
↓	falling intonation
↑	rising intonation

Once the material has been transcribed, the researcher needs to become very familiar with it. This is a process known as **immersion**, and is one of the most demanding parts of undertaking this type of study. It involves reading and rereading the transcripts, playing the tapes over and over again, and generally going through the material repeatedly, over a period of several days or even weeks. This takes real time, but it's an important part of the analysis, because it is only through the immersion stage that the researcher becomes aware of some of the deeper levels of meaning in the material.

The next stage usually involves developing some coding categories – often determined by the area of interest of the study. For example, if you were exploring the way that people use gardening as a leisure activity, your material might throw up a number of different issues concerning people's relationships with gardens, ways of perceiving gardening, social contrasts between gardeners and others, and so on. These are examples, of course – they wouldn't inevitably be the categories involved, because the categorisations emerge from the data as the researcher becomes familiar with the material. The familiarisation process will show relationships and groupings which wouldn't be apparent on a first reading.

The purpose of the coding categories isn't to classify the material, but to provide the researcher with a guide for the analysis, and a way of asking particular questions. The analysis itself will be different depending on the goals of the researcher, the purpose of the study, and the context in which it is being undertaken. Gill (1996) argued that one useful way of seeing discourse analysis is in terms of four main themes: 'discourse', 'construction', 'action orientation' and 'rhetorical organisation'. These are briefly described in Table 12.5.

Table 12.5 Themes of discourse analysis

Discourse	relates to the way that discourse analysis can refer to all different types of talk and texts, no matter whether they are written or spoken.
Construction	refers to the way that discourse analysts regard discourse as a constructive process, during which social meaning is constructed and negotiated.
Action orientation	concerns the way that discourse is a social act in its own right, not something which has an abstract, independent existence. People engage in discourse in order to do something – to blame, to present themselves in a good light, to affirm a relationship, and so on.
Rhetorical organisation	refers to the way that a great deal of discourse is concerned with establishing one viewpoint as opposed to another.

Source: Gill (1996).

The emphasis in a typical discourse analysis is on how meanings are constructed and different arguments are contrasted. So it is often useful to look at the material in terms of the **rhetorical themes** which are involved. These might be revealed by the use of different metaphors, such as whether a particular topic is represented as a 'battle' or as a co-operative venture. Alternatively, they might involve the confrontation of different ideologies. Not all forms of discourse analysis involve rhetorical analysis, but it is often a good way for someone who is new to the method to begin to become familiar with the way that it operates.

> **Interpretive repertoires**
> The concept of **interpretive repertoires** is an important one in discourse analysis. The interpretive repertoire includes all of the different aspects of the discourse which contribute towards a particular understanding. So it includes rhetorical themes, but also things like the ways in which arguments are phrased, or the kinds of logic the person is using. For example, in one well-known study Gilbert and Mulkay (1984) showed that scientists used very different forms of discourse when they were talking informally than they did when they were making formal statements in publications or conference presentations. Their informal discourse was much more definite and assertive, while the formal statements were very tentative and cautious.
>
> In a different study, Sherrard (1997) looked at the way that people talk about aesthetic taste, and showed that the same people would use a number of different interpretive repertoires, depending on the point in the conversation and the social action which was being performed – whether the person was trying to counter someone else's argument, make a new point, amplify something they had already said, and so on. The discourse contained a number of inconsistencies as people spoke about their attitudes, but it was these inconsistencies which provided the basis for the analysis.

What do these three terms mean?

interpretive repertoires

social representations

iterative cycle

Discourse analysis, then, involves exploring data in terms of the ways that things are expressed, and also the interpretations and shared meanings which become apparent to the researcher. So conducting a discourse analysis would begin with immersion in the data and the emergence of some coding categories; but as it proceeds, it is likely to involve identifying key metaphors and other rhetorical themes, and then to move on to the analysis of the interpretive repertoires which are being brought to bear on the data.

One of the things to remember, though, is that the various themes or repertoires which emerge during discourse analysis are not just ways of illustrating speech. People don't use discourse to provide simple descriptions – even if that is what they think they are doing at the time. They use it to achieve social goals – to make a point, to justify an action or a viewpoint, to blame someone else, and so on. As an example, Table 12.6 lists a number of strategies identified in a discourse analysis conducted by Van Dijk (1987), which were used by racists as justifications for their nasty beliefs. The purpose of using discourse analysis to identify strategies and repertoires is to develop a better understanding of the way in which that discourse is being used to perform social acts.

Table 12.6 Verbal strategies used as social justification

1. **Credibility-enhancing moves** in which the person makes statements designed to show that they 'know' what they are talking about.

2. **Positive self-presentation** in which the person denies being racist but provides reasons for disliking that particular minority group for what they claim as 'good' reasons.

3. **Negative other-presentation** in which the disliked group is described as engaging in negative or illegal behaviour.

Source: Van Dijk (1987).

Essentially, then, discourse analysts are concerned with looking at the ways that social actions occur through the transmission of information and the shared interpretations of those meanings. But that isn't limited to conversations or interviews: the approach can apply just as well to other types of material. In 1994, for example, Parker reported a discourse analysis of the packaging of a tube of children's toothpaste, showing how this type of approach could draw out the layers of hidden and not-so-hidden social meanings in the way that the product was packaged.

Analysing visual material

The data used in discourse analysis usually take the form of transcripts of conversations; but this isn't always the case. What has become known as the discourse approach has been used to analyse written texts, politician's rhetoric and even visual images. Other forms of qualitative analysis, too, have been used to explore visual images. Here we will look at two methods: a discourse analysis and a thematic analysis.

Analysing visual discourse

Beloff (1997) reported a study in which she used discourse analysis techniques to discuss the various types and levels of message encapsulated in a series of self-portraits produced by the artist Cindy Sherman, in much the same way as another discourse study might explore the types and levels of message encapsulated in a conversation.

Beloff recommended that the best way to begin this type of study is to read widely in the field. There are a number of texts about reading images, and these are good background for someone who wants to explore this type of work. The next step is the 'immersion' stage, in which the researcher will need to spend a lot of time with the images in question. One of the best ways is to obtain copies of them, and pin them up around the room you spend most of your time in. This will allow you the opportunity to become very familiar with them, and also to study them meticulously.

The studying process needs to be very thorough, and to include making detailed written notes about the different features of the images. It is important to make sure that all of the content is included – background as well as foreground. Beloff also recommends imitating or reproducing the stances or gestures of any people in the images, to see what kinds of feelings the artist may be trying to convey. It is worth asking other people to do this too, if you can, to see whether their experience is different from your own.

The next stage in the analysis is to go back to the question of what it all means – what the artist is trying to convey, whether the message includes any metaphors or symbols, or whether the artist is being ironic and in fact means the opposite of what is being implied on the surface. It's also useful to consider questions like why the pictures were made in the first place, and for whom. All of these issues need to be put into writing, beginning with a plain description and then following up with a series of interpretations which go beyond the surface of the image.

Once the first draft has been made, it is time to put it through an iterative analysis, adding in other material and revising it accordingly. Beloff recommends trying your first draft out on friends, to see how they respond. Disagreements, or additional information from other people, can give you more material for your analysis – although Beloff warns against automatically accepting them at face value. They, too, are material which requires reflection. It is also useful to bring in other psychological information at this time, by reading up on the kinds of topics which have been raised by the initial analysis. All of this will contribute to the rewriting of both the plain description and the interpretive one.

Discourse analysis, like many other types of qualitative research, is an iterative process, and requires the researcher to go through the same cycle several times over. As you read through your analysis you may want to rewrite bits of it, or bring in other interpretations. The final product will never be definitive – there will always be more that could be said – but it needs to be something which you are reasonably happy with. In Beloff's words, your analysis should be something: 'that you will be able to defend with spirit and pleasure' (Beloff 1997).

Thematic qualitative analysis of visual material

Discourse analysis, of course, is not the only way of analysing visual material. Finn (1997) carried out an analysis of the sectarian murals in Belfast, analysing the messages they contain in terms of social representation theory, and the way that social meanings are encapsulated in the images and themes of the murals. Different studies require different methods, and Finn pointed out that there are some circumstances where even quantitative methods can be useful in the analysis of visual material – in particular, where there is a well-defined and extremely precise topic of interest. Usually, though, qualitative methods are more useful for this type of material.

Within qualitative methodologies, though, there is a choice, and not one single answer for all visual material. For Beloff's study of self-portraiture, discourse was a good way of exploring the artist's dialogue with the viewer. For Finn's study, which involved the visual images set against a backdrop of long-term social conflict, a thematic analysis using social representation theory was more appropriate, since the theoretical background which was used was more able to encompass issues of power, control and social conflict.

Using a theoretical background of this type means that the researcher needs to have become familiar with the theory, and also with the relevant context to the study. Visual images can't be taken as sufficient material in their own right: they need to be set in their historical and social contexts. So the researcher needs to do a lot of reading and information seeking, in order to identify the social representations on which the visual representations are based.

Those social representations will give a framework for the analysis, and allow the researcher to treat the images as a kind of 'visual rhetoric'. You need to look at how the visual metaphors, themes and ideas in the images can be seen as reflections of the social representations involved; and what else the images include. Finn points out that there will almost always be contrary themes in the data, too, and these will suggest other ways of 'seeing' the situation.

Since this is a theory-led investigation, it is also important to consider what evidence would negate the interpretation which is being produced. Once this has been established, the next step is to go through the data again looking for cases which would invalidate the interpretation. This shouldn't happen just once: you need to do it several times, exploring different ways that the interpretation might be challenged. It is an important process, which will strengthen the interpretation as the interpretation is adjusted to accommodate different features of the data.

The interpretation also needs to be tested against the literature, to see whether the conclusions which have been reached from the analysis of the visual material are congruent with those in other research on the topic. If it isn't, then it will need to be either re-evaluated or well defended. Each point which is being made in the analysis should be illustrated by an aspect of the visual image. Since the visual images are the primary data on which the analysis is based, they need to provide the main evidence. But it is also important to construct verbal descriptions of these points – word-pictures which will describe the relevant image or part of the image.

There will, of course, always be alternative ways of analysing the material, and it is worth conducting two or three re-analyses or the same material. It may seem tedious, but the richness of this type of material will repay the effort. As Finn (1997) remarked: 'Every visual representation is a fragment of some social vision: every visual representation tells you something of at least one good story'.

In the next chapter, we will be looking at some more specific forms of qualitative analysis: methods which are often combined with the quantitative approaches that we will be exploring in the final chapters of this book. And we will also be taking a closer look at the whole nature of the quantitative–qualitative distinction.

Self-assessment questions

1. *What are the main differences between conversation analysis and discourse analysis?*

2. *What special features need to be included in a transcript produced for the purpose of conversation analysis?*

3. *What four concepts does Potter put forward for exploring reliability and validity in discourse analysis?*

4. *What are rhetorical themes, and how are they used in discourse analysis?*

5. *Outline the iterative cycle involved in a discourse-based analysis of visual images.*

Concepts in use

1. *How might the concept of conversation analysis be useful to a health psychologist studying doctor–patient communication?*

2. *Show how the concepts of turn-taking organisation, sequence organisation, repair organisation and turn construction might manifest themselves in a conversation between two friends. Choose a specific subject of conversation, and base your examples on that.*

3. *Give a specific example of discourse analysis in psychological research. What was the topic of the original discourse, and what were the main insights obtained from it?*

4. *What would be the similarities and differences between a discourse-based analysis of army recruiting posters and a thematic qualitative analysis of the same material?*

5. *How might a knowledge of social representations inform a thematic analysis of images of urban and rural landscapes?*

13

Protocol analysis and other techniques

Protocol analysis
Vignette analysis
Repertory grid analysis
The qualitative–quantitative divide

In this chapter, we will be looking at some specific techniques which also come under the heading of 'qualitative analysis' – although, as we will see, some of them blur that distinction a little. We begin by looking at protocol analysis, which is an approach used widely in cognitive psychology and some other areas. From there we will go on to look at repertory grid analysis, which is a widely used technique which manages to combine qualitative and quantitative approaches. The third method we will be looking at is vignette analysis, which we touched on in Chapter 8, but which should really be categorised as a qualitative technique.

These approaches to qualitative analysis all raise questions about the nature of qualitative research, and in particular the hard and fast distinction between qualitative and quantitative techniques. So, in the final part of this chapter, as a conclusion to our discussion of qualitative analyses, we will look at some of the challenges to the qualitative–quantitative distinction, and see how it is not nearly as clear-cut as it appears on the surface.

Protocol analysis

Protocol analysis is another form of qualitative analysis which is used in conjunction with established psychological theory, and in hypothetico-deductive research. It has its origins in information-processing theory, which looks at the way that the human mind works in terms of how it deals with information – both incoming information and the information which has already been stored in memory.

Ericsson and Simon (1984) proposed that it is possible to record and analyse some aspects of the individual's information processing, by asking them to 'think aloud' as they carry out a task. While this doesn't allow a researcher to identify every aspect of the information involved in carrying out a task, it does nonetheless give a researcher important information about what the person is attending to at any given moment.

The main assumption of protocol analysis is that of **serial processing** – the idea that, when we are dealing with a particular task or problem, we process one strand of information at a time. That information involves bringing relevant aspects of the task into working memory – the part of the information-processing system which involves conscious attention. By asking people to monitor their conscious thoughts, and to say aloud what comes into their minds while they are carrying out the task, researchers aim to get a record of how the working memory deals with information, and so gain insight into the way that cognitive processing is taking place.

One of the important issues here, then, is that the reports need to be **concurrent** rather than **retrospective**. In 1977, Nisbett and Wilson reviewed a large number of studies showing that when people were asked to report their decision-making processes, the reports which they gave were highly inaccurate and often didn't refer to the experimental stimuli. But Ericsson and Simon (1984) argued that the studies they had reviewed almost all involved retrospective reports – participants were asked to make the decision, and then say what had promoted them to make it. This, they argued, was what had produced the inaccuracy. In order to gain accurate information from protocol analysis, Ericsson and Simon argued, it is important to collect what goes through working memory at the time that the participant actually carries out the task. Recalling it from memory afterwards is a completely different thing, and involves other cognitive processes which are much less direct.

Collecting protocols

The protocols which are used in protocol analysis are the verbal statements or utterances which people make while they are carrying out a particular task. These have to be recorded in detail by the researcher, which means that the situation needs to be one which lends itself to the use of audio-recording. The situation also needs to be one in which the person carrying out the task can think aloud freely – as Green and Gilhooly (1996) pointed out, it wouldn't be practical to use this method to collect information about how doctors make diagnostic decisions, or at least not in real-life situations. Patients might not take kindly to hearing their doctors report all of the different thought processes they went through as they made their diagnosis!

But a similar situation which involved actors instead of real patients might be more practical.

Collecting the data for protocol analysis, then, involves establishing a research situation in which information can be easily and accurately recorded, yet the participant is able to carry out the task without interference. It also involves using participants who are able and ready to engage in this kind of limited introspection. If the task is challenging, it often happens that people will fall silent as they concentrate on it, so it is sometimes necessary for the researcher to prompt the participant, to keep them talking. Green and Gilhooly (1996) describe how participants need to be carefully briefed beforehand so that they can expect this, and how it is best to use a neutral reminder such as 'keep talking' rather than anything which might prompt their thinking into particular channels. Sometimes, too, it's best if the researcher isn't actually present, in case they 'cue' the participants by their facial expressions.

All this, of course, is quite expensive and takes a great deal of careful planning. It is also very time-consuming, which means that protocol studies, like many other forms of qualitative analysis, often have relatively few participants. Once the data have been collected, it needs to be fully transcribed for the analysis, and this too is very time-consuming, which limits the number of participants which are practical in the study.

> **What do these three terms mean?**
>
> *protocols*
>
> *serial processing*
>
> *connectionism*

Segmentation

The first step in dealing with the transcribed data is for them to be segmented, and for each segment to be coded. Segmentation and encoding are closely linked, since the coding categories used for the data will affect how it is divided up into segments. So we need to begin by looking through the data and developing a set of coding categories. Table 13.1 gives some examples of the types of coding categories which might be involved.

Table 13.1 Examples of coding categories

Q	Questioning	Segments which involve asking questions about the task or the relevant procedures
P	Planning	Segments which involve working out what to do next
E	Evaluation	Segments which involve assessing the value of a particular strategy or action
D	Description	Segments which consist of descriptions of actions or steps
F	Fillers	Segments which involve filled pauses or thinking time
O	Other	Segments which don't fit into any of the other categories

However, the initial set of coding categories isn't likely to be the same as the final one. Once it has been worked out, the next step is to take a section of the data and to divide it into segments, coding each one. This will inevitably mean that new codes need to be developed, existing ones need to be refined, and the 'Other' category needs to be sorted out to see if it has grown too large. If it has, it is probably including another category which ought to be named and coded separately. As in other forms of qualitative analysis, the development of coding categories is an **iterative** process, which involves cycling backwards and forwards between the data and the categorisation scheme.

Once a final set of coding categories have been developed, the whole set of protocols needs to be segmented. Some research projects have the information segmented independently by more than one person. This is useful for two reasons: first, because it allows the researcher to compare how clear the categories are; and second, because it gives the researcher a reliability check. Comparing the same data segmented by two different people independently will show up whether the coder is operating in an idiosyncratic manner, and how much consensus there is on the coding categories.

Interpretation

Once the data have been encoded, it is possible to use them for a number of purposes. For example, Gilhooly *et al.* (1988) used protocol analysis to look at differences between experts and novices in map reading; a different research team led by Gilhooly (Gilhooly *et al.* 1995) used protocol analysis to explore medical diagnosis, and Sloboda (1985) used protocol analysis to explore the process of musical composition. The variety of these studies shows just how useful this analytical method can be.

The purpose of the study affects how the protocols are interpreted. For example, in Sloboda's (1985) single-person study of musical composition it was the range of protocols involved, and how they throw light on the individual's cognitive processing, which was the focus of interest. In the map-reading study, however, the focus of interest was on the comparison of the expert and the novice group. As a result, the analysis looked at the types of categories that each group used, and how much they used each type.

Protocol analysis has its limitations, of course. One set of criticisms of the method is theoretical – there are other cognitive models, such as **connectionism**, which suggest that we may deal with several different 'strands' of information simultaneously; and these question the value of the kind of data derived from protocol analysis. As we saw, protocol analysis assumes serial processing – that the train of thought passing through the individual's mind as they carry out the task reflects how they are actually dealing with the material. But connectionism sees the mind as using multiple processing strands simultaneously, so it challenges that assumption.

Nonetheless, as a method of qualitative analysis, protocol analysis allows researchers to deal with much more complex meanings than would be possible if all analysis were restricted to quantitative techniques. As a result, it is often used by cognitive researchers to enhance or supplement experimental methods. But equally, it is sometimes used as an analytical technique in its own right, for exploring complex cognitive data.

Vignette analysis

In Chapter 8, we looked briefly at the process of developing vignettes, as a research method. Vignette analysis is a technique which enables researchers to bring together several experiences, including the interpretations of more than one observer. As we saw in Chapter 8, a vignette is a relatively short paragraph, of less than 200 words, which summarises one person's view of the key issues in a particular case. Miller *et al.* (1997) drew up a checklist of questions which are useful in developing the vignette (Table 13.2) and in making sure that everyone who is drawing up a vignette has roughly the same goals.

Table 13.2   Questions to address while composing vignettes

1. What objectives do you have in mind?

2. Have you clearly defined the terms which you are using?

3. What are the facts of the case and what are the problems?

4. What can be deduced or concluded from the given information? Briefly explain by reference to the text.

5. Are there any detectable underlying themes? If so, support them with examples of frequently occurring events or behaviour. Do similar themes show up in other case material?

6. What is your overall impression of the case? How do you arrive at this conclusion?

7. What analogies would best capture the essence of the case, or any part of it?

8. Do there appear to be any role changes or reversals of role among the main characters in the drama?

9. In a sentence or two, how might matters turn out in the future?

Source: Miller *et al.* (1997).

Vignettes are usually constructed using interview data as the raw material, and at least two people draw up a vignette for each interview. Usually one of the vignettists will have been the original interviewer and the other, or others, will be someone who did not participate in it. Original interviewers bring their own memories to the analysis; while people who do not know the original interviewees and are working purely from recorded interviews or transcripts can often produce new insights into the material.

A vignette analysis, therefore, often involves the comparison of several vignettes of the same case, drawn up by different people who are involved in different ways. This makes it a very useful form of qualitative analysis for real-world research, particularly in situations which involve teams of professionals, such as health-care teams. Miller *et al.* (1997) showed how a vignette analysis was useful in exploring the experiences of families of drug addicts, because it was able to bring together a range of viewpoints while still focusing on the key issues.

What do these three terms mean?
segmentation
encoding
retrospective

Analysing the vignettes

Bringing together vignettes from different people inevitably raises questions about the levels of description which researchers use. Some people like to approach a vignette by looking at the subjective experiences of the participants, while others interpret what is going on in terms of underlying motives and strategies, and others focus strictly on observable behaviour. These different analytical styles are part of what add depth to the approach: human social behaviour is always more complex than can be described using just one style or level of explanation.

The analysis of the vignettes involves identifying the themes and issues which recur in the course of the vignettes. These might be content-based themes, such as the nature of care in a health-service team, or the management of the team. Alternatively, they might be themes which reflect positive or negative aspects of the case, such as sources of emotional support or strength, or anxieties about the future. Another common exercise is to identify the various metaphors and analogies which have been used by the vignettists. Looking at whether someone's role is described as the 'little mother', or whether a situation is described as a 'battleground' can often give an insight into the way that the problem is perceived.

One important source of differences between vignettists is the **analytical style** which is manifest in the vignettes. Miller *et al.* (1997) identified four different levels of abstraction which emerged from their study: descriptive, deductive, thematic and speculative. These are described more fully in Table 13.3. Looking at the material in these terms can help the researchers to interpret and integrate the different viewpoints, so that in the end they are able to produce a coherent picture.

Table 13.3   Levels of abstraction in vignette analysis

The descriptive style	This is the most basic, consisting essentially of factual material without any particular inference or abstraction.
The deductive style	This involves drawing conclusions or inferences from the material, such as inferring underlying or recurrent patterns of interaction.
The thematic style	This involves the researcher standing back from the material even more, in order to identify consistent themes such as complexity of relationships, or recurrent concerns with anger or love.
The speculative style	This involves high-level abstractions, such as the development of hypotheses about unconscious motives and needs.

Source: Miller *et al.* (1997).

A vignette, almost by definition, is one person's subjective view of what needs recording. Condensing understanding into 200 words or less inevitably means that some things must be left out. Each vignettist has to choose what is important and what can be left out, and this inevitably raises the question of **commonality** between accounts. If all researchers identify the same key issues, that is a strong indicator of their importance. But sometimes, two or more descriptions don't seem to fit together very well. This isn't necessarily a problem: it can be useful data in itself – a bit like a photograph of an object taken from different angles. There may be little in common between the various images, but combining them helps to provide a three-dimensional picture of the object.

Vignette analysis, then, can be used as a research method in its own right, or as a way of supplementing other research methods. It is particularly strong in real-world research dealing with complex issues, because of the way that it helps to broaden and deepen understanding of the issues. Vignettes can also be used to highlight particular features of special cases, or to highlight general features occurring across several cases. But it is the way that they deal with complex social perspectives, and bring together different social analyses, which gives them their particular strength.

Repertory grid analysis

There are other types of qualitative analysis which attempt to look at issues from the point of view of the participant. Most psychologists

What do these three terms mean?

vignette

levels of abstraction

commonality

using these methods see their great strength in their ability to deal with depth of meaning in ways that would be impossible with statistical techniques. By allowing the researcher to describe a phenomenon from the point of view of those experiencing it, it becomes possible to understand some of the more complex dimensions of social living.

In his study of the experience of pregnancy, reported in Chapter 8, Smith (1997) used a range of methods for collecting the case-study data, including **repertory grid analysis**. Repertory grids are a technique based on personal construct theory, which enable a researcher to explore the personal mini-theories, or constructs, which an individual uses to explore and make sense of their world. Although making sense of your own world is a phenomenological process, and not one which is done in exactly the same way by anyone else, it is still possible for researchers to begin to understand it. Repertory grid analysis is a tool which researchers can use to explore individual personal construct systems in an orderly manner.

Developing a repertory grid begins with eliciting the constructs which the person uses. This is done by taking significant **elements**, grouping them in threes, and identifying how any two of them are similar and different from the third. An element, in this context, is something significant. Most of the time, repertory grids are used to explore how participants construe their social worlds, so most of the time the elements of a grid analysis are other people. But repertory grids are also used in marketing research and other contexts, and in such cases the elements might be something inanimate, such as cars, or even something intangible, such as different types of holiday, or hobbies. For the purpose of this discussion, though, we will talk about a repertory grid in which the elements are other people.

The very first step, then, is to identify the elements which will be used in this part of the analysis. This is usually a set of eight or ten individuals, all of whom matter personally to the research participant. They don't necessarily have to be liked, but they do need to be personally important. These people are then given code numbers or letters. So the initial document in a repertory grid analysis would look something like the one in Figure 13.1.

Figure 13.1 Coding names for a repertory grid analysis

A Mummy	E Gran
B Janet	F Jonathan
C Simon	G Caroline
D Daddy	H Sally

The second step is to take these elements in groups of three, and identify in what way any two of them are similar, and different from the third. A common way of doing this is to ask the participant to complete sentences, as shown in Figure 13.2. This produces a set of **bipolar constructs** – constructs with two opposite ends, such as kind–cruel or energetic–passive. But what is important is that it is the participant, thinking about those real people, who has produced the descriptions and the words which are used to express them.

Figure 13.2 Identifying constructs for a repertory grid analysis

(A B C) ..*A*.. and ..*C*.. are ..*thoughtful*.. while ..*B*.. is ..*careless*......

(D E F) ..*F*.. and ..*E*.. are ..*placid*.......... while ..*D*.. is ..*energetic*......

(G H A) ..*H*.. and ..*A*.. are ..*economical*.... while ..*G*.. is ..*generous*......

In the third step, the grid itself is constructed. The elements are listed down the side of the grid, so they form the rows. The constructs are listed at the top of the grid, to form the columns (Figure 13.3). Usually, though, only one end of the construct is listed as the column heading – its opposite end isn't included. Some people, though, like to name the other end but keep it in brackets, or italics, so that they know it isn't the one which has been marked on this grid.

Figure 13.3 A repertory grid

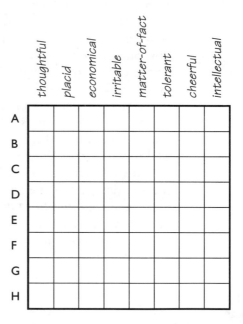

Once the grid has been constructed, the participant works along the rows, thinking about each person (or element), and ticking constructs if the named end of the construct applies to that person. If the opposite end applies, the person puts a cross in the grid instead of a tick. Since the exercise usually identifies some fairly fundamental constructs which people use, it is generally possible to apply the constructs to each of the persons in the grid, even if the person didn't originally think of

Figure 13.4 A completed repertory grid

	thoughtful	placid	economical	irritable	matter-of-fact	tolerant	cheerful	intellectual
A	✔	✘	✔	✔	✔	✔	✘	✔
B	✘	✔	✔	✔	✘	✘	✔	✘
C	✔	O	✘	✔	✘	✘	✘	O
D	✘	✘	✘	✘	✔	✔	✔	✘
E	✔	✔	✘	✔	✔	✘	✘	✔
F	✔	✔	O	✘	✘	✔	✔	✔
G	✘	✘	✘	✔	✔	✔	✘	O
H	✔	✘	✔	✘	✘	✔	✔	✘

them that way. Occasionally, though, a construct simply doesn't apply in that context – either positively or negatively. In those cases, the participant enters a zero on the grid (Figure 13.4).

Once a repertory grid of this kind has been developed, it can be used for a number of purposes. For a clinical psychologist, the insights it provides can provide a useful basis for therapy. Research psychologists use them rather differently, and in fact it would be unethical to use research data for therapeutic purposes, unless it was a research project undertaken by a qualified clinical psychologist and with the participant's full consent. Smith (1997) used them in his study of pregnancy, as a way of extending his and his participants' understandings of their experiences. And other psychologists have used them in similar ways, to highlight how people understand and experience specific issues.

Repertory grids are one of the analytical techniques which fuzz the edges of qualitative and quantitative analysis. What they effectively give us is a systematic way of understanding someone's phenomenological world, and, as such, they are a valuable qualitative tool for the psychological researcher. But by providing a systematic, symbolic chart in what amounts to a digital code, they are converting qualitative information into quantitative data. The nature of the information they are dealing with, the way it has been elicited, and the way that meaning is expressed, all mean that this is generally accepted as a form of qualitative analysis; but a strict definition of the term might conclude otherwise. In fact, as we shall see, the distinction between the two types of analysis really isn't all that clear.

The quantitative–qualitative distinction

In fact, each of the techniques we have looked at in this chapter raises questions about the qualitative–quantitative distinction. The distinction is mainly concerned with the way that we conduct the analysis of our material, and the way that we summarise what we have found. Data provided by different research methods can take a number of different forms, and some of these are to do with quantities, while others are to do with the qualities of the data. So in its very simplest form, the difference could be expressed by saying that quantitative analysis involves describing data in terms of numbers, while qualitative analysis involves describing data in terms of words. But this would be an over-simplification.

Quantitative analysis does indeed involve describing and summarising data using numbers. It is concerned with obtaining specific numbers – statistics – which will express the mathematical relationships or properties of the data which have been obtained by the researcher; and we will be looking at some explicitly quantitative methods in the remaining chapters of this book. By contrast, qualitative analysis involves looking at data from the point of view of its meanings and implications, and very often it does so by using verbal descriptions. However, quantitative analysis can still give us information about meanings and implications, while some forms of qualitative analysis may provide richness of meaning by a process which uses numbers at some stage.

In fact, there is a considerable overlap between qualitative and quantitative analysis, even though people often refer to them as if they were polarised opposites. Hammersley (1992) examined seven different definitions of the quantitative–qualitative distinction which can be found in the social science literature (Table 13.4). Each of them seems to be talking about an absolute distinction, or dichotomy, on first sight. But examining them closely shows that, actually, the distinction isn't as sharp as all that. In fact, what we seem to be describing is more like the two ends of a change of emphasis, rather than two opposite approaches.

> **What do these three terms mean?**
>
> *personal constructs*
>
> *repertory grid*
>
> *phenomenological*

Table 13.4 Issues in the quantitative–qualitative distinction

Data	Inductive and deductive
Settings	approaches
Meanings	Description or prediction
Natural science	Idealism or realism

Source: Hammersley (1992).

Data

The first definition is that the two are distinguished by the data which they use. According to this view, quantitative analysis involves numbers, whereas qualitative analysis doesn't. Strauss and Corbin (1990), for example, defined qualitative analysis as analysis which doesn't involve numbers or counting. But Hammersley pointed out that it isn't really that simple. Qualitative analysis often involves concepts like 'more', 'fewer' or 'frequent', and these are quantitative statements.

In fact, Hammersley argued, the real issue here isn't about numbers or words, but about precision. Qualitative analysis does involve amounts, or numbers, but they are not as precisely specified as they are in quantitative analysis. And on the other side of the apparent divide, using numbers doesn't always mean precision – sometimes quantitative analysis can make data look much more definite and exact than they really are. So what seemed to be a clear case of polarised opposites actually turns into a continuum, when we look at it more closely – a continuum which is really about the degree of precision which our data express.

Settings

The second definition of the quantitative–qualitative dichotomy which can be found, particularly in the social science literature, is the idea that qualitative research takes place in 'natural' settings, while quantitative research involves artificial ones such as laboratories. Laboratories provide controlled environments in which behaviour is carefully prescribed and can be measured using quantitative research tools. But because the 'natural' setting is closer to the way that people live their everyday lives, the information obtained from it is richer, and contains more of the symbolism and other forms of meaning that we deal with in everyday life. So research in these settings is generally qualitative.

There is, of course, the argument that a court of law, a shopping centre, or a classroom is actually no more 'natural' than a psychological research laboratory. Any environment created by human beings influences, if not determines, the way that people act; and in that respect they are all pretty well equivalent. But Hammersley points out that there is another argument too, which is that this definition is really concerned with the amount of control which the researcher has over the data. The idea is that laboratory research involves very tightly controlled, precisely measured data, while research conducted in a shopping centre or a school classroom involves more variability and is less rigorously controlled. Yet this, like the previous definition, is an illusion. Research can take place in 'natural' settings yet still be tightly controlled, as both organisational and consumer psychologists are aware. Or a research project may take place in an 'artificial' setting while the researcher is nonetheless gathering qualitative information.

What this definition really describes, then, is a continuum of control over the data – not a simple quantitative–qualitative dichotomy. At one extreme, some types of quantitative research do involve rigorous control, while at the other, some types of qualitative research aim to impose as few constraints on their participants as possible. But even there is a lot of variability. Most psychologists who use quantitative analysis do try to exert control over their data, but some collect it in naturalistic settings and look for ways of collecting the data which can handle the imprecision involved. Most psychologists who use qualitative analysis look for ways of collecting their data which allow their research participants as much freedom of expression as possible, but others find it more helpful to use research formats like repertory grids, which do exert some control or constraint over the data. What seems at first sight to be an 'either/or' dichotomy is actually a continuum, with lots of intermediate points between the two extremes.

> **What do these three terms mean?**
>
> *elements*
>
> *bipolar*
>
> *introspection*

Meanings

A third definition of the quantitative–qualitative distinction is the idea that quantitative research tends to focus on behaviour, while qualitative research focuses on meanings. This definition has a long history within psychology – it is, for example, closely linked to J.B. Watson's rejection of introspective research in the first half of the twentieth century, and his insistence that in order to be scientific psychologists should only study objective, observable data – in other words, behaviour. Watson's 'scientific' approach went hand in hand with an emphasis on quantification and statistical analysis of behaviour.

But although the behaviourists made claims to being the only 'real' scientific approach in psychology, there had been a great deal of systematic, well-designed research carried out before, much of which had involved quantitative analysis, while still being concerned with experience and mental life. Inspired by the psychophysicists Weber and Fechner, Wilhelm Wundt and others showed how it was possible to measure attention and other 'mental' experiences using quantitative techniques, as well as qualitative ones. Their influence, though not as dominant as behaviourism, remained in European and British experimental psychology throughout the twentieth century.

Yet again, when this apparent dichotomy is examined more closely, we find a continuum rather than a strict division. While behavioural studies may lend themselves more to quantitative analysis than to qualitative, this is not always the case. We saw in the last chapter how conversational behaviour can be analysed qualitatively, even though it is strictly behavioural data which have been collected. And while

EXERCISE 13.1	Coding protocols

Try collecting a set of protocols of people solving arithmetical problems. Begin by developing a set of four relatively straightforward (but not too easy) division and multiplication problems. Then ask a friend to solve them, and to think aloud as they do so, so that you can tape-record what they say. Their thinking aloud should reflect the way that they went about solving the problem.

Do the same thing with another friend, and compare the two sets of protocols. Were they the same?

Now try coding the protocols, by developing a set of coding categories which will describe the type of mental activity that each protocol reflects.

You might find it interesting to compare your final coding categories with those developed by a friend working on the same material. Did you agree?

Finally, show your coding categories to the two people who produced the original protocols. Did they think the coding represented what they were actually thinking at the time?

studies of social meaning and experience generally lend themselves more to qualitative analyses, this too is not always so. Doise *et al.* (1993), for example, developed quantitative approaches for the study of social representations, which are directly concerned with the shared meanings and explanations of everyday life.

Natural science

The fourth distinction between quantitative and qualitative analysis which can be found in the social science and psychological literature says that quantitative analysis is based on the idea that natural science should be a model for social research, while qualitative analysis rejects the natural science paradigm and is concerned with other, more critical or discursive forms of enquiry. Like the other distinctions, there are many examples to be found illustrating this; but also like the others, there are enough points in between the two extremes that closer examination reveals a range of values, rather than a simple dichotomy.

Part of the question lies in the definition of natural science that is involved. We looked at some of these issues in Chapter 1, where we saw that different ways of defining a science lead to different assumptions about the 'proper' ways of investigating and analysing information. If we take a definition of science as being the development of mathematical models of the natural world, that by definition implies that quantitative analysis is essential. If, on the other hand, science is defined in terms of the practices of the scientific community, as Kuhn (1962) suggested, or in terms of theory building and refutation, as Popper (1959) argued, then the door is open for the use of both quantitative and qualitative analyses.

The most important aspect of the question, however, is to do with **positivism**. The 'founding fathers' of psychology, such as Wundt (1862) and James (1890), adopted the philosophical approach of **scientific empiricism** – the idea that natural science approaches could be applied to the psychological domain. But this became transmuted into the idea that only empirical facts are important, which is the approach known as positivism. Social researchers have long rejected this idea, and the growth of qualitative analysis in both psychology and the other social sciences reflected that rejection of positivism.

There is, however, a difference between rejecting positivism and rejecting the whole natural science model. Wundt's scientific empiricism has been a model for many researchers who have also used qualitative techniques, although there are fewer examples of critical or discursive psychologists who have adopted the natural science framework. Increasingly, we find that qualitative analysis has been used in a range of different contexts, and adopting a range of different philosophical perspectives (Hayes 1997b). There are even forms of qualitative analysis, such as protocol analysis, which sometimes occur within a positivistic framework. So using the acceptance or rejection of the natural science model as a way of distinguishing between quantitative and qualitative research is not as clear-cut as it might seem on the surface.

Inductive and deductive approaches

Hammersley's fifth definition of the qualitative–quantitative divide is the idea that the two are distinguished by the methodologies which they adopt. Specifically, quantitative research is perceived as using deductive approaches, while qualitative research is perceived as using inductive methods (see Chapter 1). This idea is frequently linked with the previous point, since the model of natural science involved in such discussions associates it invariably with deductive approaches.

But this is again an over-simplification. As we saw in Chapter 1, there are many natural sciences, and they adopt a wide range of different approaches to research. Astronomy, for example, offers relatively little scope for hypothesis-testing, and many of its insights have been developed using inductive methods. The same applies in geology, biology and even nuclear physics. Their methods are very different from the idealised deductive experimentation assumed by social scientists, yet their 'scientific' nature has never been called into question. Moreover, the inductive methodologies which they use are not invariably linked with qualitative research – indeed, most are associated with quantitative, rather than qualitative, forms of analysis. Nor do they involve absolute commitment to one model rather than another: it is common in biology, for example, to find that some areas are investigated by a combination of inductive and deductive methods.

The use of inductive or deductive methodology, then, is less of a dichotomy than it may seem, and it is also much less tightly linked to the use of qualitative methods than one might assume by looking at the social science literature. As with everything else, there are extremes to be found, and some researchers using qualitative methods see them as inextricably linked with inductive methodologies. But the source of that linkage lies in the nature of the material they are investigating, and their perceptions of the research which they are undertaking. It is not an inevitable property of the use of qualitative as opposed to quantitative methods.

Description or prediction

The sixth meaning of the qualitative–quantitative distinction which can be found in the social science literature seems at first sight to have more relevance for sociology and anthropology than for psychologists. It is concerned with the overall research aim. The idea is that qualitative research is more likely to be associated with the identification of cultural patterns, while quantitative research is more concerned with scientific laws. Some research psychologists maintain a similar perception, by perceiving the distinction as to do with whether the research goal is description or prediction, and seeing qualitative research as associated with description, while quantitative research is perceived as associated with prediction.

It is a moot point whether the aim of research psychologists – even those using 'hard-core' quantitative methodologies – is still prediction. Many see themselves as being concerned with the description of psychological processes, rather than the prediction of behaviour. But in any case, it is possible for both qualitative and quantitative analyses to be used for either function. Some users of qualitative methods aim to cultivate understanding through description (e.g. Smith 1997). Others use qualitative analysis as a way of investigating predictive laws or principles (e.g. Hayes 1997a); and yet others see the iterative processes involved in qualitative approaches to description as leading on to the development of more general laws (e.g. Pidgeon and Henwood 1997). Again, an apparent dichotomy disguises a range of possibilities.

Idealism or realism

The seventh definition of the quantitative–qualitative divide is concerned with the underlying **epistemology** within which the research is located. Epistemology is concerned with the nature of knowledge, and with what counts as knowledge in a given context or framework. It is sometimes argued that quantitative methods are associated with **a realist** epistemology – that is, an approach to knowledge which argues that the real world exists, is directly knowable, and causes our personal experiences. Qualitative methods, by contrast, are associated with an **idealist** epistemology – an approach to knowledge which argues that all of our experiences come from our sensory inputs and mental representations, and that the real world is irrelevant.

In philosophical terms, pure idealism challenges the notion that any real world exists at all, taking the view that objects only exist while they are perceived; but idealism in social science tends to be less concerned with that issue, and more with the idea that our subjective experience is the only important reality. And for many psychologists, studying the richness of experience from a phenomenological point of view, qualitative methods do appear to be much more suitable than quantitative ones. But the distinction is not absolute – some researchers adopt a phenomenological stance while still using quantitative methods, while others locate their work within a realist epistemology while still using quantitative approaches.

Overall, then, it seems that the distinction between qualitative and quantitative research is less clear-cut than it might seem at first glance. But really, whether a psychologist chooses to conduct qualitative or quantitative research, or a combination of both, is entirely to do with their judgement about what that particular research topic requires. As psychology becomes more and more concerned with everyday life, getting to grips with social meanings and how people interpret their experience has become more and more important. Very often, traditional quantitative techniques simply aren't appropriate for looking at this. But many psychologists continue to investigate psychological processes and mechanisms, and how they manifest themselves, and these matters very often lead them to adopt quantitative methods as the most suitable for investigating their particular topic.

This brings us to the end of our explorations of qualitative research methods – although there are many more ways of carrying out qualitative research which we have not had the space to look into here. As we saw earlier, some qualitative approaches can complement quantitative methods, and can be used quite easily within the hypothetico-deductive research framework. Others represent an inductive approach to methodology, rejecting positivistic approaches to research and offering an alternative way of obtaining information about human beings.

What do these three terms mean?

the quantitative–qualitative divide

natural science paradigm

inductive methodology

EXERCISE 13.2   **Developing a repertory grid**

Repertory grids have been used in many different contexts, one of which is consumer-based marketing research. In that context, it is often used as a way that researchers can find out how different products are perceived.

Try carrying out a repertory grid analysis on different makes of car. Begin by selecting eight noticeably different makes, such as Fiat, Volvo, Renault, Ferrari, BMW, etc. Label each make with a letter from A to H. These are your elements for the grid.

Taking them in groups of three at a time, ask a friend to complete eight sentences, all taking the following form:

****** and ******** are _____, while ********* is _____

The sentence is completed by putting a car make where the asterisks are, and a description where the dotted lines are. Use the following groups of three for the sentences:

ABC, DEF, GHA, BDG, CEH, AFG, BEH, FCD

The descriptions are the personal constructs which you will use for the grid.

Compile the grid, with the elements along the top and the constructs along the sides, and put a tick or cross wherever it applies, and a zero if it is irrelevant. If you're not sure what should go in a particular space, you can ask the friend who provided the constructs in the first place.

If you like, you can do this more than once, taking the data from several different people and compiling a grid for each one.

Try using your repertory grid to write brief, contrasting descriptions of how two of the car makes are perceived. Did the grid give you any surprises?

In the next chapter, we will go on to look at ways of analysing quantitative data. These range from ways of describing information using numbers or images, to ways of making generalisations about whole populations on the basis of the numbers obtained from a sample of respondents. We begin our exploration of quantitative techniques with a discussion of some of the underlying principles and assumptions involved.

Self-assessment questions

1. *What is the information-processing approach adopted in protocol analysis?*

2. *Why is it important to use concurrent rather than retrospective reports in protocol analysis?*

3. *Outline two strengths and two weaknesses of vignette analysis.*

4. *In what way is a repertory grid both qualitative and quantitative?*

5. *Describe three of the major qualitative–quantitative distinctions, and explain why they have been challenged.*

Concepts in use

1. *How might the techniques of protocol analysis be useful to a traffic psychologist studying how people learn to drive?*

2. *What problems would you expect to encounter in applying protocol analysis to the training of ice skaters? How might you overcome these problems?*

3. *Give a specific example of how repertory grid analysis can be used in real-world research. If you like, you can draw your example from your knowledge of existing psychological research.*

4. *Taking each of the four different levels of abstraction described in the text, explain how each one might apply to vignettes describing a particular individual's teaching style.*

5. *Show how a combination of qualitative and quantitative analytical methods would be useful in studying the relationship between violence on television and people's anxieties about the state of society.*

14

Introducing quantitative analysis

Levels of measurement. Scaling data and standard scores
Descriptive and inferential statistics
The normal distribution. Probability and significance testing

Our investigation of analytical techniques is now ready to move from qualitative analysis to quantitative. Qualitative techniques, as we have seen, are approaches to data analysis which focus on the meanings of the information which has been received, and which attempt to draw out those meanings as part of the analytical process. Quantitative techniques, by contrast, are methods of analysis which involve the manipulation of numerical data and, at least in psychology, very often include calculations of probability.

The form of analysis that we use is closely linked with the research method that we have used to collect the data in the first place. We have looked at a variety of different methods of gathering information. Some of these, such as laboratory experiments and observations, are very tightly controlled, and limited in the number of possible outcomes which they allow. The information they give us, too, is very clearly defined and specific. Other research methods, such as interviewing or field observations, are more open to outside influences, and the information that they provide is more variable and unpredictable. Table 14.1 lists a number of different types of information that we might want to discover as part of a psychological research project. It isn't an exhaustive list, but it does give an idea of the range. In each case, some research methods would be appropriate for gathering that type of information, while others would not.

Table 14.1 Types of information

feelings	e.g. emotions, social anxieties
reactions	e.g. brain activity, galvanic skin responses
responses	e.g. decisions, perceptions
activities	e.g. habits, skilled behaviours
knowledge	e.g. factual information, beliefs and opinions
intentions	e.g. plans for action, personal resolutions
evaluations	e.g. appraisals, judgements
descriptions	e.g. experiences, accounts of perceived events

Types of data

As we have seen, there are some tricky issues which come up when we try to draw hard and fast distinctions between quantitative and qualitative research. In practice, though, we usually assume that the two are distinguished by the type of **data** which they involve. Incidentally, 'data' is the word we use to describe information that we obtain from our research. A single piece of information would be called a 'datum', but we use the plural noun, 'data', because we almost never come across just one item of information at a time.

Quantitative analysis is concerned with making sense of data which are expressed in terms of quantities. But that data can come in several forms. Sometimes what we obtain from a research project is a very precise measurement – a measure of reaction time, for example, or of the exact degree of error caused by an optical illusion. But sometimes quantitative data are less precise than that. We might, for example, conduct a diary study which involves counting the number of absent-minded errors someone makes during the day. That would give us quantitative data, but they wouldn't be as exact as our measures of reaction time.

In a different study, we might want to investigate people's colour preferences in different contexts. We could express the data that we obtained from this study by arranging them in order, from most popular colour to least popular. That would still give us quantities: that one colour was liked more than any other, or that another colour came third in the ranking. But those quantities wouldn't be precise ones. Or yet another study might give us data which were simply about categories. We might, for example, conduct an observational study of children playing, and count up how many times they showed co-operative behaviour, how many times they engaged in a personal, self-absorbed activity, and how many times their behaviour showed conflict with others. That, too, would give us quantitative information, but of a kind which is quite different from something like an exact measure of reaction time.

These different ways of measuring information, then, all give us quantitative data, but each one is of a different type. On the surface, they may look very similar – after all, the data can all be expressed in terms of numbers. A measure of reaction time can be expressed in terms of the number of milliseconds, which gives us a number that we can use in our analysis. We can count the number of errors made on a particular day, and get a number from that. We can rank colour preferences in order and give them numbers, with the most popular getting the rank of 1, the second of 2, and so on. And we can assign numbers to categories, calling one type of behaviour category 1, another type category 2, and so on.

But those numbers don't necessarily all mean the same thing. If a single piece of data is the number 4, we can only know what that means if we know the kind of **measuring scale** which was being used to obtain it. Looking at a list of numbers, and knowing that a '4' means 4 milliseconds tells us one thing. Knowing that it refers to an instance of category 4 behaviour shown by children in a playgroup tells us something quite different. So one of the first things we need to do when we are about to use quantitative analysis is to identify just what kind of numbers we are dealing with, and what sort of measuring scale is involved.

Levels of measurement

Stevens (1946) identified measurement in psychology as using four different types of measuring scale. We refer to these different scales as different **levels of measurement** (Table 14.2). These levels of

Table 14.2 Levels of measurement

Ratio scales	Scales with equal intervals and an absolute zero.
Equal-interval scales	Scales in which the difference between consecutive measuring points on the scale is of equal value throughout.
Ordinal scales	Scales in which the items can be ranked in order.
Nominal scales	Scales which consist of arbitrary categories, which cannot be ranked.

measurement have a direct influence on the way that we conduct our analysis, because some of them are more amenable to mathematical operations than others. The four types, arranged in order from most precise to least precise, are: ratio scales, equal-interval scales, ordinal scales and nominal scales.

Ratio and equal-interval scales

Ratio scales are types of measuring scale in which all of the numbers on the scale are equally far apart, and there is also an absolute zero, where we begin counting, which means that we can't have minus measurements. That may sound complicated, but in actual fact, ratio scales are the numbers that we deal with most of the time. Measurements of length, for example, use a ratio scale. Something may be 1, or 5, or 97 centimetres long; but it can't be −5 centimetres in length. There is an absolute zero, and we can't go below that. Moreover, the numbers on the scale are arranged as equal intervals, the same as in the next level of measurement. Ratio scales are the most precise form of numbers that we can obtain, but a lot of the time psychological research gives information which isn't nearly so exact.

Equal-interval scales are sometimes referred to as 'interval scales', but the two terms mean the same. In an equal-interval scale, the numbers on the measuring scale are equal distances apart, as they are with a ratio scale. But it doesn't have an absolute zero. Perhaps the most familiar example of this type of measuring scale are the ones we usually use for temperature. If we measure the temperature of water in degrees Celsius, we can see that the difference between 3 and 4 degrees is 1°, and the difference between 97 and 98 degrees is also 1°. Those degrees are the same amount, and the intervals on the measuring scale – the thermometer – reflect those equal amounts. What we don't have, though, is an absolute zero, because if we are measuring in Celsius, we can have temperatures which are below zero.

Having an absolute zero may not seem that important, but it makes a lot of difference to how we can use the numbers. In both equal-interval and ratio data, we can be sure about differences – that a difference of one unit will be the same amount, regardless of where it occurs on the scale. That means that we can add and subtract measurements accurately, in both scales. But we can only multiply or divide measurements if we are using a ratio scale. We need an absolute zero to do that.

For example: if we measure a piece of wood and find that it is 2 cm long, and then measure another and find that it is 6 cm long, we can say, correctly, that the second piece is three times as long as the first. But if we measure the temperature of a jug of water and find that it is 2°C, and then measure another jug and find that it is 6°C, that is

> **What do these three terms mean?**
>
> *datum*
>
> *measuring scale*
>
> *levels of measurement*

quite different. We can say that the second jug of water is 4°C warmer than the first, in the same way that we can say that the second piece of wood is 4 cm longer than the other. But it would be completely inaccurate to say that the second jug of water is three times as warm as the second. Compared to the amount of heat energy that water is capable of holding, the two temperatures are really very similar, and one is certainly not three times that of the other.

Perhaps it is time to look at these using more psychological examples. Imagine an experiment in which we were measuring the time that someone took to recognise a word written in a peculiar script. In one condition, Condition A, a research participant recognises the word in just two seconds; but in the other condition, Condition B, which has far more distractions, the same research participant takes six seconds before they have worked out what the word is. Assuming that the other results were similar, it would be valid for us to say that the research participant took three times as long in Condition B than in Condition A.

Now imagine a second experiment, in which we were looking at the relationship between habituation and temperature. In Condition A, we ask our research participants to handle very cold items first, and then to adjust the temperature of a piece of metal until it has reached room temperature. In condition B, we ask them to do the same thing, but we give them very hot items to handle beforehand. Imagine, too, that the research participant adjusted the metal to 10°C in condition A and 20° in Condition B. We could subtract the temperature of the metal in Condition A from the temperature in Condition B, and the difference between the two would tell us a lot. But we could not say that the temperature obtained in Condition B was twice that of Condition A, because it wouldn't be true.

What do these three terms mean?

ratio scale

equal-interval scale

absolute zero

Plastic interval scales

In psychological experiments, there is a third type of interval scale, which Wright (1976) referred to as a **plastic interval scale**. This is the type of scale produced when psychologists develop standardised instruments for measuring mental characteristics (see Chapter 6). Intelligence tests, attitude scales, aptitude tests and other forms of psychometric test all involve summing the responses to sets of items, and taking the number of appropriate responses as indicating how the person has scored on that particular set. Psychometric tests usually contain several measuring scales, and each test item contributes to one of these scales.

Stevens (1946) and many psychologists subsequently, assumed that psychometric scales can be treated as **equal-interval data**. But this is terrifically controversial, because each item on a test is different, and

continued

some questions may carry more weight than others. Asking someone if they sometimes feel shy in company, for example, isn't as powerful an indicator of introversion as asking them if they ever avoid going to parties because they feel self-conscious. Nonetheless, those who develop the scales, and many of those who use them, argue that such differences average out, and are unlikely to influence the test outcomes as a whole. Also, many tests involve converting the test items to standard scores for the scale as a whole, and this, in the opinion of those psychologists, justifies treating the scales as equal-interval data.

The reason why this matters is that the alternative is to treat these scales as **ordinal data** – and ordinal data are much less powerful. Although there are several statistical tests which can be used with ordinal data, there are many more which are suitable for equal-interval data; so the data can be treated in more complex ways, giving more interesting kinds of conclusions. Some psychologists argue that this is a case of **GIGO** – 'Garbage In, Garbage Out' – because if the data are inappropriate for the statistical test, what emerges is just nonsense, no matter how definite or exact it may appear. But that has not stopped many psychologists from treating psychometric test data as if they were equal-interval, and using parametric statistics.

Fife-Schaw (1995) suggested that the best way to deal with this problem is to conduct two analyses on this type of data – one using ordinal tests, and the other using tests suitable for equal-interval data. If the measuring scale really can be approximated to equal-interval data, then the two should produce similar answers and it is reasonably safe to use the stronger tests. But if the answers are very different, then it is safest to use the ordinal data test results.

Ordinal scales

Ordinal scales are measuring scales for which we cannot be certain about the size of the intervals of the scale. We can say that one item on the scale is more or less than another, but we can't say by how much. For example, if we ask people to rank a series of colours in order of preference, we might be able to say that one particular person liked blue more than orange, and also that they liked orange more than red, and red more than purple. But we couldn't make statements about the size of that preference. We couldn't say, for example, that the person liked blue exactly twice as much as they liked orange, or even that they preferred blue to orange by exactly the same amount that they preferred red to purple. It doesn't work that way, because the measuring scale of 'preference' simply isn't that exact.

So with ordinal scales, all we can really do is **rank** the scores – put them in order, from highest to lowest. We can assign the most popular the highest number, and then give all of the others lower numbers which indicate their place in the ranking. For example, in the previous example we could say that blue had a rank of 4, orange had a rank of 3, red had a rank of 2 and purple had a rank of 1. Then we could go on to collect similar rankings from other people, and that would tell us some things – like that a colour which had a lot of high-ranking scores was more popular than one which had a lot of low-ranking scores.

Often, the results we obtain from a psychological experiment really give us ordinal data even though they look equal-interval. And ordinal data can still tell us quite a lot. There are some useful statistical tests we can do on this sort of data, which can tell us things about how probable or typical our results are, or how closely they correlate with something else, such as the amount of education someone has had, or whether they also chose those colours to wear. We will be looking at some of these in Chapters 17 and 18. But those tests are not as powerful as the tests we can use with equal-interval data, so many psychologists prefer to assume that they have equal-interval data if they possibly can.

> **What do these three terms mean?**
>
> *ordinal data*
>
> *test power*
>
> *ranking*

Nominal scales

Nominal scales are the lowest level of measurement. Effectively, they are simply categories, which can't even be ranked in order. For example, we might find that we had nominal data in an observational study of children's play, if we were looking at the different types of activity children engaged in. Our observations would be likely to fit into a number of categories – co-operating with others, conflicting with others, engaging in solitary activity, approaching others, or some other set of categories which mirrored what we were interested in more effectively. Then we could count up how many examples of each type of behaviour we had in each category.

But we would not be able to organise those categories in any meaningful way. We couldn't, for example, say that 'solitary activity' was 'more' than approaching others, or that 'playing with objects' should rank higher than 'co-operative play'. All we could really do is to name the categories, and count examples of each. There are also some simple descriptive statistics we could do, which we will be looking at in the next chapter; but still, at the end, we would be left with the categories, and how many items of our data set fall into each one.

Test power

Nominal data, then, are the weakest form of data in terms of how much you can do with them; and ratio data are the strongest. Ratio data can undergo just about any arithmetical manipulation. Equal-interval data, as we have seen, can undergo quite a lot but not everything – not multiplication and division, for instance. Ordinal data can be ranked, and nominal data cannot really be manipulated at all. The result is that statistical tests which have been performed on ratio data are considered to be more powerful than those performed on data which correspond to a lower level of measurement. The **power** of a test is all about how likely it is to describe the data fully (in the case of descriptive statistics), or about how likely it is to make correct inferences about the population (in the case of inferential statistics). We will be coming back to the idea of descriptive and inferential statistics later in this chapter.

Scaling data

Many psychological studies give us raw data which aren't really very usable, because the measuring scale is not very precise, or has some other kind of flaw. Sometimes, these can be converted into data at a higher level of measurement – so that the researcher can analyse them more effectively. Various ways of scaling data can result in scores which give a clearer representation of what one person's result implies when compared with the results from other people.

When many of the early psychophysics scales were developed, for example, researchers found that just dealing with the raw scores and trying to plot them on a chart gave a very jagged-looking image, which didn't really represent the systematic changes they were trying to summarise. But if they took the logarithm values of the scores, instead of the scores themselves, that would produce a much smoother curve, which seemed to express the relationship between, say, the perceived loudness of a sound and its physical energy, much more clearly.

There are lots of other ways that we can scale data for effective comparisons. Nowadays, one of the most common approaches to scaling is to convert scores into **mean scores**, or sometimes into percentages (scores out of 100). That allows us to tackle problems which might come up when we want to compare, for example, the results from different groups of people or different groups of tests. We will be looking at how to calculate mean scores in the next chapter.

Another possibility is converting the information into **standard scores**, which are also sometimes called z **scores**. These describe how far the person's original score was from the mean, or average score, obtained by everyone in that group. Standard scores express this in terms of standard deviations, which are ways of describing a data set that we will be looking at in the next chapter. In that chapter, we will also look at how to calculate a z score.

Whichever scaling method is used, the result is that the original data become converted into a form which is much closer to an equal-interval scale, and which will allow the researcher to use more powerful statistics. Whether the scaling is actually justified, or whether it simply results in more precisely described rubbish, depends to some extent on how carefully the data were collected in the first place and how sensitive the measuring instrument was; and also, sometimes, on your point of view.

Descriptive and inferential statistics

As we will be seeing in the next few chapters, there are many different types of quantitative analysis. Some of them simply allow us to describe our data – to summarise it, so that it is possible for someone else to see clearly just what it is that we have found from our study.

Descriptive statistics

Statistics which describe data are, unsurprisingly, known as **descriptive statistics**, and they allow us to summarise our data. When we have finished gathering quantitative data in a research project, no matter which research method we have used, we will probably end up with data which consist of lists of figures. Lists of figures aren't much help to anyone – we need something which will allow us to grasp the essential features of the data quickly and easily. And this is what descriptive statistics do.

Descriptive statistics come in the form of either numbers or images. Numerical descriptive statistics, in their turn, are also of two kinds – numbers which give us a typical score, and numbers which tell us something about the whole set of scores. An arithmetic **average**, for example, is a number which summarises the data. It tells us what a typical score for this particular data-set would be. A **range** tells us what the highest and lowest score in a set is, so it gives us a picture of what the whole data-set is like. Both of these are numerical descriptive statistics, because they are ways of describing the data. But data can also be summarised using pictures or images. A graph, for example, is also a way of summarising data, but this time by presenting it as a kind of picture, which allows us to see at a glance the highs and lows in the data-set.

There are several different kinds of descriptive statistics, and we will be looking at them more closely in the next two chapters. But there are other kinds of quantitative analysis too. In particular, there are statistics which allow us to go beyond our data, so that we are not just describing what we have found, but can make inferences about the likelihood of these findings – about the probability that our findings would turn out the way they have. These are known as **inferential statistics**, and we will be looking at them in Chapters 17–19.

The normal distribution curve

Inferential statistics are possible because research data are very rarely random. In most cases, the entire set of possible data which could be collected has a characteristic **distribution**, which tells us what we could expect. If we were doing a physics experiment, for example, looking at the release of heat radiation from metal at different temperatures, our study would give us particular findings. Those findings would vary slightly, as a result of all sorts of subtle factors – atmospheric pressure, humidity, the purity of the metal, the rate of heating, and so on. So our results wouldn't always be totally consistent. But they wouldn't be entirely random either – we would know roughly the range of findings that we might expect, so we would be able to tell if a particular finding seemed very peculiar or unusual. In other words, we would know the distribution of the possible data that we could obtain.

There are many different distributions, all with special properties. One of the most common in psychology is the **Gaussian distribution**, which was named after the mathematician who first described its mathematical properties. This distribution is so common in psychology that it has another name, which is the **normal distribution**. The normal distribution forms a bell-shaped curve, in which the majority of the scores occur in the middle, and the further away from the middle we get, the fewer scores there are. If we were looking at recognition scores, for example, and we were able to obtain all of the possible scores for how quickly people recognised a drawing of a cat, we would find that a few people would take a very long time to recognise it, most would take an average amount of time, and a few would recognise it very quickly. What we would get, when we drew our findings on a graph, would be a normal distribution curve (Figure 14.1).

> **What do these three terms mean?**
>
> *nominal scales*
>
> *raw data*
>
> *scaling*

Figure 14.1 A normal distribution curve

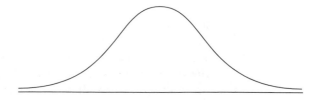

Properties of the normal distribution

A distribution, as I said before, describes the entire set of possible data related to a particular topic. It's a kind of ideal concept, which we can know about but not measure directly. In reality, of course, we couldn't obtain all of the possible scores for an entire population. All we can really do is to **sample** that population – to obtain the scores of a smaller number of people. We looked at the principles of sampling in Chapter 2, and at how important it is to try to make sure that the sample is as representative of the population as possible.

In fact, we can tell how typical our sample is, if we know about the population, and in particular if we know the two crucial measurements of the normal distribution curve. Those two crucial measurements are the mean and the standard deviation. We will be looking at these in more detail in Chapter 15, because they are both descriptive statistics. The mean is the typical, average score and it is at the highest point of the curve, while the standard deviation describes how the scores are spread out around the mean. If we know these two measurements for the population as a whole, then we know everything we need to know about the normal distribution that it represents. We could even re-draw the distribution curve, if we wanted to. And that puts us in a position to know quite a lot about our particular sample.

A normal distribution curve has some reliable mathematical properties. Thanks to Gauss, and some others, we know that the first normal standard deviation falls at the point where the curvature changes – where the curve of each side becomes convex rather than concave. We also know that 68 per cent of the scores fall within one standard deviation either side of the mean. And that 95 per cent of all of the scores fall within two standard deviations either side of the mean (see Figure 14.2). And so on. We can use this information to infer things about our sample – and it is this inference which is the basis of inferential statistics.

Figure 14.2 Probabilities and the normal distribution

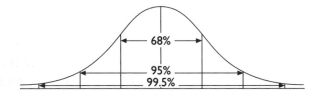

Inferential statistics

Inferential statistics, then, go further than just describing data. They use the properties of the normal distribution curve, or of other types of distribution, to make inferences about the data. The inferences they make are judgements of probability. Knowing the mean and standard deviation of a normal distribution curve, for example, would allow us to find out exactly how **typical** a sample was of the population as a whole, and how probable it was that we would get the research results that we did. So as well as describing our data, we could make judgements about representativeness, and how unusual or extreme our scores were.

We don't always know the mean and standard deviation of the population in advance, but some statistical tests are able to use the distribution of the scores obtained from the research to calculate what they would have been – or at least, to calculate what they are likely to have been. Other tests can look at the data obtained from two sets of scores, and assess how likely it is that they have come from one single normal distribution, or whether it is more likely that they have come from two separate ones. We will be looking at this more closely in Chapters 17–19. But the important thing about inferential statistics is that they can tell us about **probability** – about how likely it is that we would have obtained the results we did, just by random chance.

> **What do these three terms mean?**
>
> *descriptive statistics*
>
> *inferential statistics*
>
> *normal distribution curve*

Probability and significance testing

There are several different kinds of inferential statistics. Some of them are distribution tests, which tell us how likely it is that we have obtained our results just by chance or random factors. Some are difference tests, which tell us how likely it is that the differences between two (or more) sets of scores have come about by chance or random factors. And some are correlation tests, which tell us how likely it is that the similarities between two sets of scores have come about by chance or random factors.

In Chapter 17, we will be looking at two-sample difference tests, which are inferential tests that we use when we have two sets of scores, and we need to find out whether they are really different or not. In Chapter 19 we will be looking at analysis of variance, which is the test we use when we have more than two sets – for example, when we have three or four conditions of the independent variable in an experiment, and not just two. It is more complicated, but the principles underlying the test are effectively the same as for a test involving two sets of scores.

What these tests are really doing is looking at the sets of scores, and making a judgement about whether they are likely to have come from just one population, or whether they might have come from two entirely different populations. As we saw in Chapter 2, a **population** is the whole number of instances of a particular set – people, animals

EXERCISE 14.1   **Levels of measurement**

The list below describes several different types of quantitative data which might be obtained as part of a psychological study. For each one, state whether it would represent ratio, equal-interval, ordinal or nominal data.

Self-ratings of emotional reactions to spiders
Estimates of levels of skill in sport
Jury judgements of guilty or innocent
,Self-ratings of shyness
Ratings of violence at a football match
Electrical recordings of brain activity
Time taken to make risky decisions
People's perceptions of an ambiguous picture
Number of items recalled from a list
Rating scales describing social opinions
Recordings of galvanic skin reactions to spiders
Price estimates for attractive pieces of jewellery

or events – while a **sample** is a selected group, or subset, of those instances. When we use these terms in statistics, they have the same meaning, but the word 'population' then means the whole possible set of scores which that situation could have produced; while the word 'sample' means the set of scores that we have actually obtained from our study.

It may be that our two sets of scores both come from the same population. In fact, this is the basis for the **null hypothesis**. The null hypothesis for any two-sample difference test is that any differences between the two sets of scores have come about as a result of sampling error. It means that one group of scores has been taken from one part of the distribution, while the others have been taken from another part. They look different, but both of them really belong to the same set. But it is also possible that there are actually two populations involved, and that our sets of scores, even though they look quite similar, have actually come from two different populations. If those populations overlap, that can happen even if the actual scores don't look very different at all. We will be looking at this again in Chapter 17.

The **alternate hypothesis** for a study states that the two sets of scores have actually come from two different populations. The null hypothesis, as we have seen, states that they have really come from one population, and that any differences between them have come

---

EXERCISE 14.2   **Art and emotions**

You have decided to conduct an investigation of people's emotional responses to the paintings in a small exhibition set up in your local art gallery. You ask your participants to walk round the gallery with a small tape-recorder, talking about their reactions to each of the paintings as they come across them.

You have transcribed the recordings and, as a preliminary analysis, you have conducted a simple content analysis on the material, using different emotions as the categories and counting how often each one is referred to by your respondents.

What type of data have you obtained from this study?

Are there ways you could make these data more powerful? If so, what are they?

What ethical considerations would you need to address in designing and carrying out this study?

How might you present the results of your study if you were describing it in a report?

---

from sampling error. This is why we need to state both the null hypothesis and the alternate hypothesis very clearly from the beginning of any analysis – so that we can be clear just what our test results mean.

Obviously, though, we can't be absolutely certain about this. As a general rule, samples which have come from the same population will be fairly similar to one another, while those which have come from two different populations will be different. But, as we've seen, that isn't always the case. We can sometimes have a situation in which the two samples are very similar, but have really come from two populations; or we can have a situation in which they are very different, but have really come from the same population.

All we can really do in a situation like that is estimate probability. Although these extreme situations are possible, it is actually much more likely that two very different sets of scores have come from two different distributions; and that two very similar sets of scores have come from the same distribution. So what an inferential test tells us is **probability** – it gives us a number which expresses how likely it is that the two sets of scores have come from different populations. That number is always expressed as a decimal fraction, and it tells us how likely it is that the null hypothesis of the study will hold true.

Interpreting probability statements

If you're not used to mathematical notation, probability statements can seem a little odd at first, but really they are just a convenient shorthand. We can see this more clearly if we look at the different parts of a probability statement. We'll take **$p < .01$** as our example.

The first item in the statement is p. This stands for the probability that the null hypothesis should be retained. In practical terms, this is very similar to saying that our findings have happened as a result of chance; but if we want to be strictly technical about it, it is sampling error which originally allowed chance to get a foot in the door. We always use the small letter 'p' for probability, not a capital letter.

The symbol '$<$' means 'is less than'. If you forget which way round it should be, think in terms of reading across the page – it is small on the left, and then it opens out widely to the right. So the thing on the left, in this case p, is smaller than the thing on the right, which is the decimal fraction .01.

The decimal fraction gives the size of the probability. If you want to make sense of it, one of the best ways is to turn it back into an ordinary fraction. For example, .1 is one-tenth, or 1/10, and this means 'one out of ten'. Similarly, .05 can be written as 5/100, and this means 'five in a hundred', which works out the same as 'one in twenty'. In our example, .01 means 1/100, which means 'one in a hundred'.

Some people like to put a zero in front of the decimal fraction, but that isn't really accurate. It isn't necessary, either, because you can't have a probability higher than 1 anyway. A probability of 1 would mean that something happened every single time, and nothing can happen more often than that!

Taking all these together, then, we can now see that the statement

$$p < .01$$

means 'the probability of the null hypothesis being true is less than one in a hundred'. So it implies that we can be 99 per cent certain that the results did not come from sampling error, and that there really was a difference between our two scores. It doesn't automatically mean that our hypothesis was correct, because there might be a different explanation for that difference. But it does tell us that the difference is likely to be real.

Significance levels

The decimal fraction that we obtain from our research, then, tells us the likelihood of the null hypothesis being true, and that in turn tells us how much confidence we can have in our findings. That is why these measures of probability are sometimes called **confidence levels** – they are a precise measurement of the level, or degree, of confidence we can have in the results. More commonly, though, they are referred to as **significance levels**, because they tell us whether the differences or correlations that we have observed in our data are actually important or not.

There is no fixed significance level which all researchers use. It depends entirely on what we are researching, and how accurate we believe our measures are in detecting subtle differences. When we are conducting any research project – in just about every science, not just psychology – we need to decide what probability we will find acceptable. If we were investigating a completely new phenomenon, for example, we would need to set a fairly low significance level, because we wouldn't know if our measures were the best ones to use. So we would use a fairly low level, like $p < .05$, because that would give us a fair chance of detecting something if it was there.

If we were looking at something really controversial, though, we wouldn't think that $p < .05$ was rigorous enough. In medical studies, for example, researchers generally use much higher significance levels, because they don't want to take chances of getting a false positive result. The same applies in parapsychological studies: there is so much controversy in that area, that researchers don't usually find $p < .05$ to be adequate. They need to use a stricter confidence level instead. Table 14.3 shows some of the more common significance levels, and explains what they mean in ordinary words.

Table 14.3 Some common significance levels

$p < .05$	There is less than one chance in twenty that the null hypothesis is correct.
$p < .01$	There is less than one chance in a hundred that the null hypothesis is correct.
$p < .005$	There is less than one chance in two hundred that the null hypothesis is correct.
$p < .001$	There is less than one chance in a thousand that the null hypothesis is correct.
$p < .0001$	There is less than one chance in ten thousand that the null hypothesis is correct.

Type I and II errors

Setting your significance level too low, then, can lead you to a false positive result, where the null hypothesis is rejected when really it ought to have been retained. This is known as a **Type I error**, and it can have dramatic consequences. For example, if we were testing a new drug, and we set a low significance level, we could end up believing that the drug was really effective when it actually wasn't. Quite by chance, we could have obtained samples which seemed significantly different, but really came from the same population. If our research could lead to the marketing of that drug among the general population, then a false population like this could have dramatic effects.

Alternatively, if we set our significance level too high, we can end up with a result which appears negative, when it shouldn't be. This is a **Type II error**. Suppose we were looking to see if a particular pollutant – asbestos, for example – had an effect on a population living near to an asbestos factory. There would be a great many factors influencing how susceptible people were: factors to do with lifestyle, genetics, length of residence, and all sorts of other things. Even things like whether a family has a tradition of taking a walk in the country on Sundays can influence the development of emphysema. So the pollutant could be having quite a strong effect, but those effects could be hidden among lots of other factors. A research study which set the significance level too high could easily miss those effects, and end up with a Type II error, concluding that the pollutant hadn't had any effect when really it had.

Significance, then, is the basis for the probability judgements that we make about our data. In the next chapter, we will be looking at some of the ways that we can summarise our data sets using numbers – by finding typical scores, and scores which describe how 'spread out' the data are. These are useful in their own right, but they are also important when we come to make probability judgements about our research findings.

> **What do these three terms mean?**
>
> *Type I error*
>
> *Type II error*
>
> *significance level*

Self-assessment questions

1. *Outline the four main levels of measurement used by psychologists.*

2. *What is a plastic interval scale, and why does it matter?*

3. *What do we mean when we talk about the power of a test?*

4. *Distinguish between descriptive and inferential statistics.*

5. *What are the special properties of the normal distribution curve?*

Concepts in use

1. *Give a specific example of ordinal data arising in a psychological study. If you like, you can draw your examples from your knowledge of existing psychological research.*

2. Imagine you have just conducted a study of people's sleeping patterns. What level(s) of measurement would be involved in collecting data about preferred bedtimes and hours spent sleeping?

3. A psychologist conducts a study of music and revision habits among students, and announces that she can be 99 per cent certain that classical music enhances revision, but only 95 per cent certain that other types of music do so. How would you express this finding in formal symbolism?

4. How might the concept of standard scores be useful to a set of research psychologists studying popularity?

5. Describe a real-life situation in which you would prefer to make a Type II error with your data than a Type I error. Contrast this with a real-life situation in which you would prefer to make a Type I error, and explain why.

15

Numbers as descriptive statistics

Measures of central tendency
Measures of dispersion
z scores
Summary tables
Content analysis

When we undertake research which provides us with quantitative data, those data come to us as lists of numbers. We obtain numbers, or scores, each time one of the participants in our study completes a task we have asked them to do; and since quantitative studies usually involve quite a lot of participants, those numbers come to us as long lists. But long lists of numbers are not easy for anyone to understand. So the first analytical task that we have to carry out on our data is to convert those lists of numbers into a form which allows us to see – and to grasp – what we have found more easily. This is the purpose of descriptive statistics.

Descriptive statistics, as we saw in the last chapter, are statistics which allow us to describe our data. They don't draw conclusions about probability, or allow us to infer how typical those scores may be. Instead, they give us an image of the data, allowing us to collect our information and present it clearly. Sometimes that image takes the form of more numbers – ones which summarise the information that we have found. But sometimes descriptive statistics take the form of graphic images, showing in pictures what the data are like. We will look at numerical descriptive statistics in this chapter, and graphical descriptive statistics in the next.

Numerical descriptive statistics, then, are ways of summarising research findings by using numbers. There are three main types of numerical descriptive statistics. The first ones we will look at are known as **measures of central tendency**. These are single numbers which are typical of, or represent, the data that we have obtained. The second group are **measures of dispersion**, which are single numbers or pairs of numbers which express how spread out the scores are, and how similar they are to the measure of central tendency. And the third type of numerical descriptive statistic is perhaps the simplest of all: the **table of results**. We will look at it in the final section, even though it is the most straightforward, because tables of results usually involve measures of central tendency and dispersion, so it makes sense to know what these are first. Also, tables of results are a kind of half-way point between numerical statistics and pictorial images of the data, which is what we go on to look at in the next chapter.

Measures of central tendency

Measures of central tendency, as we have seen, are single scores which represent a whole set of data. There are three different measures of central tendency – the mean, the mode and the median – and which one we choose depends on the **level of measurement** of our data. We looked at levels of measurement in the last chapter, so look back at Table 14.2 for a quick reminder of the most important points. It may also help to remember that when it comes to statistical analysis, we tend to group equal-interval data and ratio data together, so anything which applies to equal-interval data is also the one to use if you have obtained ratio data from your study.

What do these three terms mean?
descriptive statistics
measures of central tendency
measures of dispersion

The mean

The first measure of central tendency is one which you are already likely to be familiar with: the arithmetic **average**, or **mean**. The mean, as you may have learned in school, is calculated by adding up all of the scores, and dividing the result by the number of scores that there are in the set. It's a reasonably straightforward procedure, but it gives us a good opportunity to begin to become a bit more familiar with some of the shorthand symbols which we use when we are doing statistics.

We need the shorthand because it would be very cumbersome to have to express everything in words all the time. For example, we use one symbol, the capital letter N, to stand for 'the number of scores there are in the set'. That means we don't have to write it out all of the time. We use another letter, the Greek capital letter sigma, which looks like this Σ to mean 'the sum of'. We use a single small letter x to refer to 'the scores' which we are dealing with. And we use the letter X with a bar across the top of it, $\bar{X}$ to refer to the mean.

The first thing you do when you want to work out a mean, then, is to count how many scores you have. This gives you N. Then you add up the scores, and doing that gives you Σx. Once you have obtained those two numbers, you calculate the mean by dividing the second number (Σx) by the first one (N). We can write that in shorthand by arranging it as a fraction, with the number which is doing the dividing on the bottom and the number that is being divided on the top.

All this means that, by using these symbols, we can describe the whole process much more quickly than we can in words, as shown in Formula 15.1. It may seem long-winded when you're only talking about calculating a mean, but it is a good idea to get used to using these symbols, because you will come across them quite often in the next few chapters. They can seem quite intimidating if you don't know what they mean; but once you do know them, they are really very straightforward.

Formula 15.1	**Calculating the mean**

$$\bar{X} = \frac{\Sigma x}{N}$$

Reminder
$\bar{X}$ = the mean
Σ = the sum of
x = the scores
N = the number of scores in the set

The median

As you can see, calculating a mean involves adding up and dividing numbers. So we can only use a mean as a measure of central tendency if we have equal-interval or ratio data. If we have ordinal or nominal data, we can't calculate a mean, because we couldn't add our scores up. For that reason, there are two other measures of central tendency: one which we can use when we have ordinal data, and one which we can use if we only have nominal data.

The measure of central tendency which we can use if we have ordinal data is known as the **median**. Put simply, this is the middlemost score of the data-set – the one which falls in the centre, if all of the scores are set in order. There isn't a generally agreed shorthand for the median – you will find that most of the statistical terms are only used with equal-interval or ratio data – but when they need a shorthand for it, most people follow Guilford (1956) by using **Mdn** – that is, a capital letter M with lower-case d and n.

The median is pretty straightforward to calculate, as long as you can rank your data properly. Worked Example 15.1 shows a good way of doing ranking. It is not particularly difficult: it is just a matter

Worked example 15.1　How to do ranking

Here is the basic data set we are working with:

5,6,11,12,14,13,7,8,9,9,8,9,15,14,12,14,6,10,9,8

There are 20 scores, so they will fill 20 ranks. There are always the same number of ranks as there are scores.

The easiest way of working out the ranks is to draw 20 pigeonholes labelled from 1 to 20. These are the available ranks.

1	2	3	4	5	6	7	8	9	10	11	12	13	14	15	16	17	18	19	20

The next step is to put the scores into the pigeonholes, in order from the lowest to the highest. Put each score in a pigeonhole, even if it is the same as another score:

1	2	3	4	5	6	7	8	9	10	11	12	13	14	15	16	17	18	19	20
5	6	6	7	8	8	8	9	9	9	9	10	11	12	12	13	14	14	14	15

Take the ranks which apply to the same-value scores, and average them. Leave the ranks that apply to single scores alone.

1	2.5		4		6			9.5				12	13	14.5		16		18		20
1	2	3	4	5	6	7	8	9	10	11	12	13	14	15	16	17	18	19	20
5	6	6	7	8	8	8	9	9	9	9	10	11	12	12	13	14	14	14	15

Now you can see clearly which rank belongs to each score:

1	2.5		4		6			9.5				12	13	14.5		16		18		20
5	6	6	7	8	8	8	9	9	9	9	10	11	12	12	13	14	14	14	15

of arranging the scores in order of size, and making sure that scores of the same size get the same ranking. The only slight complication in calculating a median comes when there is an even number of scores in the data set, so that there isn't a single figure in the middle. When that happens, we calculate the median by working out the figure which would be half-way between the two middlemost scores. We do this by adding those two scores, and dividing them by 2.

The mode

The **mode** is even more straightforward than the median. It is, quite simply, the most commonly occurring score in the data-set. Guilford

(1956) uses the shorthand **Mo** to refer to it. We can work out a mode simply by counting how many scores we have obtained in each category of our data, and seeing which of those totals is the highest. If you think about it, when you have purely nominal data, the mode is the only type of central tendency you could use, because all you know about the data is what the categories are, and how many examples you have in each. You can't calculate a median, because you can't rank the categories in order; and you can't calculate a mean because you can't add the categories together. So the mode is all that is left.

But that doesn't mean that we only ever use the mode for nominal data. We can use it with higher levels of measurement too. And sometimes, the information that it will give us is actually more useful than the mean or the median. For example: supposing you wanted to know what a typical salary in Britain was. You could work out the mean – the average salary. But the answer you would get would seem higher than it ought to be if it were really typical, because there are a few people who earn astronomical salaries, while most people earn much less. Adding up all of the scores would mean that those astronomical salaries were included too, and that would make the mean higher than we would expect of a 'typical' salary. In a situation like that, it would be more representative to use the mode, because that represents the type of salary that happens most often.

> **What do these three terms mean?**
>
> *mean*
>
> *mode*
>
> *data-set*

Skewed distributions

The example of salaries which I have just given is an example of a **skewed distribution**. In the last chapter, we looked at the normal distribution and some of its mathematical properties. Sometimes, we get a distribution which is nearly normal, but not quite, because it has a lot of scores at one end or the other. We refer to those distributions as 'skewed' because they are unbalanced: one end of the distribution is longer or more spread out than the other. A skewed distribution still has some predictable mathematical properties, so it is still useful for statistical analysis, but there are also noticeable differences.

One of the major differences concerns where the mean, mode and median fall in the distribution. In a normal distribution curve, the mean, mode and median all fall in the same place. The highest part of the curve is the mode, of course – it's higher because it has the most scores. But it is also the middlemost point – the median – and if we calculate the mean, that comes at that point too. But in a skewed distribution, the mean, mode and median are spread out.

If the tail of a skewed distribution is stretched out to the right, we say that it has a **positive skew**. In that case, the mode will still be at the highest point, of course, but the mean will be far off to the right, and the median will be in between the other two. If the tail of a skewed distribution is stretched out to the left, we say that it has a **negative skew**, and in this case the mean is over on the left while the mode is on the right. Figure 15.1 shows examples of central tendency in normal and in positively and negatively skewed distributions.

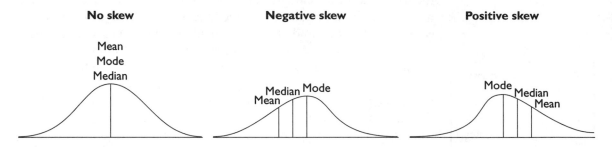

Figure 15.1 Central tendency in normal and skewed distributions

There are more examples of skewed distributions in human behaviour than you might think. For example, we might believe that something like the speed of serving a tennis ball would produce a normal distribution curve: some people would do it slowly, most would be average, while others would be pretty fast. But in fact, it's a skewed distribution, because there are some high-powered athletes who have trained themselves until they are able to hit tennis balls at speeds of well over 100 mph. The distribution has a positive skew. The same goes for kicking a football, and a great many other types of human behaviour.

A mean, as we have seen, wouldn't be typical of that data. So if we have a skewed distribution, we are often better off using the mode, instead of the mean. Any measure which can be used for a lower level of measurement can also be used for a higher one, so we can use a mode with equal-interval data, even though we can't use a mean with nominal data. And sometimes, it is a useful thing to do. So whenever we are choosing a measure of central tendency to describe our data, we need to make sure that it is appropriate for what we are actually studying, as well as being appropriate for the level of measurement that we have obtained.

Measures of dispersion

A measure of central tendency, as we have seen, allows us to identify the most 'typical' score in our data. But if we really want to describe what we have found, we need to get an idea of just how typical that measure of central tendency is. We do this by calculating a **measure of dispersion** – a number which tells us about how the scores are distributed, and whether most of them are very similar to our measure of central tendency, or not.

You can see this if you look at Figure 15.2, which gives an example of two normal distributions, each of which has exactly the same mean. One of them, though, involves scores which are all very close to the mean; while the other involves a much wider range of scores. Knowing the measure of central tendency tells us something, but it doesn't really describe the data fully – it can't tell us the difference between those two sets of scores, for example. To do that, we need another measure, which will tell us how much the scores vary – that is, how different they are from our measure of central tendency.

Figure 15.2 Normal distributions with the same means

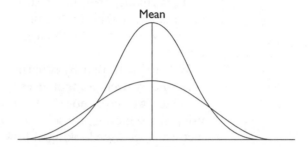

Standard deviation

Like measures of central tendency, some measures of dispersion are more suitable for some levels of measurement than others. The measure of dispersion which we use when we have equal-interval or ratio data is known as the **standard deviation**. The standard deviation can tell us a great deal about the shape of the normal distribution curve – in fact, if we know both the mean and the standard deviation, and we could draw accurately enough, we could draw the exact curve.

Figure 15.3 shows two normal distributions with the same means. This time, though, the standard deviations have been marked. In a normal distribution curve the first standard deviation occurs at the point where the curvature changes – which it switches from being a convex curve, coming down from the mean, to being a concave curve, reaching out towards the extreme ends of the deviation. So we always know exactly where on the curve the first standard deviation will be. Every other standard deviation is exactly the same distance away from its neighbour, and we also know about the proportions of the

Figure 15.3 Normal distributions with different standard deviations

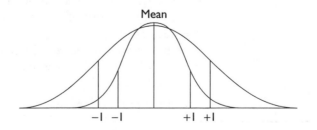

scores which are contained inside those standard deviations. So knowing the mean and the standard deviation tells us just about everything we need to know about any particular normal distribution curve.

When we are calculating a standard deviation, what we are really trying to do is to find a kind of average score which tells us how different our scores are from the mean. So we begin by subtracting each of our scores from the mean for the whole set of scores. This gives us d, which stands for 'the difference from the mean'. The problem, though, is that some of these differences will be positive (when the score is smaller than the mean), and some will be negative (when the score is larger than the mean). If we add them together, it will come out all wrong, because the negative scores will cancel out the positive ones.

We deal with that by squaring each of the scores – by multiplying each one by itself. So that gives us a whole list of scores, which we call d^2. Once we have those, we can add them up, and we describe this using the symbol Σ for adding up a whole list of numbers, which we met when we were looking at how to calculate the mean. This gives us Σd^2. What we want to do then is to average it – divide it by the number of scores there are, which you may remember is always called N.

Now, we need to remember how we dealt with the difference scores by squaring them. That made the whole sum larger than it should be, so we need to correct that. We do that by taking the square root of the answer, which brings everything back to its proper proportions.

Formula 15.2 shows the whole procedure in mathematical language. Really, it only describes what we have just looked at in words, and what it gives us is the basic formula for calculating a standard devia-

> **What do these three terms mean?**
>
> *median*
>
> *skewed distribution*
>
> *standard deviation*

Formula 15.2

The standard deviation
The standard deviation for the population as a whole looks like this:

$$\sigma = \sqrt{\frac{\Sigma d^2}{N}}$$

Reminder
σ = the standard deviation of the whole population
$\sqrt{\ }$ = the square root of
Σ = the sum of
d = the difference between each score and the mean
d^2 = the difference between each score and the mean, multiplied by itself (squared)
N = the number of scores in the set

tion from a set of scores which cover the whole population. The symbol σ (little sigma) means the standard deviation of a whole population, so it assumes that the set of scores we have used is complete, reflecting all of the population.

In practice, though, when we have carried out a research study, our scores don't cover the whole population. They are just a sample of it, and might not be exactly representative. So we use a different symbol, s, to refer to the standard deviation; and we correct the formula just a little bit, by using $N-1$ instead of N. The new version of the formula, shown as Formula 15.3, is an estimate of the standard deviation of the population as a whole, based on a sample rather than a complete collection.

Formula 15.3

Versions of the standard deviation
The usual formula looks like this:

$$s = \sqrt{\frac{\Sigma d^2}{N-1}}$$

Sometimes you may find that the formula which other textbooks give for the standard deviation looks different from the one we have just used. It might look like this:

$$s = \sqrt{\frac{\Sigma(x - \bar{x})^2}{N-1}}$$

Although the two formulas look different, they are actually exactly the same. It's just that instead of using d as a shorthand, the second version tells you exactly how d should be calculated.

The bracket around $(x - \bar{x})$ means 'do this first'. So what it means is: begin by taking the mean ($\bar{x}$) away from each score (x). Which is exactly what we did when we calculated d. So $(x - \bar{x})$ is just another way of writing d.

Reminder
s = the standard deviation
$\sqrt{}$ = the square root of
Σ = the sum of
x = each score
$\bar{x}$ = the mean
$(\;)^2$ = what is in the bracket multiplied by itself (squared)
N = the number of scores in the set

Formula 15.3 also contains another important message, which is all to do with not being frightened by strange symbols. Each symbol is just a shorthand. It isn't anything mysterious or magical – it's just a quicker way of saying something. Don't panic when you see these symbols: just look at the reminder list to see what each one means and tackle the formula a little bit at a time, doing the brackets first. If you approach it that way, you'll soon find that you can deal with quite complicated formulas without getting lost or muddled. There are small reminder lists in each of the chapters dealing with formulas, which will tell you the important things you need to remember.

The variance

There is a simpler measure of dispersion which we can use for equal-interval data, known as the **variance**. This is a figure which also tells us how much the scores are spread out around the mean, but it doesn't have the same mathematical properties as the standard deviation, so we usually prefer to use the standard deviation instead. You may sometimes come across references to the variance of a measure, though, so it's as well to know what it is. Also, we will be coming back to it again in Chapter 19.

In fact, we have already looked at how to calculate a variance. We use the symbol s^2 to describe it, and the formula is given in figure 15.8. If you look closely at Formula 15.4, you'll see that it is exactly the same as the formula for the standard deviation, except that we don't take the square root. So the variance is the square of the standard deviation, which is why we call it s^2. And, in the same way as we do when working out the standard deviation, if our scores represent just our sample data, we use N on the bottom line of the fraction, but if we want to calculate a variance which is based on a sample, but estimate what it would be for the whole population, we use $N - 1$.

Formula 15.4   **Calculating a variance**

$$s^2 = \sum \frac{d^2}{N-1}$$

Reminder
s^2 = variance
$\sum$ = the sum of
d^2 = the squared difference between each score and the mean
N = the number of scores in the set

z scores

We can use standard deviations to calculate standard scores which are known as **z scores**. A *z* score simply tells us how many standard deviations above or below the mean a particular score is. For example, in a set of scores with a mean of 30 and a standard deviation of 5, a score of 35 would be one standard deviation above the mean. So it would have a *z* score of +1. A score of 25, on the other hand, would be one standard deviation below the mean. So it would have a *z* score of −1.

Z scores are really very easy to calculate, as long as you know the mean and standard deviation. You could do it by drawing the distribution, and counting how many standard deviations away from the mean your particular score is. But it is actually easier to do it mathematically. You begin by finding the difference between the score you are interested in, and the mean, by subtracting the mean from the score. If your score is higher than the mean, this will give you a positive number, and if it is lower, it will give you a negative number. Then you divide that number by the standard deviation. Formula 15.5 shows all that in mathematical shorthand.

Formula 15.5	**Calculating a z score**

$$z = \frac{(x - \bar{x})}{s}$$

Reminder
z = the z score
x = the original score
$\bar{x}$ = the mean
s = the standard deviation

Z scores are useful when we need to compare results which have been obtained using different measures. For example, we might want to compare how well someone does on a computer aptitude test with how good they are at maths. Just knowing the scores doesn't help. For example, suppose that Janet gained 75 per cent in a computer aptitude test and 73 per cent in a maths test. Those scores look pretty similar. But if we learn that the mean score in the computer aptitude test is 70 per cent with a standard deviation of 5, while the mean score in the maths test is 80 per cent with a standard deviation of 7, they begin to look very different. In one case, Janet has scored above the mean, but in the other, she has scored below. She has a *z* score of +1 for the computer aptitude test, but a *z* score of −1 for the maths test.

Suppose Janet then took a third test, about understanding statistical concepts. This one was marked out of 40, and she gained a score of 33. Again, we couldn't tell just from the scores what that would really mean. But if we know that the mean for this test is 28, and the standard deviation is 5, we are in a better position to interpret her results. By working it out, we find that she has a z score of +1 for the statistical test. Janet, being a practical sort of person, has obtained just about the same result for computer aptitude and for statistical understanding, and those results are noticeably higher than the results she obtained for maths. The z scores show us the similarities, even though the actual scores are very different.

Parametric statistics

The standard deviation and the z score both assume that the data have come from a population which follows a normal distribution. As we have seen, the normal distribution curve has mathematical properties which allow us to draw a number of conclusions about our data. We couldn't draw those conclusions if the data were from a population with a different distribution. So we can only really use these particular statistics if we have reason to believe that the data fall within the parameters of a normal distribution curve. For this reason, they are known as **parametric statistics**.

In Chapter 17, we will be looking at statistical tests used for comparing two different groups of scores. You will find that there are different types of tests to do similar tasks: parametric tests and non-parametric ones. The parametric versions are more powerful, because they can make more assumptions about their data. But the non-parametric tests are the ones we have to use if we can't assume that our data comes from a normally distributed population, or if our data have been measured using an ordinal scale.

The range

If we have ordinal data, we can't calculate standard deviations or z scores, and we have to use a different measure of dispersion. All we can do with ordinal data, you may recall, is to rank it, setting it in order from smallest to largest, or along some other continuum like least preferred to most preferred. The measure of central tendency for this type of data is the median, which is the middlemost point. So the measure of dispersion needs to be something which expresses how spread out the scores are, around that middlemost point.

In fact, there are several measures of dispersion we can use for ordinal data. The most basic one is the **range**, which is, quite simply, the spread of the scores from the highest to the lowest. We calculate a range simply by subtracting the lowest score from the highest one. Subtractions usually assume that we have equal-interval data, but this one is permissible because we don't then perform any mathematical operations on the number which we get as a result.

For example, if we performed a study in which people were asked to rate photographs for degree of attractiveness, by giving them marks out of 10, we clearly couldn't pretend that we had equal-interval data. Our data would be ordinal, because the points on the scale are subjective, and all we would really know was that a photo which received a score of 6 had been rated more highly than one which received a score of 4. But it would be OK to describe the range of scores – to say 'the median score for this group of photos was 6.5, and the range was 4', because that would let us know what the highest and lowest scores were without assuming that the data were equal-interval.

The problem with the range is that it is easily distorted by a single extreme score. Suppose there was a photo which almost everyone in the study rated as attractive, giving it ratings of 9 or 8. However, one person gave it the lowest rating, of 1, because the photo reminded them of someone they really didn't like. That could mean that the range of scores for that photo extended to 8, when in fact all of the scores except one fell within a range of 2 or 3. We saw earlier how a mean score can become distorted by a few extremely high or low values. A range can become distorted in the same way.

The interquartile range

The way that we deal with that problem is to use the **interquartile range** instead. Quartiles are the points which separate the four quarters of the set of scores, and the interquartile range is calculated by cutting off the top and bottom quarters. The first quartile comes after the first quarter, or 25 per cent, of the scores. It is the point which marks the boundary between this quarter and the next, in the same way that the median marks the half-way boundary. The second quartile is the median – the point which separates two quarters of the scores from the other two quarters. The third quartile comes after the next quarter of the scores, marking the three-quarters point. Worked Example 15.2 shows a set of scores which have been arranged in order, and the interquartile points marked.

When we are calculating the interquartile range, we begin by ranking all the scores in order, and calculating the median. The median marks the dividing point, so that we can separate the scores into two sets: half below and half above the median. Then we divide each half into two sets, in exactly the same way – by finding the half-way point between the end score and the median. The interquartile range

What do these three terms mean?

equal-interval data

standard scores

z scores

Worked example 15.2   Quartiles in a data set

If we use the same data set that we used for ranking in Worked Example 15.1:

$$5,6,11,12,14,13,7,8,9,9,8,9,15,14,12,14,6,10,9,8$$

The first step is to arrange the scores in order of size

$$5,6,6,7,8,8,8,9,9,9,9,10,11,12,12,13,14,14,14,15$$

The next step is to find the mid-point of the scores (the median). With 20 scores, it will lie between the 10th and 11th score.

$$5,6,6,7,8,8,8,9,9,9 \quad (\text{mid-point}) \quad 9,10,11,12,12,13,14,14,14,15$$

To find the quartile points, we find the mid-point of each of the two halves. This has divided the data set into quarters, and shown us where the quartiles are.

$$5,6,6,7,8 \quad (Q_1) \quad 8,8,9,9,9 \quad (Q_2) \quad 9,10,11,12,12 \quad (Q_3) \quad 13,14,14,14,15$$

is the middle 50 per cent of the scores, from the first quartile to the third.

The semi-interquartile range

I mentioned earlier that the standard deviation is a parametric statistic – that it should really only be used when we can assume that our scores have come from a normal distribution. That leaves us with the question of what kind of measure of dispersion we should use if we don't feel that we can make that assumption. The one which is most similar to the standard deviation without making all those assumptions about the data is known as the **semi-interquartile range**.

The semi-interquartile range has an imposing name, but it is actually pretty straightforward to calculate. It is, as its name suggests, exactly half of the interquartile range. So we work it out by first calculating the interquartile range, in the same way as in the last section; and then by dividing that in half. The symbol that we generally use to refer to the semi-interquartile range is Q, and the formula for calculating it is given in Formula 15.6.

We can use the semi-interquartile range in much the same way as we use a standard deviation. Figure 15.4 shows how the semi-interquartile range fits as a measure of dispersion in a skewed distribution. It isn't the same as a standard deviation, as we can see, but it can serve much the same sort of purpose, in giving us a reasonably straightforward description of our scores which isn't badly distorted by a few extremes.

What do these three terms mean?

semi-interquartile range

variation ratio

normal distribution

Formula 15.6 **Calculating the semi-interquartile range**

$$Q = \frac{Q_3 - Q_1}{2}$$

In other words, we subtract the first quartile from the third quartile, and divide the result by 2.

Reminder
Q = the semi-interquartile range
Q_3 = the third quartile
Q_1 = the first quartile

Figure 15.4 The semi-interquartile range in a distribution

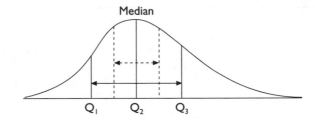

The variation ratio

The final measure of dispersion that we will look at is known as the **variation ratio**. This is the measure of dispersion that we use if we have nominal data, which can't be fitted into conventional calculations, and can't even be ranked. Nominal data usually take the form of categories, such as colours, character traits, types of animal, and so on. As we saw earlier, the only practical measure of central tendency for this type of data is the mode. The mode tells us the most commonly occurring score, or category, and it also tells us how many of the scores are in that category.

The variation ratio supplements that information by telling us what proportion of the scores are not modal – in other words, the ratio of scores in the 'mode' category to scores which are in other categories. (Incidentally, it is *very* important not to confuse the variation ratio with a different statistical test, the F test, which is sometimes referred to as the variance-ratio test. We will be coming back to the F test in Chapter 19.)

The way that we calculate the variation ratio is by adding up the number of scores which are not modal, and dividing them by the total number of scores. This gives us a decimal fraction as an answer, something like 0.6 or 0.3; and the size of that decimal fraction will tell us how much variation there is among the scores. Formula 15.7 shows this expressed in symbols.

Formula 15.7

Calculating the variation ratio

$$Variation\ ratio = \frac{\sum non\text{-}modal\ scores}{N}$$

Reminder

$\sum$ = the sum of

N = the number of scores in the set

If the variation ratio is large – close to one – then we can tell that most of the scores are not modal, so even though the mode is the largest category, it doesn't contain most of the scores. If the variation ratio is less than 0.5, it tells us that most of the scores are in the modal category, and that it is only a minority which are in the other categories. So the variation ratio is a very good way of telling us just how typical our mode is, if we have nominal data.

We have seen, then, how different measures of central tendency and different measures of dispersion do different tasks. We need to choose the measure which suits our data best, and which will tell us the information that we need to know. When we are deciding which measures to use, we have to take into account the level of measurement, and also the job that the measure is expected to do for us.

Summary tables

Summary tables are used in almost all kinds of quantitative research. They are ways of summarising more than one set of data, so that the similarities and differences produced by variables or factors can be seen as easily as possible. Summary tables often use measures of central tendency (generally the mean) and measures of dispersion (often the standard deviation, but sometimes the semi-interquartile range, depending on the data).

The convention used for summary tables in research papers is to list the variables of the study along the left-hand side, so that they form the rows of the table, and the statistical measures along the top,

What do these three terms mean?
summary table
categorisation
non-modal score

so that they form the columns. The combination of rows and columns gives us a series of **cells**, and it is these which contain the information about the data. For example, if we were drawing up a table which reported a study of two different methods of teaching children to read, we could have the two teaching methods as the rows of the table, and the mean scores and standard deviations obtained from our test results at the top (Figure 15.5). Reading along a row would tell us how a single method scored; reading down the 'mean' column would tell us whether the means of the two groups were very different; and reading down the 'standard deviation' column would let us compare the standard deviations, to see if they were very different too.

Figure 15.5 A summary table

Methods of teaching reading: results from a reading accuracy test

	Mean	Standard deviation	N
Method A	15.3	3.7	106
Method B	16.2	4.1	120

The great advantage of summary tables is that we can use them to summarise absolutely huge amounts of data, because there is no limit to the number of rows or columns we can use, and because a single cell in the table can sum up a very large number of scores. But there is, of course, a limit to how much information a human being can grasp at one time, so unless there is a very good reason for it, it is a good idea to limit the number of rows and columns to a small number. It makes them much easier to read.

Content analysis and summary tables

Content analysis is a way of using summary tables to describe qualitative data – that is, data which don't appear in the form of numbers but as words or other kinds of meaningful information – in a quantitative form. But content analysis isn't qualitative analysis, even though it is used with qualitative data. Instead, it is a way of converting that data into quantitative information – of describing it using numbers.

There are many types of data which are suitable for content analysis. It could be used in a study of the use of children in television advertisements; or in an interview study investigating people's experiences of parenthood. It could be used to identify recurrent themes in a series of paintings at an exhibition, or to analyse the content of children's reading books, or to look at reports of football hooliganism in the

EXERCISE 15.1   **Central tendency and dispersion**

A consumer psychologist is planning a diary study to look at how often people visit supermarkets. From a pilot study of 20 research participants, she has obtained the following data:

Participant	Visits
1	8
2	17
3	16
4	9
5	6
6	8
7	22
8	15
9	16
10	36
11	8
12	6
13	13
14	38
15	8
16	8
17	40
18	12
19	11
20	8

(a) Work out the mean, median and mode for these scores, and write them in the table below:

Mean	
Median	
Mode	

(b) Which measure of central tendency do you think would be most suitable to use to describe these data? Why?

(c) Is this distribution positively or negatively skewed? What possible reasons can you think of for why this skew has occurred?

media, or to make sense of observational studies of children's playground behaviour. In other words, it can be used for all sorts of different types of information, and psychologists have often used it as a way of making some sense out of complex topics.

The essence of content analysis is **categorisation**. A content analysis describes a set of data in terms of a set of categories, and how many examples have been counted in each category. Effectively, content analysis consists of setting up a series of categories and counting up how many examples of each category can be identified in the data. That information is then usually presented as a summary table, with the categories forming the columns, and the set of data forming the rows. The numbers which appear in the cells of the table are the **frequencies** – the result of counting up how often that category occurs in the data set.

What content analysis does, then, is to turn qualitative information into quantitative data, by converting it into numbers. In doing to, it describes the information, which is why it is included in this chapter on descriptive statistics. But it also opens the way for a researcher to perform additional statistical tests on the material, if that seems appropriate. The most commonly used one is chi-square, because a content analysis gives us nominal data. We will be looking at the chi-square test in Chapter 17.

EXERCISE 15.2	Conducting a content analysis

Conduct a content analysis on the following passage. Begin by identifying some suitable categories, such as 'success', or 'physical actions', and then count how often these categories come up during the course of the passage.

When you have completed the analysis, draw up a summary table of your findings.

'So it was a mess', thought Frieda. 'Well, the whole thing is completely out of my hands. There's absolutely nothing I can do about it now, and worrying won't help.' She climbed down from the platform, and moved into the darkness at the side of the hall. A smattering of polite applause followed her, but she sensed that the audience had already forgotten. They were waiting for the main event. The applause quickly subsided into a hum of expectant voices. Suddenly, the curtains twitched, and out leaped the maestro. He twirled his cape and his cane, pirouetting about the small podium like a whirling dervish. The audience clapped and roared approval in a deafening explosion of sound. 'Such showmanship', Frieda marvelled. 'That's what it's all about.'

The problem, of course, is that whenever we do a content analysis, it is important to be sure that the categories we have chosen are appropriate ones for our data. That generally means that we need to spend a lot of time examining the data and our research interests, so that we can be sure that the categories reflect what we are interested in. But if the data are very complex and meaningful – like pictures in an art exhibition, for example – using content analysis always means that we lose a great deal of the information. We need to do a proper qualitative analysis if we want to retain any of that richness in the data. Content analysis isn't a substitute for qualitative analysis, but it does give us a general, if rather simplistic, way to look at qualitative information.

We have seen, then, that we can summarise quantitative data in quite a few different ways. We can provide measures of central tendency and dispersion for just about any kind of data; and we can summarise our findings in tables of results and using content analyses. But we can also summarise our data by converting them into pictures or images, and this is what we will look at in the next chapter.

Self-assessment questions

1. *Which measures of central tendency and measures of dispersion are best suited to describe ratio data?*

2. *Why is it often better to use a mode as the measure of central tendency to describe a skewed distribution?*

3. *Why do parametric statistics have that particular name?*

4. *What does a z score describe?*

5. *In what sense can content analysis be described as both qualitative and quantitative?*

Concepts in use

1. *Imagine that you are an interior decorator collecting information about people's colour preferences. You have collected your data by asking people to mark different colour combinations on a scale of 1 to 10. What would be the best measure of central tendency and measure of dispersion to describe your data, and why?*

2. *How might the concept of z scores be useful to a group of research psychologists studying how people of different ages match up to age-related standards of physical abilities?*

3. *A sports psychologist is collecting information about how quickly athletes respond to the starting pistol. What level of measurement is this, and what descriptive statistics would be useful to describe it?*

4. *From your knowledge of existing psychological research, give a specific example of a mean or pair of mean scores in a study.*

5. *Imagine that you have carried out a study of the popularity of different brands of sports clothing. What type of summary table might you use to describe the data you have obtained?*

16

Descriptive statistics in visual images

Graphs
Bar charts
Pie charts
Scattergrams
Other graphical representations

In the last chapter, we looked at how we can use numbers to describe our results. But numbers always need to be interpreted, no matter how clearly they are presented. Even tables of results require us to read through the numbers, and to work out what they mean. Sometimes it is much quicker to convert the information into a picture instead. Graphical representations do much the same job when we are trying to understand numerical data as metaphors do when we are trying to understand complex verbal ideas. By converting the information into an image – either a verbal image or a picture – we are able to make comparisons with things we already know, and so grasp important features of the information more quickly.

There are a number of different forms of graphical representation; and, as with measures of central tendency and dispersion, which one we choose depends entirely on what kind of information we have and what we want to use it for. Sometimes we are looking at how a single measure varies or fluctuates over time, or in response to a single changing variable, and for that we would use a **graph**. Sometimes our data are arranged in categories, and what we want is an image which will tell us, quickly, how many scores we have in each category. For that, we would use some kind of **bar chart**. Sometimes we are interested in proportions, or shares, and we want to use a graphical representation which will tell us what sort of share of the whole is formed by each type of score; we would use a **pie chart** to look at these. And there are other types of graphical representation, too, which psychological researchers use in their research reports, and which we will look at in this chapter.

What do these three terms mean?

graphical representations

continuous variable

descriptive statistics

Graphs

Graphs are one of the most well-known ways of describing data as a kind of picture. We use a graph to show how a particular measure varies in response to some other continuous variable. That sounds complicated, but really it isn't all that difficult. You are probably familiar with the kind of graph which medical people use to record temperature. This type of graph has a horizontal dimension, or axis, stretching along the bottom, and a vertical axis stretching upwards. The actual measurements of temperature are recorded in the form of a continuous line, which goes upwards, downwards, or straight along the area in between the two axes. That line really consists of several separate points joined together; and each point represents the person's temperature at a particular time.

Figure 16.1 shows the temperature graph of a normal human being taken over a period of 24 hours. We could simply make a list of the temperature measurements; but presenting it as a graph, like this, allows us to see some interesting patterns in the data. For example, it shows very clearly how the body's temperature is lower during the small hours of the morning, how it rises as the person wakes up, and how it dips again in the early afternoon – the siesta time for many human societies. The graph shows the pattern clearly, but it would be much harder – not impossible, but much harder – to identify this type of information just from looking at lists of numbers.

Figure 16.1 A temperature graph

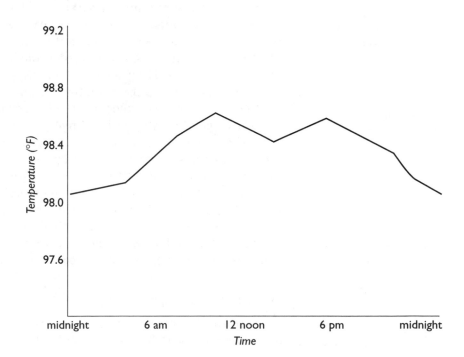

Axes and co-ordinates

The line along the bottom of the graph is known as the *x* **axis**. In a standard temperature graph, it represents time, so the various points along it are the times when the person's temperature was taken. The line up the side of the graph is known as the *y* **axis**. This represents the temperature itself – higher levels describe higher temperatures, while lower levels represent lower temperatures. So the lower down the line is on the graph, the lower the temperature is.

Every point on a graph has a set of **co-ordinates**, and these are the numbers which indicate whereabouts on the graph the point should be drawn. We indicate co-ordinates by putting them inside a bracket, and putting the *x* value first, followed by the *y* value. They are also usually written in italics. So the co-ordinates of a temperature reading of 98.5 taken at 4.30 p.m. would be shown as (1630, 98.5). The 1630 represents the time, which is the *x* co-ordinate, and tells you how far along the graph that point should be drawn; and the 98.5 indicates the temperature, which is the *y* co-ordinate and tells you how high up that point should be. Once you know the two co-ordinates, you can enter the point on the graph.

Calibration

Whenever we are drawing up a graph, or any similar type of descriptive statistic, we need to think very carefully about the way that we will portray our measurements. In particular, that means thinking about the *x* and *y* axes of the graph, and the measurement intervals that they will show. In our temperature graph, for example, it would have been pointless to show the *y* axis with zero at the bottom, and going up by one-degree intervals. The changes in body temperature are so small that they wouldn't show up if we did that. In the same way, we wouldn't want to have measuring intervals which were so large that they completely exaggerated every little change (Figure 16.2).

Drawing up a graph, then, involves exercising judgement to choose a set of intervals which will show up any patterns there are in the data, but which will also let us see those patterns in perspective. This process is sometimes known as **calibration**, because it is similar to the way that measuring instruments are adjusted to make sure that they are measuring correctly. It isn't exactly the same, but we use the word as a kind of metaphor, which helps us to describe what we are doing when we select an appropriate range of intervals for a scale.

When to use a graph

If we are going to use a graph to describe our data, it is important that the data are of the right kind. A graph takes the form of a continuous

---

What do these three terms mean?

x *axis*

y *axis*

co-ordinates

Figure 16.2 Calibrating
the *y* axis

A graph with the y axis range too high

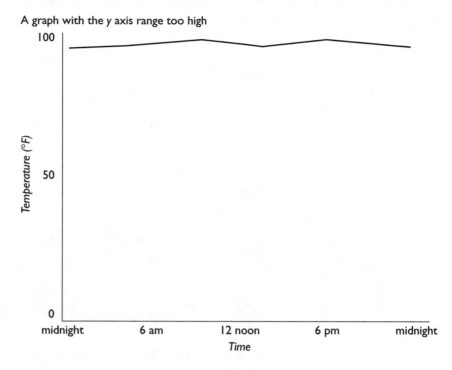

A graph with the y axis range too low

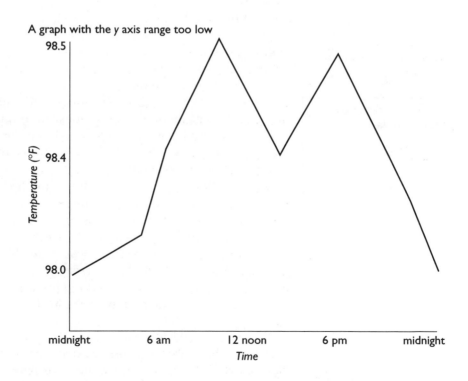

Figure 16.3
Measurement points
on a graph

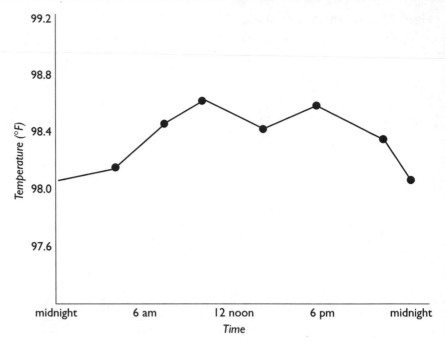

line, which joins up different points (Figure 16.3). The points represent
observations – measures taken at a particular time, or from a particular
population. Each observation is one separate item of data in a data-
set. But the fact that two observations have been joined by a line makes
an assumption. It assumes that there has been a relatively smooth and
continuous change between those observations. The line indicates the
measurement we would have obtained if we had taken a third observation, in between the two.

    You can see from this that we should only use a graph if we
can assume that there is a continuous variation between the different
observations we have made. We know that temperature is a continuous variable: it can't stop in between measures, so it is reasonable
to connect one measure and the next with a line. But if we had done
an investigation of private study hours on different days of the week,
we couldn't make any such assumption. We could indicate a point
for Monday, and a point for Tuesday; but it would be silly to join
those points with a line, because there isn't a half-way point between
them. Suppose that our average measure for Monday was three hours,
and our average measure for Tuesday was two hours. Drawing a line
between those observations would imply that we were likely to study
for two-and-a-half hours in between Monday and Tuesday, and that
is clearly nonsense.

    When we are deciding whether to use a graph, or some other measure
like a bar chart, then, we need to take into account the nature of the
data, as well as what we are wanting to illustrate. Graphs are useful

**What do these three
terms mean?**

calibration

scaling

standard scores

Hiding theory in graphs

Sometimes researchers use a graph instead of a bar chart to make a theoretical statement – to say things about the data which aren't really in the numbers, but which they believe to be true. Perhaps the best example of this is in the way that levels of processing experiments are sometimes portrayed. These are studies which ask people to deal with information in different ways: by simply looking at it and describing what it looks like (visual condition); by looking at it and saying what it sounds like (auditory condition), or by looking at it and thinking about its meaning (semantic condition). When those people are asked to remember the information afterwards, they remember least from the visual condition, more from the auditory condition, and most from the semantic condition.

Figure 16.4 Hidden theory in graphical images

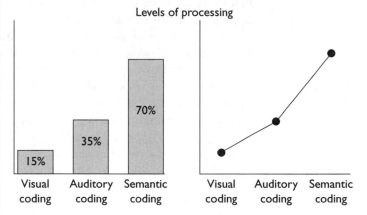

There are three conditions in the study, so the logical way to portray the data is to present them as a bar chart, indicating the amount remembered from each condition. But some psychology textbooks present it as a graph instead (Figure 16.4). The reason for this is to do with the theoretical explanation for the findings. Craik and Lockhart, who introduced this theory, suggested that the three conditions represented different levels for processing information – different amounts of mental 'work'. The semantic condition was a deeper level than the auditory one, and that in turn was deeper than the visual one. If the conditions represent different levels, then there are going to be points in between – different degrees of depth. So illustrating those findings by using a graph is actually illustrating the theory, not the findings.

Whenever you see a graph, therefore, it is as well to ask yourself whether it is really illustrating a continuous variable. If the researchers appear to have used a graph when a bar chart seems more appropriate, try to find a reason why they have done that. It can sometimes tell you some important things about the assumptions they are making about their data – and there may be times when you don't wish to go along with those assumptions. Becoming aware of them is the first step.

to illustrate continuous variables and how they change, over time or in respect to each other; but we can only use them accurately if both our x axis and our y axis are continuous variables too. If we have categories instead, we need to use a different type of graphical representation; and the most popular of these is a bar chart.

Bar charts

A bar chart, in some ways, is the simplest of all types of graphical representation. We use bar charts when we have data which belong to different categories, and we want to compare how many times, or how often, each category is represented in our set of scores. So the first thing we need to do when working out a bar chart is to establish exactly what our categories are.

That is simple enough if our data fall naturally into categories. For example, if we were looking at how many hours students spend in private study on different days of the week, we would naturally have seven categories – Monday, Tuesday, Wednesday, Thursday, Friday, Saturday and Sunday. Because the days of the week represent a nominal measuring scale, the categories are very straightforward. And we would have the same N for each category – the same number of students, because each one we asked would have told us about each day of the week, so our data would simply be the number of hours of reported study on each of those days. We would show that by the height of the bars on the chart – the more hours, the higher the bar (Figure 16.5).

Figure 16.5   A bar chart

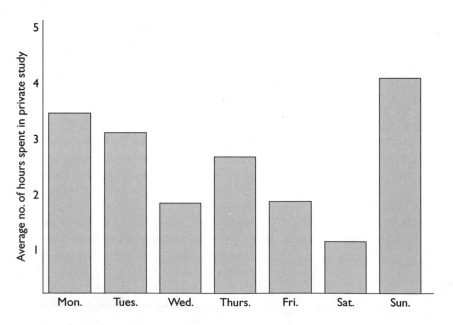

Sometimes, though, the categories of data are not so clear. If we were looking to see whether older students spent more hours in study than younger students, for example, we would have a ratio scale, representing the age of the students concerned. But we still might want to summarise our results using a bar chart – remember that we can use statistics suitable for lower levels of measurement with higher levels as well. In that case, we would need to decide on the categories in our chart – perhaps by dividing the ages of students into five- or ten-year groups.

The problem then would be that we would be likely to end up with a different N in each category. The odds are, for example, that we would have more students in the younger categories than in the older ones. So if we just counted up the number of hours reported by each group, it would seem as though younger students spent far more hours studying, when really it would just mean that we had more of them. So to get a bar chart of our data which actually told us what we wanted to know, we would need to **scale** our data for each category, so that it would give us a standard score which we could use to compare one category with another (we looked at this idea in Chapter 14). In this example, we would probably do it by converting the information into mean scores first. That way it wouldn't matter so much how many people we had in each group, because the mean score takes that into account beforehand.

The calibration of a bar chart is just as important as it is for a graph. For example, imagine that we were doing a study which was investi-

Figure 16.6 Calibrating a bar chart

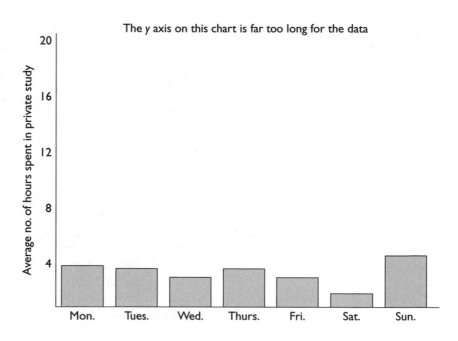

gating gender differences in general knowledge, by asking men and women 100 general knowledge questions. We would find differences between the two groups, since no two groups of people are exactly alike. But the way that we presented our findings on a bar chart could make those differences seem much more important than they really were. Figures 16.5 and 16.6 show two ways of presenting the same set of findings. One of them seems to suggest that the differences are very large, while the other implies that they are not particularly big at all. The calibration of the y axis of the bar chart makes all the difference.

Types of bar chart

The two diagrams I have given show vertical bars going upwards in the bar chart; but that doesn't have to be the case. It is quite common to find bar charts which present their bars horizontally, or even going up and down across a central line. The bars don't actually need to be bars, either. If you watch news programmes or financial programmes, you often see bar charts which are composed of sets of different images, such as human figures or currency signs (Figure 16.7). They are still bar charts, and still convey the same information, but the designers have decided that they need to be presented a little more attractively if people are going to take notice of them. Or they might have decided that presenting them in elaborate and pretty ways will distract us from noticing the main information – who knows?

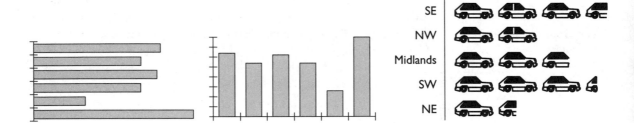

Figure 16.7 Types of bar chart

Bar charts can be very useful for different types of data. We can even draw up three-dimensional bar charts, when we have more than two variables that we want to describe. The height of the bars still represents the amount of the main variable – the one that we are really interested in – but we can represent two other variables on the other two dimensions. In a three-dimensional diagram, whether it is a graph or a bar chart, the x axis is still the one which stretches from left to right; and the y axis is still the vertical one, which stretches upwards. The third dimension, which stretches away from the observer, is known as the **z axis**. So the overall co-ordinates of an observation, on a three-dimensional chart, have three dimensions: x, y and z. We need

Figure 16.8 A three-dimensional bar chart

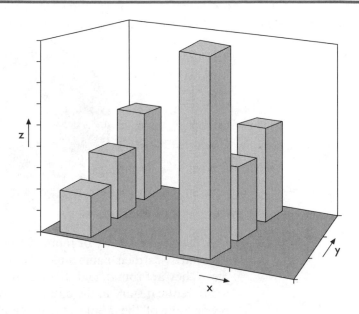

all three bits of information before we can draw the bar on the chart correctly (Figure 16.8).

You may occasionally hear bar charts referred to as **histograms**. That will sometimes be correct, but the term is often used wrongly. A histogram is indeed a bar chart; but a bar chart is not always a histogram. It is only a histogram if the proportions of the bars correspond exactly to the proportions of the scores that they are representing. So the area of the bar needs to be in exact ratio to the amount of the scores which the bar is representing. This means that a histogram needs to be very carefully measured, and has to be drawn up very precisely. Most of the bar charts used to report psychological research, though, don't need to be that exact. We tend to use other forms of analysis to give us exactitude, and just use graphical representations to give an overall image of the data rather than a precise measurement.

What do these three terms mean?

graph

bar chart

histogram

Pie charts

A bar chart is a way of representing scores obtained from different categories – of research participants, of experimental conditions, or of some other variable. We can use them to illustrate all of the scores that we have obtained, or just the scores of selected groups. But bar charts only tell us about size – which group has scored more than another group. What they don't tell us is proportion – that is, what share of the total is represented by any particular group or category. If we want to know about proportions of a whole set of scores, we need to use a **pie chart**.

Figure 16.9   A pie chart

% of courses run by a further education college

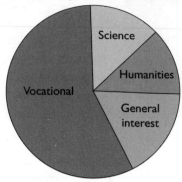

A pie chart is a way of representing a complete set of information. Pie charts, as their name suggests, are charts which look rather like pies. They are round, and divided up into slices. Each slice represents a different category in the data, and the size of each slice tells us what proportion of the whole that category takes up. A category which represents a quarter of the scores would have a slice which represented a quarter of the whole circle. A category which included two-fifths of the scores would have a slice which represented two-fifths of the circle. And so on (Figure 16.9).

Pie charts can be used with nominal data, but they can be used with ordinal or interval data too, because we can always reduce that to categories if we want to. But we do need to know the whole set of information that we are trying to represent. For example, if we wanted to describe a student population in a particular university, we could only draw up a pie chart if we had the complete set of data, and knew the proportion of the student population in the different schools or faculties. If we only had the information about one or two faculties, a pie chart wouldn't work, because we wouldn't know what proportion of the whole that information was.

As a general rule, we tend to use pie charts as very general summaries of large amounts of data. They are often used to describe the research participants in psychological studies – it is a useful way to see what a sample of research participants was like – and they are also often used to summarise survey responses. And pie charts are particularly useful when we have data which take the form of percentages. Since percentages are, by definition, numbers out of a hundred, it is relatively straightforward to convert them into chunks of a circle.

Drawing up a pie chart

Calculating and drawing a pie chart is not very difficult. First, we need to draw a circle with a radius – a straight line from the centre to the edge. It doesn't really matter which way the radius points, but it will be the starting point from which we can draw the slices of the 'pie'. Then we need to work out how large each of our slices needs to be. We need to identify the categories we are going to represent, and list the scores belonging to each of those categories. We also need to know the complete total of scores produced by all of the categories, so that we can work out how large a slice of the total each category should have.

Once we know the total scores, and the score for each category, we need to divide up the circle so that each slice is in proportion to one category's data. There are two ways of doing this. One is to guess – we know what half a circle look like, so if our data are close to a half of the total we can work out, by eye, approximately where the lines should go. We know how large a quarter of a circle should be, so we can guess that too. If the 'shares' of the circle indicated by our data are reasonably straightforward, we can work out the whole thing by approximation.

The other way is to work it out precisely. For this, we need just a little algebra, but not very much. We know that there are 360° in a circle, and that the whole circle is equivalent to our total set of scores. We can use that information to work out fractions, which are equivalent to one another. One of these fractions is the number of degrees required by a slice, which will be a fraction of 360. The other fraction is our category's scores, which will be the same fraction of the whole set. We can work out the value of the second fraction, because we know our category's scores, and also those of the whole set. The formula to work it out is:

$$\frac{x_1}{\sum x} = \frac{a}{360}$$

In this formula, x_1 is the score for the category we are trying to draw; $\sum x$ is the total scores for all of the categories, and a is what we are trying to find out – that is, the number of degrees the slice for this category should have in the diagram.

Putting all of the figures into this gives us two fractions, with only one unknown bit, and we can work this out using simple algebra. The answer that we obtain will tell us the size of the slice needed in the diagram, in degrees. We then need to work out the sizes of each of the other categories. By the time we have finished, the total number of degrees – the sum of the degrees needed by each category – should add up to 360. That's your check – if it doesn't, either there is an error somewhere in the calculations, or one of the categories has been missed out or included twice.

Working out the formula is not nearly as difficult as it might appear. Imagine that you have carried out a study with 60 research participants, and that you are drawing up a pie chart to indicate what their

The types of diagram described in the chapter are suitable for use with different levels of measurement. Several of them can be used with more than one level of measurement.

Indicate which of the four levels of measurement – nominal, ordinal, interval or ratio – are suitable for use with each diagram, and which are not, by putting a tick or a cross in the relevant box.

diagram	nominal	ordinal	interval	ratio
bar chart				
frequency polygon				
graph				
ANOVA interaction diagram				
histogram				
pie chart				
scattergram				
box-plot diagram				
stem and leaf diagram				

occupations were. Fifteen of them were students. So what size of slice should the category 'students' have on the pie chart? Putting the numbers into the formula, we have:

$$\frac{15}{60} = \frac{a}{360}$$

If you are familiar with simple algebra, you will be able to work this out for yourself. If you're not sure, or can't quite remember how to do this, Worked Example 16.1 shows the stages you need to calculate the answer. Use it as a model for other calculations. Just put different numbers into the first fraction – numbers which represent the size of the category and the size of the whole – but leave the 360 in the second one. And remember to use a calculator for any complicated bits of arithmetic!

Worked example 16.1   Calculations for a pie chart

We begin with the formula

$$\frac{x_1}{\sum x} = \frac{a}{360}$$

And put in the numbers, giving

$$\frac{15}{60} = \frac{a}{360}$$

Then we begin working it out. The first step is to take the bottom line of one of the fractions, and multiply it by the top line of the other fraction. This get rid of one of the fractions, and gives us:

$$15 = \frac{60 \times a}{360}$$

Then we look at the fraction on the left side, and cancel out what we can. In this case, we can cancel out the 60s, giving us:

$$15 = \frac{a}{6}$$

Finally, we multiply the bottom line of the right-hand fraction by the number on the left. This gets rid of the last fraction, giving us:

$$(6 \times 15) = a$$

Which works out as

$$a = 90$$

So we know that this segment should be 90° in size.

Once you know how many degrees each slice should be, you can draw them into your pie chart. Decide which category you are going to do first, and use the radius you drew at the beginning as your starting point. Use a protractor to mark another radius the correct number of degrees (the correct number is the number needed by the category you are drawing). Do this for each of the other categories, and this will divide up the whole circle. Shade the different sections with different markings or colours, so that they can easily be told apart, label the chart and provide a key to your shadings or colours, and your pie chart is complete!

Scattergrams

Scattergrams are used to illustrate correlations. We will be looking at inferential correlation tests in Chapter 17, which are used to describe correlations in terms of numbers, and at regression analysis, which looks at how correlations can be used for prediction; but a scattergram gives us an image, or picture, of the correlation. Essentially, a correlation is a measure of how two different variables relate to one another – how they co-relate. A scattergram shows that co-relation on a diagram.

The diagram that we draw for a scattergram is like a graph or a bar chart, having an x and a y axis at right angles to one another. In this case, though, the x axis represents one variable, while the y axis represents the second variable. The points on the scattergram are obtained by taking related measurements of the two variables. They might be related by being taken at the same time, or by coming from the same research participant, or in some other way; but they always represent a pair of scores. Each of these paired measurements is plotted on the scattergram, using a cross or an asterisk. And that's the scattergram. There's no need to join up the points with lines, because that wouldn't make any sense – each pair of measurements is independent of the others.

Interpreting scattergrams

What is interesting is what scattergrams can tell us about the relationship between the two variables. If there isn't any relationship between them, then the points can appear pretty well anywhere on the scattergram – there won't be any pattern, or shape, to how they are scattered about. If there is an exact one-to-one relationship between the pairs of scores, then the pattern will be in a straight line. If whenever a score is high, its pair is also high by the same proportion, we will get

Figure 16.10   Perfect correlations

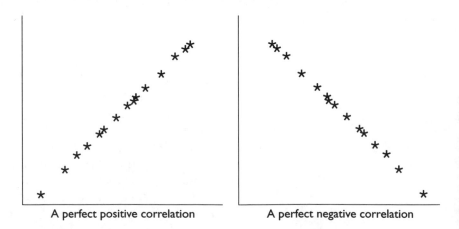

A perfect positive correlation   A perfect negative correlation

a line that runs from bottom left to top right. Alternatively, if whenever a score is high, its partner is low by the same proportion, we will get a line which runs from top left to bottom right on the scattergram (Figure 16.10). These are known as **perfect correlations**.

Perfect correlations, though, are actually rather rare. In reality, there will be some variation in the relationship between the scores. But we can still see some patterns to those relationships, if we plot the scores on a scattergram. For example, if there is what we call a **positive correlation**, the scattergram will look like the one in Figure 16.11. As you can see, a positive correlation means that high scores on one variable tend to happen along with high scores on the second one. (Incidentally, there's no causality here – one score being high doesn't *cause* the other to be high: it just happens to be so, and it's vitally important not to mistake correlation for causality. We will come across this issue again later in this book.)

Figure 16.11 A positive correlation

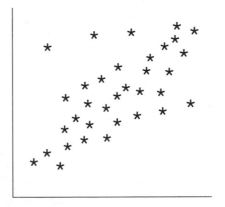

A correlation can also be negative. With a **negative correlation**, a high score on one variable is usually associated with a low score on the other one. In that case, the scattergram will look like the one in Figure 16.12. The scores will fall in the general direction of top left to

Figure 16.12 A negative correlation

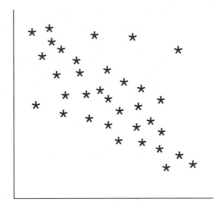

bottom right on the diagram, instead of going from bottom left to top right as they do with a positive correlation. Negative correlations are just as common as positive ones, and they are also just as important, statistically.

Notice, though, that not every pair of scores on these scattergrams goes in exactly the same direction. In most sets of data, there will be scores which are different from most of the others. So sometimes it is useful to draw an oval-shaped boundary around most of the scores, because that can show up the correlation more clearly (Figure 16.13). Sometimes, too, researchers find it helpful to draw a line on the diagram, which is known as the **line of best fit**, and is a kind of summary of the correlation. The line is placed in such a way that it would form the long axis of an oval which encompasses most of the scores, if we were to draw one. The closer a correlation is to being perfect, the more closely the scores will seem to be clustered around the line of best fit. If the line has been calculated exactly, it is called the **regression line**, and we will be coming back to this idea in Chapter 17.

Figure 16.13   The line of best fit

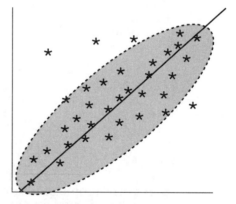

Scattergrams are extremely useful for giving us a quick, visual summary of the strength of a correlation. But as a general rule, they serve as an accompaniment to more complex statistics, not as an end in themselves. The correlation coefficient obtained from a test can indicate the precise numerical value of the correlation, and can interpret that correlation in terms of probability and chance. The regression line, when it is calculated precisely, can allow us to make predictions about pairs of scores. The scattergram is useful for illustrating both of these, but its value on its own in much more limited.

Other graphical representations

There are several other forms of graphical representation which are used commonly by psychologists. They include frequency polygons, box-plot diagrams, and stem and leaf diagrams. Each of these is used to represent different types of information, but these uses are much more specific than the general types of diagram that we have already looked at in this chapter. As a result, they are slightly less common than bar charts, pie charts or straightforward graphs.

Frequency polygons

Frequency polygons are a way of describing a set of scores which have been obtained from a research project. They give us a graphical image which indicates the pattern, or shape, of the data-set, in terms of which values of scores occurred most often, and which were the least common. In that sense, they are a little like a distribution graph, such as the normal distribution curve that we looked at in the last chapter. But they are also a bit like a bar chart, in that the measuring scale is divided into categories, or sets of scores, rather than representing individual scores as it does on a graph.

In fact, a frequency polygon is worked out in almost exactly the same way as a bar chart. Suppose for example, that we were looking at acuity of hearing in 14-year-olds and 64-year-olds. We could test several hundred research participants, but we would need a way of indicating how hearing acuity was distributed in our two samples. The first step is to organise the measuring scale into sets, or categories. So we would begin by dividing the hearing acuity scale into categories, and arranging them in order along the bottom of the chart. Suppose that we were using a continuous scale which gave us ratings from 1 to 100. We would not want 100 different categories, so we would group them into frequencies. The first might be 0–9, then 10–19, then 20–29, and so on. This would give us ten categories, which would form the x axis of our frequency polygon.

The next step would be to count up the number of scores occurring in each category. This means that we obtain the **frequency** for each category – how often each score comes up. The y axis on the graph represents that frequency: the higher the point on the y axis, the more scores there are. The frequency for each category is marked on the chart, using a dot. Then the dots are all joined using straight lines. This produces an irregular shape, which is the **frequency polygon** (a polygon is a many-sided shape), as shown in Figure 16.14.

You might notice that calculating a frequency polygon is remarkably similar to calculating a bar chart. The only real difference is that we join up dots instead of drawing bars. This makes it look a bit like a graph, and in some ways, a frequency polygon is half-way between the two. So a frequency polygon, like other forms of graphical information, needs to be carefully labelled, to make it clear exactly what it is, and what it is representing, and to avoid confusion with other forms of representation.

What do these three terms mean?

scattergram

correlation

line of best fit

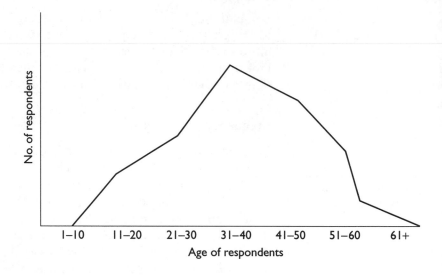

Box-plot diagrams

Box-plot diagrams (sometimes called box-and-whisker plots) are
becoming increasingly popular in research reports. They are diagrams
which take the form of a chart showing a box, or a set of boxes, each
of which has a line coming out from either side. Box-plots deal with
ordinal data. The box shows the middle 50 per cent of the scores,
which is also known as the **interquartile range** (we looked at this in
the last chapter), while the line indicates the full range of the scores.
You may find it useful to look again at the section on the range and
interquartile range in Chapter 15, to refresh your memory about these
measures.

Figure 16.15 shows an imaginary single box-plot for a group of students who have taken Cattell's 16PF personality test. The personality
factor represented by the box-plot is A, which is 'reserved–outgoing'.
The horizontal axis, or x axis of the box-plot is the measuring scale,
and the box represents the middle 50 per cent of the scores that we
have obtained on that particular measure. As we can see, the box is
not in the middle of the scale, telling us that our sample is more outgoing than most people – that our sample is **skewed**. But the left-hand
line stretches across to the left hand side, telling us that a few members
of the sample are nonetheless quite reserved. The single box-plot is a
good way of representing a set of ordinal data like this.

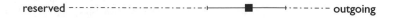

Box-plot diagrams, though, are particularly useful when we want to
describe a very large set of scores, often dealing with several different

variables, on the same diagram. Cattell's 16PF test, for example, has sixteen different personality factors, not just one. If we want to see how our sample appeared on the whole test, we can produce a box-plot diagram which shows all sixteen personality scales (Figure 16.16). The diagram can show us a full profile for this group of research participants, showing us how it may compare with other groups. So it is a very useful way of representing complex sets of ordinal data.

Figure 16.16 A multiple box-plot diagram

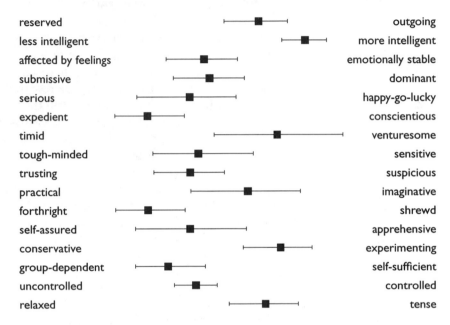

Sometimes researchers use a similar method to indicate interval data. This time, they use the mean as their central point, rather than the interquartile range, and indicate it by a dot rather than a box. Then they use the standard deviation to indicate the length of the line on either side of the dot. This form of graphical image is particularly useful for meta-analysis (see Chapter 9), when the researcher is trying to summarise the results of lots of studies investigating the same variables. An example is given in Figure 16.17.

Figure 16.17
Representing
meta-analysis

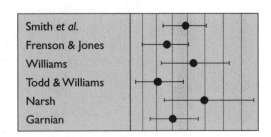

Stem and leaf diagrams

Stem and leaf diagrams are a combination of numerical and graphical representation. Effectively, they are numbers arranged in the form of a picture, and they illustrate sets of scores. But they can only be used to show two-digit variations in scores – that is, scores where the differences between them consist of just the last two numbers, because the way that they are organised, the first number of each score is part of the 'stem' of the diagram, while the second numbers form the 'leaves'.

For example, imagine that we were interested in scientific knowledge among the general population. We develop a general-knowledge quiz based on everyday scientific information, which has 100 questions, and we administer it to a group of research participants. We could illustrate our results on a stem and leaf diagram, by drawing a kind of 'tree' with a vertical 'stem', or y axis, consisting of the numbers 0–9. These numbers represent the 'tens' in our data – the first digit in each score. They are separated from the 'leaves' by a vertical line. Each 'leaf' is formed by the second digit of each score, and it goes on the other side of the line. So a score of 36 would go in the 3 part of the 'stem', and would be indicated by a 6 as the 'leaf'. A score of 74 would go alongside the 7 on the 'stem', and would be indicated by a 4.

Figure 16.18 A stem and leaf diagram

Data set

55	66	41	52	52	42	52	42	52	63
65	56	66	71	62	64	67	58	67	66
57	56	44	56	58	53	67	49	64	48

Diagram

tens	units
4	1 2 2 4 8 9
5	2 2 2 2 3 5 6 6 6 7 8 8
6	2 3 4 4 5 6 6 6 7 7 7
7	1

Figure 16.18 shows a stem and leaf diagram for a set of 40 scores. You can see that all of the leaves have been arranged in order: this is conventional, because it makes it easier to understand the diagram. You can also see how the diagram shows which are the most common results, and how the scores are distributed. If we put the 'stem' in the middle, instead of on the left-hand side, we can even use this type of diagram to compare two groups of scores – putting one group on the left of the stem, and the other on the right. Stem and leaf diagrams can be very useful ways of summarising sets of scores, because they give us quite a clear picture of the data, while still keeping the details of the scores, which is lost when we use bar charts.

ANOVA interaction diagrams

In Chapter 19, we will be looking at the statistical approach known as **analysis of variance**, or **ANOVA** for short. This is a way of analysing data from research which involves more than two different conditions or factors. There are several different types of analysis of variance, which we won't go into here, but the main distinction is between one-way ANOVA and two-way ANOVA.

A **one-way analysis of variance** can be represented quite easily using a graph or bar chart. In a one-way ANOVA, there is just one factor being investigated, but that factor may have several conditions. For example, we might use a one-way analysis of variance to investigate the relationship between age and regular exercising. There would just be one factor (age) that we were investigating, but it would have several different conditions, because the study would include people from several different age groups. Exercise would be the thing that we were measuring – the dependent variable, in statistical terms. So the graph would have the ages along the x axis, and the amount of exercise up the y axis. Alternatively, if we were very strict about our age categories we might decide to use a bar chart instead. But either way, that type of study can be easily represented using familiar graphics.

A **two-way analysis of variance**, however, presents a different challenge. In this type of data, we have two different factors that may be influencing the dependent variable. A study which looked at the effect of age on exercising might also include an investigation of educational background. So the data would consist of two factors: age and educational background; and one dependent variable, which would be the amount of exercise.

Analysis of variance investigates whether either of the factors seems to be having a significant effect. But we often find that two factors interact with one another – that they work together in some way. This is very common in modern research – in real life, it's actually very rare for people to be influenced by just one factor and nothing else. So we need to be able to represent that type of information graphically, as well as in numbers.

The ANOVA interaction diagram puts one factor along the x axis, which can be divided into two straightforward categories. In the case of age, for example, it would be 'younger' and 'older' participants. (The study does not include people over 50, so we are not talking about the very old in this investigation.) The y axis represents the dependent variable – in this case, the amount of exercising people do.

The other factor is then separated into two categories as well. In the case of education they might be something like 'little or no formal

EXERCISE 16.2   **Age and exercise**

A psychologist is investigating the amount of time people spend in sport or exercise. He has obtained the data given below, which indicate the average hours per week spent at a gym or in formal sporting activity, and the age of the participant.

What type of graphical representation would be most appropriate for representing these data?

When you have decided, explain why you have chosen that particular type of diagram, and then draw the diagram itself.

Participant	Age	Hours	Participant	Age	Hours	Participant	Age	Hours
1	18	1	11	31	0	21	42	0
2	54	1	12	45	3	22	50	0
3	36	3	13	51	2	23	19	2
4	39	2	14	57	3	24	23	5
5	26	0	15	40	5	25	40	3
6	49	2	16	33	4	26	55	2
7	47	4	17	32	6	27	24	5
8	20	3	18	21	7	28	51	3
9	23	5	19	30	3	29	58	3
10	30	3	20	35	2	30	26	0

education' and 'degree or equivalent'. Notice that the categories have ignored a whole set of classifications in the middle. This is because the purpose of this diagram isn't to summarise the whole of the results. It is to illustrate the interaction between the two factors, and that would be muddied if we tried to include everything.

The diagram is then marked with four large dots. Those dots are joined by two lines. One line and its associated two dots represent one condition of the second factor, while the other represents the other condition. In our example, one line would represent people with little or no formal education, while the other would represent people with degrees or the equivalent. The height of the dot represents the amount of exercise that group does. Figure 16.19 shows what this would look like in practice.

If we look at Figure 16.19, we can see how the diagram illustrates the interaction between the two factors. The group lacking formal education shows a high level of exercise among young people, but a much lower level of exercise among older people. However, the group

Figure 16.19 ANOVA interactions

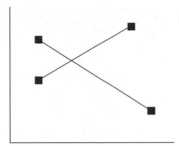

with degree-level education shows a lower level of exercise to start with, but a higher level as they get older. It implies that there is an interaction between the two factors, in that both educational background and age influence the amount of exercise that people do, but not in a straightforward way.

This type of diagram, as you may realise, represents a slightly different way of summarising research findings. It isn't about incorporating all of the data into a summary chart. Instead, it's about identifying the main trends in the data, and drawing a diagram which will illustrate those. We can use diagrams for either purpose, but it is very important to be clear about whether a diagram is a summary of all of the data, or whether it is just illustrating some significant trend but not including everything.

This chapter and the previous one have been mainly about **descriptive statistics** – statistics which allow us to describe our data, but not to do much more than that. In the next few chapters, we will be looking at some **inferential statistics** – statistics which allow us to make probability estimates from our data, and to infer how likely it is that our results are simply the outcomes of sampling error or chance, or whether they seem to have much stronger implications.

 Self-assessment questions

1. *Explain how the co-ordinates of a graph are described.*

2. *What is the difference between a bar chart and a histogram?*

3. *Distinguish between a perfect positive correlation and a perfect negative correlation. What would each one look like on a scattergram?*

4. *What information would you need to construct a box-plot diagram?*

5. *How would you calculate the frequencies for a frequency polygon?*

Concepts in use

1. *In an experimental study of noise levels and concentration, the dependent variable was accuracy in solving arithmetic problems. What would be the x axis and what would be the y axis of a graph of the results?*

2. *Imagine you have just conducted a study of people's sleeping patterns. You have a range of different times when people in your study report going to bed. How would you display this information graphically?*

3. *A researcher has used a pie chart to illustrate the proportions of leisure time which a sample of students spend in different activities. What are the advantages and disadvantages of this decision?*

4. *Give a specific example of a negative correlation. If you like, you can draw your examples from your knowledge of existing psychological research.*

5. *If you had conducted an analysis of variance looking at the effects of anxiety and learning method on test performance, how might you represent your data graphically?*

17

Two-sample tests

Sign test
Chi-square
Wilcoxon sign
Mann–Whitney U
Related t test
Independent t test

The previous two chapters were concerned with descriptive statistics – statistics which simply describe the data which have been obtained, without making any particular inferences about them. In the final three chapters, we will be looking at **inferential statistics**. Inferential statistics allow us to go beyond the data that we have actually obtained, to infer things about the population that the data have come from. They let us make judgements about whether the distinctive patterns or characteristics in our scores are important, or whether they are just likely to be an artefact, which has happened because of sampling errors or problems with methodology.

As we saw in Chapter 14, these judgements are assessments of **probability**. We can't be absolutely certain about our conclusions, because there is always room for chance or for sampling errors. We can't rule these out altogether: it is always possible that we may have drawn our sample of research participants from a particularly unusual section of the population, so that they are not representative of their population at all. So there is always some level of uncertainty in our conclusions. When we carry out inferential tests, we become able to put a figure to that uncertainty – to state just what the odds are that our results have happened as a result of sampling error. We can't rule out uncertainty altogether. But we can be pretty exact about how uncertain we are!

In this chapter we will be looking at the kind of statistics we use when we have two or more sets of scores, and we want to know whether they are significantly different. This situation happens surprisingly often in psychological research. It can happen because we have conducted an experiment, and want to see if our manipulations of the independent variable have produced an effect; it can happen because we have conducted an observational study and want to see if there are consistent differences between one set of observations and another; or it can happen because we have conducted a questionnaire study and want to see if the responses which people gave to one of our questionnaire items are significantly different than those for another. Any of these situations, and several others, can lead us to conduct two-sample difference tests on our data.

Two-sample statistical tests are examples of **inferential statistics** – statistics which allow us to make inferences about probability (see Chapter 14). There is a wide range of inferential tests available, and, like descriptive statistics, each one is appropriate for different circumstances. The test that we choose depends on the type of data that we have, on the task that we want the test to do, and on the assumptions that we feel able to make about the population that our data come from.

Some types of test make much stricter assumptions than others – assuming that the data come from a normal distribution and have a couple of other special characteristics. These are known as **parametric tests**, because they assume that the distribution of possible scores from the population lies within certain parameters. We will be looking at them later in this chapter. Some tests, though, don't make such stringent assumptions about the population. Because of this, they are known as **distribution-free tests** or, more commonly, **non-parametric tests**.

> **What do these three terms mean?**
>
> *inferential statistics*
>
> *normal distribution*
>
> *two-sample statistical tests*

Non-parametric tests

Non-parametric tests use the ordinary laws of probability to evaluate whether a particular set of findings is likely to have come about as a result of sampling error or not. Sometimes they do look at the data to see whether they seem to have come from a particular type of population, as parametric tests do; but unlike parametric tests, they don't take that for granted.

The fact that non-parametric statistics don't make so many assumptions about their data also means that they can be used with levels of measurement which are unsuitable for parametric tests. In Chapter 14 we saw that many psychological research projects give us **ordinal data**, which can't be added up or treated arithmetically but only ranked. Some studies even give us **nominal data**, which can only be categorised. While this type of data can't be used to perform complex arithmetical operations, it is still possible to examine them and make inferences about whether they would have been likely to have come about by chance. But to do that, we need special tests.

Parametric tests assume that their data are always at least equal-interval. But non-parametric tests don't make that assumption, and as a result, there are non-parametric statistics which can deal with both ordinal and nominal data. We will begin this chapter by looking at two tests which can deal with nominal data: the sign test and chi-square. Later we will go on to look at tests which can deal with ordinal data: the Wilcoxon Signed-ranks test and the Mann–Whitney *U*. In the final part of this chapter we will look at some of the assumptions of parametric tests, and at the most useful parametric test of them all – the *t* test.

What do these three terms mean?

parametric tests

distribution-free tests

nominal data

The sign test

The sign test is often just referred to as the **binomial sign test**. It is one of the easiest statistical tests of them all, and doesn't even use real quantitative information – it just uses plus and minus signs instead. We really only use it in situations where all we can say is that one of a pair of scores is higher or lower than the other, and we don't have any other meaningful quantitative information about them.

For example, if we were conducting a study on friendliness, part of that study might involve collecting information about whether people judged that they felt friendlier towards other people in the morning or in the afternoon. We wouldn't have precise quantitative data about this, but we could use the idea of 'more' or 'less' in order to conduct a sign test.

RULES TO REMEMBER

Brackets like this ( ) or like this [ ] mean 'do what is inside me first, before you do anything else'. If you have a little bracket inside a big one, do the little one first.

Any fraction – that is, anytime you see a number above another one, with a line running across between them – means 'divide the top number by the bottom one'.

A number next to another number, with nothing in between, means 'multiply these two together'.

The null hypothesis for the sign test says that there is an equal probability of one set of scores being higher than the other set, or the other set being higher than the first. Formula 17.1 gives the statistical way of expressing this. It looks complicated, but, in simple language, what it says is that there is an even chance of either set of scores being bigger than the other.

Formula 17.1   **The binomial test**

$$p(X_A > X_B) = p(X_A < X_B) = 0.5$$

Reminder
X_A = the first of each pair of scores
X_B = the second
p = probability

So to carry out the sign test, we have to look at whether the A score in a pair is higher or lower than the B score. We give each pair a sign, using plus (+) if the A score is higher, and minus (–) if the B score is the high one. But if a pair is the same, we drop it from the analysis altogether. Then, when every pair has either a plus or a minus (or been dropped), we add up all the pluses and all the minuses. Finally, we take the smaller of the two answers. This is the final answer to our calculations, and we call it x.

If the null hypothesis were true, we would expect to end up with an equal number of plus and minus signs; but in real life our findings are unlikely to be balanced so perfectly. So we need to find out what the probability is for what we have actually found, and for this we need Table A. Table A requires us to know x, which we have already calculated, and N, which is the number of pairs of scores that we have actually used in the sign test – that is, the number left over once we have dropped the equal ones from the analysis.

In Chapter 14, we looked at how we use probability to judge whether our findings are significant or not. The usual way of doing this is to say that if the probability of the null hypothesis being true is less than .05, or one in twenty, then we will accept it. The probability figure in Table A is the probability of the null hypothesis being true. So in order to regard our findings as significant, we need to obtain a probability which is less than or equal to 0.05. If it is more than that, our findings are not significant and we need to conclude that the null hypothesis is true.

The sign test, then, is as simple as adding up the pluses and minuses obtained from two pairs of scores. But it is, nonetheless, a real significance test, and it does show us something of how they can be used. Sign tests, as you can see, can be used with **nominal data**. But they are not very powerful, so it is very important that any confounding variables are minimised as much as possible. This means that it should really only be used for **repeated-measures designs** – that is, when each pair of scores has come from the same person.

> **What do these three terms mean?**
>
> *ordinal data*
>
> *two-tailed test*
>
> *non-parametric tests*

One- and two-tailed tests

In some books, you will find two versions of significance tables like Table A: one for a one-tailed test and one for a two-tailed test. This depends on the prediction that we have made about our findings. If we have simply said that one set of scores will be more than the other, without saying which one, then we have a two-tailed prediction – our findings could go either way. But if we are saying which member of the pair of scores will be larger, we have a one-tailed prediction, which only accepts differences in one direction. It makes a difference to the probabilities, which is why there are sometimes two versions of the table.

For example, if we predicted that there would be a difference between mornings and afternoons in people's friendliness, but we didn't say which was the friendlier time, we would have made a two-tailed prediction. It could go either way. But if we predicted that people would be more friendly in the afternoon, it would be a one-tailed prediction. In that case, we would have to ignore findings which went in the opposite direction, and that would affect our probabilities.

All inferential tests can be used with either one- or two-tailed hypotheses, and that always affects the probabilities. So we always need to be very clear beforehand just which type of hypothesis we are testing.

The tables I have provided in the back give the significance levels for two-tailed hypotheses unless they have both versions. If your hypothesis is one-tailed, then your results will be twice as significant. So a significance level of $p < .05$ obtained for a two-tailed hypothesis would be a significance level of $p < .025$ for a one-tailed hypothesis. Bear this in mind when you look significance levels up in the tables.

Chi-square for two samples

Sometimes we have two sets of scores which have come from two different groups of people. If we have nominal data and an independent-measures design, we can use the test known as the **Chi-square** to calculate whether we have significant differences between our two samples – see Formula 17.2.

We begin by arranging the categories of our data in a grid, so that that rows represent the two samples, and each column represents one of the categories. The numbers in the grid are known as the **frequencies** – they describe how often each category has occurred in the complete set of data. Then we look to see whether the frequencies that we have actually observed are the same as the ones we might have expected to find, if the null hypothesis was true.

What do these three terms mean?

one-tailed test

significant difference

frequencies

Formula 17.2   **The chi-square test**

$$\chi^2 = \sum \frac{(o - e)^2}{e}$$

Reminder
$\sum$ tells you to 'add up these numbers': it means 'the sum of'
o means 'the observed scores'
e means 'the scores expected if the results had been purely random'

In real life, no two groups of people are exactly the same, and even if the population as a whole shows certain characteristics, it is always possible that we have selected a group of people who don't. In which case, it would be our sampling which produced the differences, and not any real effect from our study. So, as with all inferential tests, we have a **null hypothesis**, which predicts that any differences we might have actually found have come about by sampling error, and not because those differences are reflected in the population as a whole. Using the chi-square test, we can judge whether the observations we have actually obtained from a study are likely to have happened just by chance; or whether they seem to support the idea that there really are some differences between the samples, or between the different categories.

For example, if we were looking at colour preferences among a sample of girls and boys at junior school, the measure we would collect would be their favourite colour. So our data would consist of a table of colours, with how many research participants had chosen each one. One row of the table would represent the boys and the other would represent girls. The numbers in the table would be the frequencies that we had observed in our study. We would look to see if there were significant differences between the boys and the girls by applying chi-square, and seeing whether those frequencies were different from the ones that we might have expected.

The test uses the formula:

$$\chi^2 = \sum \frac{(o - e)^2}{e}$$

In this case, o is the observed data (the numbers in each category); e is the expected data (the numbers we would expect to find if the null hypothesis were true), and $\sum$ means we need to work out the answer separately for each of our categories, and then add them all up. This gives us the value of the statistic known as chi-square, or χ^2. There are several ways of working out chi-squares of this sort, but one of the clearest is to draw the cells separately as you work them out, see Worked Example 17.1.

Worked example 17.1   A chi-square test

The data set (i.e. the observed scores) is as follows:

	red	blue	green
girls	6	12	14
boys	15	19	2

The formula is

$$\chi^2 = \sum \frac{(o-e)^2}{e}$$

So first, we need to find out the totals, by adding up rows and columns:

	columns			totals
rows	6	12	14	**32**
	15	19	2	**36**
totals	**21**	**31**	**16**	**68**

Now we work out the expected score for each of the cells. The best way is by drawing the cells again, so you don't forget.

o = observed scores
e = expected scores

We calculate the expected scores, or *e*, by using the formula

$$e = \frac{\text{row total} \times \text{column total}}{\text{overall total}}$$

Expected scores

9.88	14.59	7.53
11.12	16.41	8.47

Now we work out the $(o-e)$ scores, by subtracting the expected score from the observed score, again, separately for each cell in the table:

$(o-e)$

−3.88	−2.59	6.47
3.88	2.59	−6.47

Then we square the $(o-e)$ scores:

$(o-e)^2$

15.05	6.71	41.86
15.05	6.71	41.86

We divide them by *e*:

$$\frac{(o-e)^2}{e}$$

1.52	0.46	5.56
1.35	0.41	4.94

And we add them up, giving us our final value of chi-square:

$$\chi^2 = 14.24$$

Once we have obtained the χ^2 statistic, we need to find out what it means. Some values of chi-square would mean that we would have to retain our null hypothesis, while others suggest that it could be rejected. Roughly speaking, the bigger the value of χ^2 is, the more likely it is to be significant. But for us to say that it has reached an acceptable level of significance, we need to know its **critical value**. This will vary, depending on how many categories we have in our study and what level of significance we find acceptable.

Table B gives values of chi-square for the significance levels of $p < .05$ and $p < .01$. The rows in table B represent **degrees of freedom**. We calculate the degree of freedom appropriate for our particular study by using the formula:

$$df = (r - 1) \times (k-)$$

In this formula, df means 'degrees of freedom'. The term 'r' means the number of rows that we have. The 'k' term means the number of columns that there are in the table. So we calculate the degrees of freedom by subtracting one from the number of rows, subtracting one from the number of columns and multiplying those two numbers together.

Then we use this number to look up the critical value of χ^2 in Table B. If our value of chi-square is more than the critical value, then we can say we have achieved that level of significance. If it is less, then we have to conclude that our data is not significant, and we need to retain the null hypothesis.

Degrees of freedom

Degrees of freedom are really about how much freedom there is for variation in the data. We know, in a study of this kind, what the total number of observations is. We also know how many categories we have. But the data can vary quite a lot between those categories, and lots of those variations won't be statistically significant. So it matters how many different possibilities for variation there are.

The best way of visualising this is to look at it in terms of a real data set. Imagine that we had a set of twenty-four possible scores, which would fall into four categories. There are all sorts of possibilities for the first category of a set: it can have any frequency at all – as long as it isn't more than 24, of course. So that frequency has freedom to vary, until we know what it is. Once we do know what it is, we have three categories left. This means that the next frequency has freedom to vary too. It might contain all of the remaining scores, or just one or two of them, or any number in between. Once the second category has been settled, there are two categories left, and only a certain number of scores. There is still one degree of freedom left, because

> **continued**
> the third category might contain any or all of the remaining scores. But once that has been settled, the final category can't vary at all. It has to contain the scores which are left over from the other three.
>
> That might sound complicated, but it isn't really. Imagine you were dropping 24 marbles into four boxes. You can choose how many to drop into the first box, so that's one degree of freedom in your actions. You can choose how many to drop into the second box, and that's another degree of freedom. You can choose how many to drop into the third box, and that's a third degree of freedom. But the marbles you have left over all have to go into the fourth box, so you don't have any choices left. A set of four boxes gives you three degrees of freedom. A set of eight would give you seven degrees of freedom.
>
> There are other statistical tests which also use degrees of freedom. Since they deal with different kinds of data, the ways that you work out the degrees of freedom are slightly different. But the underlying principle is always the same, so understanding this example will give you the basic idea.

Yates's correction

There is just one additional feature which is a bit special for a two-sample chi-square. It applies when we have two samples, but we also have only two categories of data, so that the data table has just four cells. This is the minimum number of cells that we would need to analyse differences between two samples, and it needs to be treated a bit specially because of the type of situations that it represents.

For example, we might want to use a two-sample, two-condition chi-square test to look at older and younger people's answers to a yes/no question in a questionnaire, or in some other situation where there were only two possible categories for respondents. But the problem is that whenever we try to classify human behaviours into just two categories, we end up over-simplifying – making things seem much more definite than they really are.

You may have found that it often isn't all that easy to give an absolute 'yes' or 'no' to a questionnaire answer. We end up choosing the one that seems to apply most often. But the real answer is often 'sometimes yes, and sometimes no, depending on other factors'. This is the **questionnaire fallacy** that we looked at in Chapter 5. And even categories which appear to be straightforward – such as girls or boys – aren't necessarily that clear-cut. Some families bring up their girls in a way which would be considered 'masculine' by others, while others expect qualities from their boys which are more associated

What do these three terms mean?

questionnaire fallacy

repeated-measures design

rankings

with femininity. Parental expectations about appropriate behaviours for girls and boys vary widely from one family to another, and these affect all sorts of aspects of development. So in a psychological study, simply dividing respondents into girls and boys may exaggerate the differences between the groups a bit too much.

Because of this, we need to adjust the two-sample chi-square, to reduce the exaggeration a bit. The adjustment is known as **Yates's correction**, and involves subtracting a half (0.5) from the value calculated for each data cell, before adding them all up. This makes the

---

EXERCISE 17.1   **Analysing communication**

A research project into health behaviours involved looking at how people understand and act on the information they are given by health professionals. As part of that project, a health psychologist collected reports from two different GPs about the treatments they advised for particular patients, and how these treatments should be used. The psychologist also interviewed the patients themselves (who had consented, of course, to participate in the study beforehand) and gathered their accounts.

The communication process, it turned out, was not that straightforward. What the GP told the patient often didn't match what the patient believed that they were told. In fact, when the psychologist compiled a set of 'accuracy scores', based on what the patients remembered and how much of it seemed to be roughly similar to what the doctor had said, they showed wide variation. The patients from one GP seemed to have misunderstood quite a lot of their instructions – their 'accuracy scores' varied between 10 per cent and 60 per cent, with only three of those 20 patients gaining scores higher than 70 per cent. Those from the other GP seemed to have understood more, but still only two patients out of the 20 in that group were able to report their instructions accurately in all respects.

The psychologist was then faced with the problem of reporting the results. Some of the information could be conveyed using qualitative reports. But it was also very important that the researcher should be able to produce some kind of quantitative analysis of the findings. Among other things, the psychologist felt that it was important to highlight the differences between the two doctors, and this could provide support for the idea that doctors might benefit from communication training. What kind of test would be most suitable for this kind of analysis, and why?

formula look like the one shown as Formula 17.3. And that means that we have to find slightly bigger differences between our observed findings and the ones we would have expected, in order to regard those differences as significant. It just cuts down the exaggeration a bit, by making all of the differences a little smaller.

Formula 17.3

Chi-square with Yates's correction

$$\chi^2 = \sum \frac{[(o - e) - 0.5]^2}{e}$$

Notes
Σ tells you to 'add up these numbers'. It means 'the sum of'
o means 'the observed scores'
e means 'the expected scores'

Chi-square can be used to look at more than two samples. You can use it with several different research participant groups, and several different measures. The calculation process is exactly the same. But it's easy to get lost if you are doing a complex chi-square; so always make sure that you can recognise what a significant result actually means – just which part of the data the significant difference comes from. You can refer to Worked Example 17.1 and follow that if you like.

Chi-square, then, is a useful test which can be applied in a number of different ways. It is probably the most important way of analysing nominal data. But if the data that we have are at least ordinal, there are other tests we can use. These tests are more powerful than chi-square, because they can take into account more of the information in the data. The two main tests for looking at differences in ordinal data are the Wilcoxon Signed-ranks test and the Mann–Whitney U.

The Wilcoxon Signed-ranks test

The **Wilcoxon Signed-ranks test**, also known as the **Wilcoxon Sign test**, is really just a more sophisticated version of the sign test. The way that it works is by comparing two sets of scores, looking to see if one set is consistently higher or lower than the other. To do this, it uses the direction of the difference between two pairs of scores, just as the sign test does; but it also looks at the size of those differences. It can do this because it is used for data at the ordinal level of measurement or above – that is, data which can be ranked. The positive or negative sign is not applied to the data themselves, as it is in the sign test, but to the **rankings** of the data.

Like the sign test, though, the Wilcoxon Sign test can only be used with data which consist of **matched pairs** – that is, sets of data in which the confounding variables which could interfere between a pair of scores have been very tightly controlled. The most practical way of doing this is by only using it when we have a **repeated-measures design** – in other words, when both the scores making up a pair have come from the same person. There are other ways of doing it – by using identical twins, or very carefully matched samples, for example – but these other methods leave more room for confounding variables to come in, so they aren't ideal.

The very first step in carrying out a Wilcoxon Sign test, then, is to arrange the scores in two columns. Then take the scores in one column away from their matched scores in the other column. It doesn't matter whether you take the A scores from the B scores or the other way round, as long as you do it the same way all down the column. This will almost certainly give you some positive answers, some negative ones, and maybe some which come out as zero because the scores were the same. The ones which come out as zero are dropped from the analysis. They don't count any more.

Subtracting one set of scores from the other gives you a new column of figures, which you should call d (standing for 'difference'). Incidentally, if you are doing your calculations by hand, you might find it easier to have your two data columns widely spaced, so that you can put any other columns you happen to calculate in between them. This is illustrated in Worked Example 17.2.

The next step is to rank all of the ds. We discussed how to do ranking in Chapter 15, so look back there if you have forgotten how to do it. Essentially, though, it involves putting all the scores in order, and then numbering each score according to its place in that order, making sure that equal scores are given the same number. Don't take any notice of whether any particular d is positive or negative when you are ranking it – just look at the number itself, regardless of whether it has a plus or a minus sign.

The plus and minus signs come back in the next stage. Ranking the differences will give you another column, consisting of ranks, which you can call Rd. The next step in the analysis is to give each of the ranks in column Rd either a positive or negative sign, depending on the d that they originally came from. Finally, you add up all of the ranks with a positive sign, add up all of the ranks with a negative sign, and take the smaller one as your answer. The smaller of the two sums gives you a statistic known as T, which you can then look up in Table C to find out whether your results are significantly different or not.

When you're looking it up in Table C, you will also need to know the N of your sample, which is the number of pairs of scores that you have used in your analysis. The ones which you dropped from the

Worked example 17.2 A Wilcoxon Sign test

Ratings of attractiveness of two architectural designs for a new college

Design A	d	Rd	Sign	Design B
5	1	1	+	6
4	−2	2.5	−	2
3	4	6	+	7
3	0	−		3
8	−6	7.5	−	2
7	−3	4.5	−	4
5	2	2.5	+	7
9	−6	7.5	−	3
5	3	4.5	+	8
6	0	−		6

The sum of the positive ranks is 14.

The sum of the negative ranks is 22.

Therefore the value of T is 14.

The number of scores used in the analysis is 8.

The value of T required for significance at $p < 0.05$ with 8 scores is 3 or lower (see Table C).

Therefore T is not significant.

analysis because they were the same don't count, so the N you use to look in the Table may not be the same as the number of research participants you had at the beginning of your study. It just represents the number of research participants who produced different results in the two conditions of your study.

Mann–Whitney U test

The Mann–Whitney U test uses ordinal data too, and it performs much the same kind of analytical task as the Wilcoxon Sign test. Unlike that test, though, it can cope with samples which have been taken from different groups. So we could use the Mann–Whitney U test if we were doing a study comparing, say, Scottish and Welsh children, or older and younger consumers.

The first step in conducting a Mann–Whitney U test is to arrange your scores in two columns, representing your two groups of participants, and to call one of them group A, and the other group B. It may sound trivial, but it is important, because the formula for the test involves a number of references to A and B scores, and if you aren't clear which is which, you could make some serious errors. Since this test is used for an independent-measures design, you may have a different number of scores in each column. That doesn't matter – unlike the Wilcoxon Sign, this test doesn't involve pairs.

The second step is to rank all of the scores, treating the whole lot as just one set. We looked at ranking in Chapter 15, so if you have forgotten, go back to that chapter to see how it is done. When your scores have all been ranked, arrange them into two columns: one column being the ranks for group A, and the other being the ranks for group B. Add up all of the ranks for group A, and then add up all of the ranks for group B, separately.

RULES TO REMEMBER

Brackets like this ( ) or like this [ ] mean 'do what is inside me first, before you do anything else'. If you have a little bracket inside a big one, do the little one first.

Any fraction – that is, anytime you see a number above another one, with a line running across between them – means 'divide the top number by the bottom one'.

A number next to another number, with nothing in between, means 'multiply these two together'.

You use these figures to calculate U, which is the statistic that the Mann–Whitney U test ends with. Actually, to be precise, you calculate two values of U, one for group A, and one for group B, so there are two versions given in Formula 17.4. Work out the two

---

Formula 17.4   **Calculating Mann–Whitney U test scores**

$$U_A = N_A N_B + \frac{N_A(N_A + 1)}{2} - R_A$$

$$U_B = N_A N_B + \frac{N_B(N_B + 1)}{2} - R_B$$

Reminder
R_A the ranks for group A
R_B the ranks for group B
N_A is the number of scores in group A
N_B is the number of scores in group B

values of U using each formula, and take the smaller one as your final result. You can follow Worked Example 17.3 if you like. Then you can look up the score in Table D, and find out if it was significant. If you look at Table D, you can see that it is arranged as a grid, rather than as a list. This is because you may have different Ns for each group, so the top row gives values for N_A and the first column gives values for N_B.

Worked example 17.3 A Mann–Whitney U test

Begin by ranking all of the scores in the data set, as if they were a single group:

Condition A	R_A	R_B	Condition B
8	16	8	5
9	17.5	8	5
7	14	1.5	2
4	5.5	5.5	4
6	11	3.5	3
6	11	17.5	9
7	14	11	6
3	3.5	1.5	2
		14	7
		8	5

When you have ranked all the scores, calculate the totals you will need for the formulas:

$N_A = 8$
$N_B = 10$
$R_A = 92.5$
(add up the A group ranks)
$R_B = 78.5$
(add up the B group ranks)

Now put the numbers into the formula:

$$U_A = (8 \times 10) + \frac{8(8 + 1)}{2} - 92.5 \qquad U_B = (8 \times 10) + \frac{10(10 + 1)}{2} - 78.5$$

$$U_A = 80 + \frac{72}{2} - 92.5 \qquad U_B = 80 + \frac{110}{2} - 78.5$$

$$U_A = 80 + 36 - 92.5 \qquad U_B = 80 + 55 - 78.5$$

$$U_A = 116 - 92.5 \qquad U_B = 135 - 78.5$$

$$U_A = 23.5 \qquad U_B = 56.5$$

The lower of the two scores is *23.5*.

The critical value required for significance at $p < .05$ is 20 or less.

Therefore U is not significant.

Converting Wilcoxon Sign to a z score

You might have noticed that Table C only deals with samples of up to 50 cases and Table D up to 20. This is because it is only with relatively small samples that the values of T (Wilcoxon Sign) or U (Mann–Whitney) are distinctive. When we have larger samples, then the probabilities for T and U tend to fall into a pattern which is like a normal distribution curve. The similarity is close enough that we can convert our results into a z score. We looked at z scores in Chapter 15, and, if you have a good memory, you may recall that they are a way of expressing how close a particular set of scores are to the mean. If you don't remember, it might be a good idea to look back at that chapter to remind yourself.

To convert a Wilcoxon Sign T score, we have to use a conversion formula, which gives us a z score. The conversion formula for the Wilcoxon Sign test requires you to begin by calculating the value of T, by carrying out the standard Wilcoxon Sign test that we have just been looking at. You use that, and the value of N that you used in your calculations, in Formula 17.5.

Formula 17.5   **Converting Wilcoxon Sign Test results to z scores**

$$z = \frac{N(N+1) - 4T}{\sqrt{\left(\dfrac{2N(N+1)(2N+1)}{3} \right)}}$$

Notes
T = the value obtained from your Wilcoxon Sign test
N = the number of pairs of scores which you used in the Wilcoxon Sign calculations

---

Don't be intimidated by the formula: even a complicated formula becomes much easier if you approach it a little bit at a time, working it out as you go. Begin by putting numbers in place of the letters, without doing anything else to them. Then do the simplest calculations, but don't do anything else. If you tackle just a little bit more in each step, and write it out as you go, you'll be surprised how easy it is.

When you have done the calculations, you just need to look at the value of z that we have obtained. If it is more than 1.65, we can conclude that our findings are significant at $p < .05$, and if it is more than 2.33 we can conclude that our findings are significant at $p < .01$, (using a one-tailed test).

Converting Mann–Whitney to a z score

Exactly the same principle applies to a Mann–Whitney U score. If there are more than 20 scores in each sample, the probabilities become very similar to those for z scores. So we can convert our findings into a z score, and work out the probability from that.

The conversion formula for the Mann–Whitney test is more complicated, because you have to begin by doing the Mann–Whitney test, and then you have to work through your data and calculate a special value called T every time you come across any tied ranks (when several numbers have received the same ranking). These Ts need to be calculated each time you come across one of these ties, and Formula 17.6 shows you how to do this.

Formula 17.6

Calculating T for Mann–Whitney conversions

$$T = \frac{t^3 - t}{12}$$

Notes

t is the number of times that particular rank has been allocated. You will need to work out several different values of T – one for each time you come across a tied rank.

The little t in the formula is the number of times that rank has been allocated – in other words, the number of scores which share the same rank. So if you have three scores of 14, the t value for that rank would be 3 and the T value would work out as $27 - 3$ divided by 12, which works out as 2. In another case, you might have four scores of 6, all of which would have the same rank. So the t value would be 4, and putting it into the formula would give you $64 - 4$ divided by 12, which works out as 5. When you have calculated all your T scores and added them up, you can use them in Formula 17.7. The probabilities for the z scores are exactly the same as for the conversion of the Wilcoxon T.

Again, don't be intimidated by the formula. Begin by putting numbers instead of the letters, and then tackle it a little bit at a time. If you write it out again at each step, just changing the one thing you have calculated, you won't get lost. Alternatively, you can use a computer package, like SPSS, and let it do the work for you. (Personally, I much prefer this option.)

Formula 17.7   **Converting Mann–Whitney results to z scores**

$$z = \frac{\dfrac{U - N_A N_B}{2}}{\sqrt{\left(\left[\dfrac{N_A N_B}{N(N-1)}\right] \times \left[\dfrac{N^3 - N}{12} - \Sigma T\right]\right)}}$$

Reminder

U is the result of your Mann–Whitney U calculations

ΣT is the total values of T calculated using Formula 17.6

N_A is the number of scores in group A

N_B is the number of scores in group B

N is the sum of N_A and N_B

Parametric tests

The tests we have looked at so far are **non-parametric tests** – that is, they don't make assumptions about the shape of the population that the data have come from. That has its advantages, as we have seen, because it means that they can handle lower levels of measurement – nominal or ordinal data. But it has its disadvantages too, because it means that they are less **powerful** than tests which can use higher levels of measurement, or which can make assumptions about their data.

Assumptions of parametric tests

What we call the **power** of a test is its ability to detect significance – how sensitive it is to what the data are actually implying. It is possible to detect significance using non-parametric tests, as we have seen, but they are a little clumsy because they don't take into account all of the possible information in the data. Ranking scores is better than simply counting how many of them fit into a category – it takes a bit more of the information into account – but it is even better to deal with scores arithmetically – for example, by calculating means or standard deviations. If we can do that, we become more likely to detect significance if it is present.

We can increase the power of a test, therefore, if we are able to make the basic assumption that the data we are using are equal-interval or ratio. That allows us to use the characteristics of the data more fully. We can calculate means and standard deviations, take

| EXERCISE 17.2 | Evaluating sports training |

A new international sports training centre has appointed a sports psychologist to conduct research into training and practice schedules for athletes. In one study, the psychologist collects data from runners who have come to the centre for advanced training. The psychologist gathers achievement scores, calculated from the difference between their mean times for a 100 m sprint on their first three days at the centre, and their mean times for a 100 m sprint during a three-day period after three weeks of training. The scores express any improvement (or otherwise) which has happened after three weeks.

The purpose of these achievement scores is to allow the athletes to monitor their own performances. But the psychologist decides to use them to compare the two sets of training schedules being used at the centre. Some athletes train using a schedule which involves three training periods spaced throughout the day. Others use a schedule which involves one prolonged period of training each day. The scores below represent the achievement scores obtained by athletes using the two main training schedules. Using an independent-measures t test, find out whether there is reason to believe that either of the schedules is preferable to the other.

Single session	Triple session
2	5
3	7
2	3
7	4
4	2
5	9
3	5
6	6
2	3
5	7

square roots, and perform other arithmetical tasks which will tell us more about what we are dealing with, whenever they seem appropriate. So having **equal-interval ratio or data** is the first assumption of a parametric test.

The second assumption concerns the distribution of the populations which the scores have come from. Parametric tests assume that the scores come from a normally distributed population. This is a slightly controversial assumption, because it has been almost habitual in psychology to assume that just about every score relating to human behaviour or experience is likely to be normally distributed among the population as a whole. Some modern psychologists are beginning to question that idea. But it is this assumption which really gives a parametric test most of its power.

We saw in Chapter 14 that the **normal distribution** has some mathematically predictable properties. In particular, it is able to tell us about probability – if we know the mean and the standard deviation of a normal distribution, we can tell where any particular score has come from, and just how likely we are to have obtained it. So we can make precise probability estimates about a set of scores if we can assume that they have come from a normally distributed population. Which is why this is the second assumption of a parametric test.

The third assumption of a parametric test is that the samples which are being analysed have roughly equal variances. This is to make sure that we are really comparing like with like. If we had one sample which fluctuated wildly – for example, where the scores ranged between 1 and 100 – it would be difficult to compare it with a sample with less variation – for example, where all the scores fell between 45 and 55 (see Figure 17.1). Even though the means of the samples might be similar, we wouldn't be able to compare them properly because the standard deviations wouldn't have anything in common. There would be so many minor differences that we just wouldn't be able to sort out the important ones from the unimportant. So having approximately **equal variances** in the samples is the third assumption of a parametric test.

Figure 17.1 Samples with differing variances

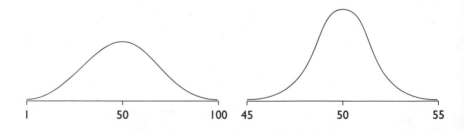

Parametric tests have their name, then, because they are dealing with data which fit within quite strict **parameters**. These parameters are summarised in Table 17.1. Data which don't fit these three assumptions should be analysed using a non-parametric test, and not a parametric one.

Table 17.1 Assumptions of a parametric test

The scores must be equal-interval or ratio data.

The samples must be drawn from a normally distributed population or populations.

The samples should come from populations with equal variances.

Abuses of parametric tests

This, though, is more controversial than it sounds. Because parametric tests are so much more powerful than non-parametric tests, psychologists have almost always used them when their data could be regarded as equal-interval, without actually evaluating whether their data fell within the other two parameters. Most of the time, the idea of a normal distribution underlying the scores has been taken for granted, and not really explored at all. Many recent researchers are beginning to question whether that is really a valid assumption to make.

That isn't the only problem. The other is that parametric tests have often been used in situations where the data aren't even equal-interval. The most common example here is in intelligence testing, where IQ scores have been used as the data for complex parametric tests, even though the difference between an IQ score of 60 and 65 couldn't in any way be regarded as being of the same value as the difference between 120 and 125; and values below 50 hardly exist in any meaningful sense. These scores are normally distributed, because the scales are constructed from the beginning to give normal distributions; but they are not equal-interval, and it is very questionable whether the arithmetical operations performed on them can be justified.

The modern solution, given all of this controversy, is that in cases where there is uncertainty as to whether equal-interval data really fit the parametric assumptions or not, it is best to use both types of test. By analysing the data twice, using both a parametric and a non-parametric test, it is possible to use the power of the parametric test in detecting significance if it is present; and also to use the **robustness** of the non-parametric test, which can cope with a wide range of variations and conditions of the data. Doing both types of test on the same data allows the researcher to get the best of both worlds, and avoid the criticisms or limitations which may arise from doing just one.

The *t* test

The parametric test which we use for analysing differences between two sets of scores is known as the *t* test. It has two versions: one which applies when we have repeated measures (in other words, when our two sets of data have come from the same people, or people so closely matched that other variables are unlikely to have influenced the differences) and one which applies when we have independent measures (in other words, different people in the two groups). The calculations for these two are slightly different, but those differences are really just arithmetical ones. The overall task which the *t* test is performing is the same, regardless of whether we use the repeated-measures or the independent-measures form.

What the *t* test is actually doing is looking at the means of two sets of scores, and at their standard deviations, and estimating whether those means are so different that they are likely to have come from different populations. The null hypothesis predicts that they have actually come from the same population, and that their means and standard deviations are only different because any sampling of a population is likely to include differences. The *t* test explores the alternative possibility: that those means and standard deviations are different because they really have come from different populations.

For example, imagine that we are conducting a study of the effects of daylight on school test performance. We have two matched tests, with questions carefully chosen to give us equal-interval data to analyse. We have two matched groups of students taking the tests, at the same time of day, and with all the other variables that we can think of having been controlled. We ask one group to do the test in a brightly lit indoor room, and the other to do the test in a room lit by natural daylight.

No matter how much we try, we are not going to get identical results from the same group, because human beings just don't work that way. There will always be individual differences. So we can expect the mean score obtained by the two groups to be different. The question is whether that difference is significant or not. It might be that it has only happened because we are dealing with real people and they always vary a little bit in what they do – that the lighting in the room has nothing to do with it. In which case, our two groups would really have come from the same population, and the differences between them would just have come from the fact that we tested two samples of people, rather than the whole population. By chance, our samples had been drawn from the same population, but in such a way that the results produced differences – much like the example shown in Figure 17.2.

On the other hand, it might be that the scores are different because natural daylight really does make a difference to how people perform.

What do these three terms mean?

population

power

robustness

Figure 17.2 Samples from the same population

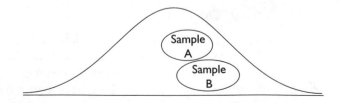

In that case, we would have two populations, not one. We would have one population of possible scores which can be obtained from indoor rooms, and an entirely separate population of possible scores which can be obtained from doing tests in rooms with natural daylight. The two populations would overlap, but they would be different nonetheless – like the example shown in Figure 17.3.

Figure 17.3 Samples from different populations

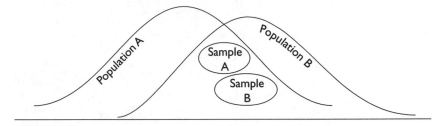

What the *t* test does is to estimate whether it is likely that the scores have actually come from different populations. It does this by looking at the differences between the means, and also at the standard deviations of the scores. If the two means are almost identical, and the standard deviations are similar, the odds are high that they have come from the same population. If they are very different, there is more chance that they have come from two different populations. The final value of *t* which is obtained from a *t* test expresses that probability.

There are two versions of the *t* test. One of them is for repeated-measures samples, and it is the slightly abbreviated version, given in Formula 17.8. In this test, we can subtract one person's scores in one condition from their scores in the other condition, and this simplifies the formula quite a lot. We use *d* to refer to those differences. And we can also know for sure that there are the same number of scores

Formula 17.8

The repeated-measures *t* test

$$t = \frac{\sum d}{\sqrt{\left(\dfrac{N\sum d^2 - [\sum d]^2}{N - 1}\right)}}$$

Reminder

$\sum$ tells you to 'add up these numbers'. It means 'the sum of'.

d means the difference between each person's scores on one test, and their scores on the other one.

d^2 means those differences squared – in other words, each one multiplied by itself.

N means 'the number of pairs of scores that you have'.

Worked example 17.4   A repeated-measures t test

Data and calculations of d values: Formula:

Condition A	d	d^2	Condition B
20			15
18			14
15			13
19			12
17			12
12			18
13			19
15			13
14			16
18			14

$$t = \frac{\sum d}{\sqrt{\left(\dfrac{N\sum d^2 - [\sum d]^2}{N - 1} \right)}}$$

Calculations:

Condition A	d	d^2	Condition B	
20	5	25	15	$\sum d = 15$
18	4	16	14	
15	2	4	13	$(\sum d)^2 = 225$
19	7	49	12	
17	5	25	12	$\sum d^2 = 215$
12	−6	36	18	
13	−6	36	19	$N = 10$
15	2	4	13	
14	−2	4	16	
18	4	16	14	

Now put the numbers into the formula:

(1) $t = \dfrac{15}{\sqrt{\left(\dfrac{(10 \times 215) - 225}{10 - 1} \right)}}$ (4) $t = \dfrac{15}{\sqrt{213.89}}$

(2) $t = \dfrac{15}{\sqrt{\dfrac{2150 - 225}{9}}}$ (5) $t = \dfrac{15}{14.62}$

(3) $t = \dfrac{15}{\sqrt{\dfrac{1925}{9}}}$ (6) $t = 1.03$

The critical value required for significance at $p < 0.5$, is 1.833. Therefore t is not significant.

RULES TO REMEMBER

Brackets like this ( ) or like this [ ] mean 'do what is inside me first, before you do anything else'. If you have a little bracket inside a big one, do the little one first.

Any fraction – that is, anytime you see a number above another one, with a line running across between them – means 'divide the top number by the bottom one'.

A number next to another number, with nothing in between, means 'multiply these two together'.

in each group, so we can just use N to refer to the number of pairs of scores. You can use Worked Example 17.4 to follow if you want to.

When you have completed your t test, you will need to find out if the value of t that you have obtained is significant. To do this, you need to know the **degrees of freedom**. For the repeated-measures t test, we look at the number of pairs of scores, and subtract 1 – in other words, we use the formula $N-1$, where N is the number of pairs of scores that we have used in the analysis. Using the degrees of freedom, we need to look up our value of t in Table E, to find out if it is significant, and if so, to what extent.

The independent-measures t test can't make the same assumptions as the repeated-measures test. We can't subtract one person's scores from those of anyone else; and we might have a different N for each group. So if you look at Formula 17.9, you can see that it ends up looking quite complicated. But don't be put off by that. Tackle it one little bit at a time, and you will find that you can work it out

---

Formula 17.9

The independent-measures t test

$$t = \frac{\bar{X}_A - \bar{X}_B}{\sqrt{\dfrac{\left(\sum X_A^2 - \dfrac{(\sum X_A)^2}{N_A}\right) + \left(\sum X_B^2 - \dfrac{(\sum X_B)^2}{N_B}\right)}{(N_A - 1) + (N_B - 1)} \times \left(\dfrac{1}{N_A} + \dfrac{1}{N_B}\right)}}$$

Reminder
$\sum$ means 'add these up'
$\bar{X}_A$ is the mean of the scores for group A
$\bar{X}_B$ is the mean of the scores for group B
N_A is the number of scores in group A
N_B is the number of scores in group B

very easily. Begin, as always, simply by putting the numbers into the formula, without doing any calculations, then work it out one bit at a time. Follow Worked Example 17.5 if you like.

If you avoid being intimidated, and look closely at the formula for an independent-measures t test, you can see that some chunks of it are actually quite familiar. It actually includes information about

---

Worked example 17.5 An independent-measures t test

Formula:

$$t = \frac{\bar{X}_A - \bar{X}_B}{\sqrt{\frac{\left(\sum X_A^2 - \frac{(\sum X_A)^2}{N_A}\right) + \left(\sum X_B^2 - \frac{(\sum X_B)^2}{N_B}\right)}{(N_A - 1) + (N_B - 1)} \times \left(\frac{1}{N_A} + \frac{1}{N_B}\right)}}$$

Calculations:

Condition A (X_A)	X_A^2	X_B^2	Condition B (X_B)
8	64	25	5
10	100	121	11
12	144	4	2
4	16	16	4
6	36	144	12
6	36	100	10
7	49	36	6
3	9	4	2
9	81	49	7
5	25	25	5
4	16	25	5
8	64	9	3
	1	1	
	49	7	

Begin by working out the expressions you will use in the formula, so that you have numbers instead of symbols:

$N_A = 12$

$N_B = 14$ $\qquad \bar{X}_A = \frac{\sum X_A}{N_A} = \frac{82}{12} = 6.83$

$\sum X_A = 82$

$\sum X_B = 80$ $\qquad \bar{X}_B = \frac{\sum X_B}{N_B} = \frac{80}{14} = 5.71$

$\sum X_A^2 = 640$

$\sum X_B^2 = 608$

Then put the numbers into the formula:

$$t = \frac{6.83 - 5.71}{\sqrt{\frac{\left(640 - \frac{(82)^2}{12}\right) + \left(608 - \frac{(80)^2}{14}\right)}{(12-1) + (14-1)} \times \left(\frac{1}{12} + \frac{1}{14}\right)}}$$

$$t = \frac{1.12}{\sqrt{\frac{\left(640 - \frac{6724}{12}\right) + \left(608 - \frac{6400}{14}\right)}{11 + 13} \times (0.08 + 0.07)}}$$

$$t = \frac{1.12}{\sqrt{\frac{(640 - 560.3) + (608 - 457.1)}{24} \times 0.15}}$$

$$t = \frac{1.12}{\sqrt{\frac{79.7 + 150.9}{24} \times 0.15}}$$

$$t = \frac{1.12}{\sqrt{\frac{230.6}{24} \times 0.15}}$$

$$t = \frac{1.12}{\sqrt{96.08 \times 0.15}}$$

$$t = \frac{1.12}{\sqrt{14.4}}$$

$$t = \frac{1.12}{3.8}$$

$$t = 0.295$$

the mean of each sample, and calculations of the standard deviation. The repeated-measures t test does the same, but in a cut-down version. As I said before, what these tests are really doing is comparing the means of the two samples, taking into account their variances, and seeing whether they are different enough that it is likely they have come from different populations.

The trick in handling a complex formula like this is to tackle it just a little bit at a time, the way that the worked example does. That way, you are only doing a very simple calculation each time, and it is very satisfying to see how it becomes simpler and smaller as you progress. When you've completed your analysis, you will need to look up the answer in Table E, to see if it is significant, and for that you need to know the degrees of freedom. For the independent-measures *t* test, we calculate it using the formula $N_A + N_B - 2$, in other words, by adding the number of scores in the first set to the number of scores in the second set, and then subtracting two. The table gives the different values of *t* which are required for different levels of significance; and our result needs to be equal to, or higher than, the number in the table for us to consider it significant at that level.

We have seen, then, that there are several different kinds of test that we can use in situations where we have two sets of data and we want to discover whether they are significantly different. In the next chapter, we will go on to look at some more parametric and non-parametric tests. This time, they will be investigating correlations, or similarities between sets of scores, rather than differences.

Self-assessment questions

1. *How does the question of whether a hypothesis is one- or two-tailed affect significance levels?*

2. *What is the robustness of a statistical test?*

3. *Why do we use different tests for repeated-measures designs and independent-measures designs?*

4. *State the three assumptions of a parametric test.*

5. *What does it mean to say that a statistical test is powerful?*

Concepts in use

Which two-sample difference test would you use to analyse each of the following:

1. *Preference ratings obtained from the same team of consumers for blue or yellow wallpapers.*

2. *The speed of mid-morning and mid-afternoon traffic on a city ring-road.*

3. *Children's preferences for musical or artistic toys, as measured by the amount of time each child spends playing with each kind of toy.*

4. *Self-ratings of exam anxiety experienced by science and arts students.*

5. *Types of foodstuff purchased by older and younger people.*

18

Correlation and regression

Correlation
Regression
Multivariate analysis

In the last chapter, we looked at tests that we can use when we have two sets of data and want to compare them, to see if they are significantly different. In this chapter, we will be looking at tests which can look at two sets of data and estimate how similar they are – not in terms of their specific values, or the actual measuring scale which has been used to obtain them, but in terms of how they vary.

In the first part of this chapter we will be looking at this from two sides. We will begin by looking at **correlation**, which is concerned **with** expressing the numerical relationship between two variables. Then we will go on to look at **regression**, which is still about correlation in many ways, but looks at it from a slightly different angle. It is useful for us to look at regression as well as correlation, because once we understand both of them, we can use the two approaches – correlation and regression analysis – to help us to make sense of several variables at a time. This is what we will be looking at in the second part of the chapter, and it will begin our exploration of analysis of variance, which we will be continuing in Chapter 19.

Correlation

A correlation test is exactly what its name suggests – a test which looks for co-relations. If we say that two variables are correlated, what we mean is that they vary in similar ways – that a certain size of score on one variable is likely to be associated with a certain size of score on the other. It might mean that a large score on one variable is likely to be associated with a large score on the other. If so, that would be a **positive correlation**. Or it might mean that a large score on one variable is likely to be associated with a small score on the other. That would be a **negative correlation**.

In Chapter 16 we looked at scattergrams, which are the way that correlations are represented graphically. Scattergrams are useful for giving us a general idea of how strong the correlation is. But the most accurate way of judging the size of a correlation is by finding out the **correlation coefficient** – the number which states, precisely, just how strong the relationship between the two variables is.

A correlation coefficient is a number between −1 and +1. Occasionally, but very rarely, we come across what is known as a **perfect correlation** – a correlation in which the two variables co-vary by exactly the same proportions. In a perfect correlation, knowing the value of one score would allow us to state exactly what the value of the other score was, because they are so exactly related. A perfect positive correlation, in which large scores on one variable were associated with equivalent large scores on the other, and small scores were associated with equivalent small scores, would have a correlation coefficient of +1. A perfect negative correlation, in which large scores on one variable were associated with small scores on the other, and small scores on that variable were associated with proportionately large scores on the other, would have a correlation coefficient of −1.

In real life, though, perfect correlations are extremely rare. There is always some variation in the way that the two variables relate with one another. A correlation coefficient is a number between −1 and +1 which describes how closely the two variables relate. The perfect correlation values of −1 and +1 represent the extreme ends of the scale, and all the other possible correlation coefficients fall in between these numbers. The closer they are to those extreme ends, the stronger the correlation; the closer they are to the middle of the scale, the weaker the correlation. So a correlation coefficient of zero, or close to zero, means that there isn't really any correlation between those two variables (Figure 18.1).

What do these three terms mean?

positive correlation

negative correlation

perfect correlation

Figure 18.1 The correlation scale

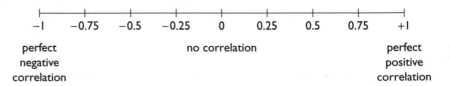

What a correlation test actually does is to look at the data and work out the exact value of the correlation coefficient. There are different correlation tests for different levels of measurement, and in this chapter we will look at the two most commonly used ones: Spearman's rank-order correlation test, which is used when we have ordinal data; and Pearson's product-moment correlation test, which is used if we have equal-interval data. They are both very straightforward to calculate, even though they might look a little complicated at first.

Spearman's rank-order correlation test

The Spearman correlation test gives us a statistic known as ρ (the Greek letter 'rho'), which is the name for the correlation coefficient obtained by this test. Carrying out this test is a bit like working through a complex recipe: it's a lot easier if you get everything ready beforehand. What you have to get ready for this test are the columns of data, and then the other columns based on those data.

Like other tests which use ordinal data, the calculations for the test are based on rankings. So the first thing to do is to arrange your pairs of scores in columns, ready to be ranked. I recommend leaving a wide space between them so that you can put the other columns in between. You don't have to do this, but it makes it easier to see where you have got to in your calculations. When you have done this, you are ready to rank each set of scores, separately. If you call the first set of scores variable A, and the second set variable B, this will give you two columns: one set of ranks for A, which you can call R_A and one set of ranks for B, which you might as well call R_B.

When you have done this, you need to find the difference between the ranks, for each pair of scores. Go down the columns, subtracting the R_A figure from the R_B one (or the other way round, if you want). This gives you a column which you should call d, standing for 'the difference between the ranks'.

RULES TO REMEMBER

Brackets mean 'do this first'.

Do smaller brackets before bigger ones.

A number next to another number with no symbol between them means 'multiply these two together'.

A fraction means 'divide the top number by the bottom one'.

Finally, you need another column, which should be called d^2, for reasons which will become obvious. To complete this column take each of your d scores in turn, and square it – that is, multiply it by itself. Put the answer on the same line, in the d^2 column. When this column is completed, you are ready to tackle Formula 18.1.

Sigma, or Σ, as you may recall, means 'add this up'. So Σd^2 means 'add up all the scores in column d^2'. N means the number of pairs of scores in the data set. So you can begin working out the correlation in the same way as always, by putting in numbers instead of the symbols. You can follow Worked Example 18.1 if you like.

Formula 18.1   **The Spearman rank-order correlation test**

$$\rho = 1 - \frac{6\sum d^2}{N(N^2 - 1)}$$

Reminder
N = the number of pairs of scores
d = the differences between the ranks

Worked example 18.1   Spearman's rho test

Begin by setting out the columns you will need.
Rank each set of scores separately

Variable A	R_A	d	d^2	R_B	Variable B
8	6.5	−3	9	3.5	21
7	5	1.5	2.25	6.5	23
9	8.5	−2	4	6.5	23
10	10	0	0	10	26
5	2.5	−1	1	1.5	20
3	1	4	16	5	22
9	8.5	0.5	0.25	9	25
8	6.5	1.5	2.25	8	24
6	4	−2.5	6.25	1.5	20
5	2.5	1	1	3.5	21
			$\sum d^2 = 42$		

Then insert the numbers into the formula:

(1) $\rho = 1 - \dfrac{6 \times 42}{10(10^2 - 1)}$ (4) $\rho = 1 - \dfrac{252}{990}$

(2) $\rho = 1 - \dfrac{252}{10(100 - 1)}$ (5) $\rho = 1 - 0.25$

(3) $\rho = \dfrac{252}{10(99)}$ (6) $\rho = 0.75$

The critical value required for significance at $p \leq .05$ is 0.648 or higher.

Therefore ρ is significant at $p \leq .05$.

What do these three terms mean?

correlation coefficient

ranked data

equal-interval data

The end result of your calculations, then, will be a value of ρ which is somewhere between -1 and $+1$ (if you get any other answer, you've made a mistake somewhere in the calculations). The closer it is to either $+1$ or -1, the stronger your correlation is.

Pearson's product-moment correlation test

The Pearson's product-moment correlation test is the one that we use if we have equal-interval or ratio data. It is a **parametric test**, which uses the means and standard deviations of the data sets in making its comparisons, so it should really only be used if the data fit the three assumptions of parametric tests which we looked at in Chapter 17. It is, however, robust enough to be able to cope if these are not absolutely perfect.

The first step in calculating the Pearson's product-moment correlation test is to arrange your scores into two columns representing the two variables that you are correlating, calling one column X and the other Y. You will then need to calculate three more columns: one called X^2, which you work out by taking each X score and multiplying it by itself; one called Y^2, which you work out by taking each Y score and multiplying it by itself; and one called XY, which you work out by multiplying the X score and the Y score together, for each pair. Once you have calculated these columns, you are ready to tackle Formula 18.2.

Formula 18.2

Pearson's product-moment correlation test

$$r = \frac{N\sum(XY) - \sum X\sum Y}{\sqrt{[N\sum X^2 - (\sum X)^2][N\sum Y^2 - (\sum Y)^2]}}$$

Reminder
$\sum X^2$ means 'add up the X^2 column'.
$(\sum X)^2$ means 'add up the X column, and then multiply the answer by itself'
$\sum Y^2$ means 'add up the Y^2 column'.
$(\sum Y)^2$ means 'add up the Y column, and then multiply the answer by itself'

It looks very complicated. But really, it is much easier than it looks: it's just a matter of dealing with it one bit at a time. Begin by looking at the top line, and putting numbers instead of letters. The first symbol is N, which is the number of pairs of scores in your data. The next is $\sum$, which means 'add this up', and the thing which follows it is

The following list describes variables which might be obtained in psychological research. There are three possibilities:

1. Some variables could only be used for a Spearman's rank-order correlation.

2. Some variables would be suitable for either a Spearman's test and Pearson's product-moment correlation.

3. Some variables would not be suitable for use in a correlation test at all.

Work down the list, deciding which of those three descriptions applies to each variable.

    colour preferences
    estimates of line lengths
    GSR scores
    IQ scores
    measures of pupil dilation
    estimates of degrees of happiness
    membership of different social groups
    observer ratings of aggression
    popularity ratings
    pulse rates
    reaction times
    signs of the zodiac

(XY). So to deal with this bit, we need to add up all of the XY scores (which is why we made a special column for them) and then multiply it by N.

Moving along the line, we come to $\sum X \sum Y$. That means 'the sum of X scores multiplied by the sum of Y scores'. So you need to add up all the scores in the X column, add up all the scores in the Y column, and then multiply those two answers together. When you have done that, you have all the numbers you need for the top line of the equation. The bottom line is similar. You can follow Worked Example 18.2 if you like.

When you have completed your Pearson's product-moment correlation test, you will obtain the correlation coefficient for your data. Again, it will be a number somewhere between −1 and +1, which describes the relationship between the two variables that you were exploring.

Worked example 18.2 Pearson's product-moment test

Begin by setting out the necessary columns, and adding them up:

Variable X	Variable Y	XY	X^2	Y^2
10	19	190	100	361
9	22	198	81	484
7	22	154	49	484
12	24	288	144	576
7	18	126	49	324
8	20	160	64	400
11	23	253	121	529
10	22	220	100	484
8	18	144	64	324
7	19	133	49	361
$\sum X = 89$	$\sum Y = 207$	$\sum XY = 1866$	$\sum X^2 = 821$	$\sum Y^2 = 4327$

Then put the numbers into the formula. Use extra brackets to tell yourself to do some calculations before others.

$$r = \frac{(10 \times 1866) - (89 \times 207)}{\sqrt{[(10 \times 821) - (89^2)] \times [(10 \times 4327) - (207^2)]}}$$

Work out the formula one step at a time, beginning with the small brackets

$$r = \frac{18\,660 - 18\,423}{\sqrt{[8210 - 7921] \times [43\,270 - 42\,849]}}$$

$$r = \frac{237}{\sqrt{289 \times 421}}$$

$$r = \frac{237}{\sqrt{121\,669}}$$

$$r = \frac{237}{348.8}$$

$$r = 0.67$$

The critical value required for significance at $p \leq .05$ is 0.63. Therefore r is significant at $p \leq .05$.

Testing correlations for significance

A correlation coefficient is a descriptive statistic – it describes the relationship between the two variables, without making any inferences about probability. But it is also possible to use correlation tests as inferential statistics, in situations where they investigate predictions about the results. For example, we might conduct a study investigating a possible relationship between students' academic achievement and the amount of exercise they do. In such a case, we would obtain a score for exercise, probably based on some kind of rating scale; and a score for academic achievement, which might be exam results or something similar.

We could make a two-tailed prediction: that there would be a relationship between the two, but that it might be either positive or negative. Or we could make a one-tailed prediction – that students who took more exercise would be likely to do better at examinations (because they were able to control their stress levels better). So once we had conducted the correlation test, we could then check it for significance.

In this case, we would have to use Spearman's test, because data from a rating scale is only ordinal. Table F gives the significance levels which would be obtained from particular correlation coefficients, depending on N, which is how many pairs of scores were used in the test. You can see, though, that Table F only goes up to N values of 30. If you have more pairs than this, it is usually considered that your correlation coefficient will be strong enough to regard it as equivalent to Pearson's r, so you can look up those significance values in Table G instead.

If you look at Table G you can see how the size of the correlation needed for significance changes depending on the number of pairs of scores. The more scores there are, the lower the correlation coefficient needs to be. This is because a small group of scores can be easily influenced by one or two particularly strong ones, giving a large correlation that has still come about as a result of chance or sampling error. But a large set will depend much more on general consistency across the group as a whole, so we can be more certain that the correlation coefficient reflects a real relationship.

The significance table for the Pearson's product-moment correlation, Table G, uses degrees of freedom to express the size of the sample, rather than N. We looked at degrees of freedom in Chapter 17, and the principle here is the same. But because we are dealing with two variables and the relationship between them, the degrees of freedom for this particular test are calculated as $N - 2$.

The coefficient of determination

There is another way of getting an idea of what a correlation coefficient actually implies. It is to look at how much of the variation in the two scores has actually been accounted for by the correlation. This is known as the **coefficient of determination**, and it is calculated, very simply, as r^2: Pearson's coefficient of correlation, multiplied by itself.

We can visualise what the coefficient of determination means by imagining one data set overlapping with another (Figure 18.2). The

---

What do these three terms mean?

inferential statistics

two-tailed prediction

one-tailed prediction

Figure 18.2 The
coefficient of
determination

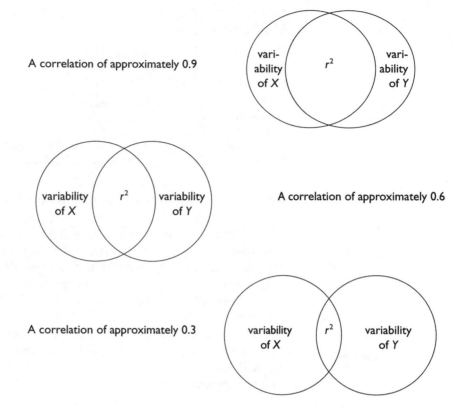

A correlation of approximately 0.9

A correlation of approximately 0.6

A correlation of approximately 0.3

area of overlap represents r^2. If the correlation is large – say, 0.9 or so – then the area of overlap will be large, and we can say that the correlation between the two variables accounts for over 80 per cent of their variability. But if the correlation is smaller, such as 0.6, it accounts for only 36 per cent of the variability, which still leaves 64 per cent unexplained. And if the correlation is 0.3, it accounts for less than 10 per cent of the variability.

This is a useful thing to do, because it reminds us that correlations don't account for everything. A correlation may be significant, but it still may not account for much of the variability in the scores. There is almost always some of the variance unaccounted for, and sometimes this is much more than we realise. Moreover, finding that two things vary together doesn't tell us that one causes the other. It only tells us that they vary together. So we always need to be a bit cautious about the implications that we draw from correlations.

Regression

Correlation, as we have seen, describes the relationship between two variables. Regression is all about using the same type of information for prediction. If we know about a correlation between two variables,

---

RULES TO REMEMBER

Brackets mean 'do this first'.

Do smaller brackets before bigger ones.

A number next to another number with no symbol between them means 'multiply these two together'.

A fraction means 'divide the top number by the bottom one'.

---

we can use the value of a score on one variable to predict the value of a score on the other. There will always be some uncertainty about this, of course – as we have seen, there is always some variability unaccounted for by a correlation. But the higher the correlation is, the more accurate the prediction in a regression analysis can be.

In Chapter 16, we saw how scattergrams can be used to illustrate correlation. We also looked at the idea of a **line of best fit** – a line which is best able to indicate the relationship between the two variables being illustrated (Figure 18.3). When this line has been precisely calculated, it is known as the **regression line**. The regression line is a straight line, indicating the relationship between the first variable, x, and the second variable, y.

Figure 18.3 The regression line

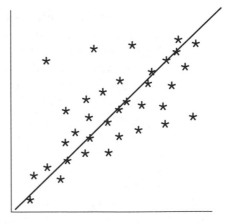

It is possible to perform a linear regression analysis by hand, but it is complex and involves a good knowledge of mathematics; so for the most part it is better to use a computer statistics package. If you are mathematically knowledgeable, and would like to know how to carry it out, one of the best explanations I have found is in Perry Hinton's *Statistics Explained* (1995). But knowing what you are doing when you perform a regression analysis, and why you are doing it, and

EXERCISE 18.2 **Coffee-drinking and exam anxiety**

Caffeine is a drug that acts directly on the central nervous system, and can stimulate physiological arousal. This is also stimulated by anxiety, so a psychologist decided to investigate the relationship between coffee-drinking and exam anxiety.

Coffee-drinking scores were measured according to the average number of cups drunk each day, and anxiety scores were self-ratings on a scale of 0–9.

The study produced the data given in the table below.

Which would be the more suitable correlation test to use with this data?

When you have decided on the appropriate test, use it to work out the correlation between the two sets of scores.

Was the outcome significant?

S	Coffee	Anxiety	S	Coffee	Anxiety
1	3	7	11	14	9
2	5	6	12	5	4
3	2	6	13	7	5
4	8	9	14	4	6
5	4	9	15	18	9
6	6	9	16	5	8
7	2	7	17	8	9
8	2	5	18	3	5
9	9	8	19	0	4
10	6	6	20	1	5

whether it is justified by your data and your research questions, is enough for most psychologists.

What a linear regression analysis is doing, then, is finding the exact value of the 'line of best fit', and using that to make predictions about particular scores. There is uncertainty in this, as I said before. In a perfect correlation, all of the scores will fall along the line of best fit, so that knowing one of the scores means you can predict, with certainty, what the other score in that pair will be. But as we have seen, most correlations are not perfect. So there will be some error – some deviation from the line – which makes the prediction of scores more of a matter of probability than of certainty. And the weaker the correlation, the more error there will be.

What do these three terms mean?

degrees of freedom

coefficient of determination

regression line

The regression line minimises the amount of error as much as possible. We can use a regression line to make predictions about scores – to say 'if the value of the x score is such-and-such, then the value of the y score is likely to be . . .'. We can even do this for scores which didn't form part of the original data-set. By tracing the regression line further, we can look at larger or smaller values of x, and use them to predict the value of y. So, if we were doing a regression analysis in our research about exercise and academic achievement, we could predict an academic outcome for someone who did much more, or much less, exercise than our particular research participants had done.

It is here that the value of regression analysis lies. By allowing us to make predictions about scores which weren't actually included in the original study, we can go beyond our limited sample data, and begin to make general observations about the population as a whole. But we do need to know how useful our predictions really are, and it is here that the **coefficient of determination** comes into play. This measure, as we saw, shows how much variability is accounted for by a particular correlation. But we can also use it to tell us how valuable an x score is, as a predictor of a y score. A high coefficient of determination tells us how certain we can be about the prediction we are making, while a low one tells us that knowing x might not actually tell us very much about y.

Linear regression, then, is a way of using correlation data to make predictions which are beyond the scope of the data-set which we originally obtained. But we can also use it as a way of exploring several different correlations at a time. This process is known as **multiple regression**.

Multiple regression

One of the great differences which computers have made to psychology, and to all of the social sciences, is that they have made multivariate analysis very much more common than it used to be. Up until now, we have explored the kind of statistics which deal with just one or two variables. These can be carried out by hand fairly easily, which is why I have included worked examples. But statistical analyses which deal with several different variables are much more complex, and if we are also dealing with large samples, then computers are really the only practical way of conducting them.

Like everything else, this has its bad side and its good side. On the bad side, it is very easy to shove a lot of numbers into a computer and conduct an analysis which is really much too complex for the data, getting results which appear to be very accurate and precise, but which actually have very little meaning. GIGO – 'Garbage In, Garbage Out' – has been the watchword of computing ever since computers were first invented. No matter how technical or sophisticated your analysis, if your data are only rough approximations, or your measuring scale is irrational, then what you will end up with will be nonsense.

The good side, though, is that making this kind of analysis more possible has enabled psychologists to deal much more fully with the complexities of human beings. Using statistics which can only explore one variable at a time inevitably encourages researchers to investigate one variable at a time, but just about everything that people do is more complex than that. We are often influenced by many factors, working together; and human events often have several causes, not just one. So we need to be able to analyse research data in ways which can show us how several variables interact, as well as being able to look at the influence of single variables. For the rest of this chapter, and the next one, we will be looking at multivariate statistical techniques, beginning with those methods which deal with correlational data.

What do these three terms mean?

multivariate analysis

GIGO

partial correlation

Partial correlation

Partial correlation is a way of exploring how the various relationships between variables can connect with one another. Quite often, we find that a topic we are exploring has more than one factor which seems to influence it – or at least, which correlates with it. But those factors also influence one another, so if we want to sort out the true relationships between them, we need to find a way of dealing with the overlap.

Let's take an example. Suppose we were interested in looking at sporting achievement. We conduct some research and find that high-achieving sportspeople tend to have high levels of achievement motivation. That seems to be a fairly straightforward correlation. But we also find that it isn't the whole story, since achievement also correlates with the amount of training that they do. So that gives us two variables: motivation and training, correlating with a third variable of sporting achievement.

The problem, though, is that these variables overlap with one another. For example, the amount of training someone does is affected to some degree by how strongly they are motivated. So some part of the correlation between training and achievement will come from that. If we want to understand what sort of a contribution training on its own makes to sporting achievement, we need to find a way of separating

Figure 18.4 Partial
correlations

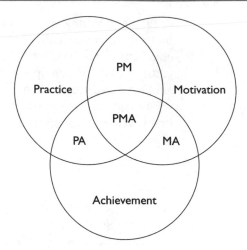

the effects of the other variable from the correlation. In statistical terms, this separation is referred to as **partialling out** the unwanted variables.

Figure 18.4 illustrates the kind of overlap between variables that we are talking about. Supposing our interest is in the influence of motivation on achievement. Some of the correlation just concerns those two variables. But part of it is also influenced by a third variable, training. We sort out the effects of the unwanted variable by performing a **partial correlation** – that is, a correlation which has been reduced down just to that part which is uninfluenced by the other variables. By calculating a partial correlation, we can find out just how important a single variable is, even when it is operating in conjunction with several other variables.

It is possible to calculate partial correlations by hand, but in reality, it is almost certain that you would want to use a computer to analyse research data using these types of calculations. Partial correlations are almost always used as part of a more complex multivariate analysis, and there is absolutely no need for most people using these tools to be able to do them by hand, when computers can do them perfectly well. Think of it as the difference between using a hand drill and an electric drill. It's possible to put up a set of shelves using a hand drill, but it's very hard work, and an electric drill makes it all much simpler. Even with an electric drill, though, you need to measure accurately and use the drill appropriately. The same applies to statistics: you do have to know what you are doing and why, and you have to have obtained proper measurements beforehand.

A partial correlation, then, is a way of distinguishing the effects of just one variable from a whole lot of others, even when they seem to be all jumbled up together. It's a useful technique in its own right, but it also forms the basis of another statistical technique we can use with correlational data: multiple regression.

Multiple regression

We saw earlier how a regression analysis allows us to predict one variable from the other. If we know the score of one particular value, we can use the regression line to calculate the probable value of the other, and we can use the coefficient of determination to express the amount of confidence we can have in this prediction. To put this in statistical terms, we use one set of scores, X, as the independent variable, and then use them to predict Y, the dependent variable.

Sometimes, though, we encounter a situation where what we are interested in actually depends on more than one variable. Foster (1993) gives the example of job satisfaction. Imagine that we have conducted research investigating the variables which seem to be associated with job satisfaction. We have found that the level of the job shows a positive correlation, and so does level of pay. Ordinary correlation tests tell us the correlation coefficient for each of these variables. But we may also want to know just how much of the variation in job satisfaction is accounted for by these two factors combined. To find this out, we would perform a multiple regression, taking job satisfaction as the dependent variable (which we call Y), and the other two factors as independent variables, which we call X_1 and X_2.

What do these three terms mean?
multiple regression
correlation matrix
eyeball test

The multiple regression analysis looks at each of those variables, and the way that they interact, in order to find their combined influence on the dependent variable. In order to do this, it looks at the original correlation coefficients, the coefficients of determination, and several other aspects of the data. It also carries out partial correlations, in order to correct for any of the variables overlapping, and to avoid counting the same variance twice.

It's a complex calculation, but you wouldn't be expected to calculate a multiple regression by hand. The arithmetic becomes very complicated – and in any case, that's what computers are for. But you are expected to know when and under what circumstances you would want to use a multiple regression, and how to choose the variables you are regressing. If you do want to understand the detailed mathematics of a multiple regression, Hinton (1995) gives a very clear and thorough explanation.

The first step in conducting a multiple regression, even by computer, is always to look at your data and decide which of the several factors you are investigating is your dependent variable. The dependent variable in this context is the one you are interested in: the one which is (or may be) affected by the other factors. Once you have identified your dependent variable, you then identify which of the other variables you are interested in.

Incidentally, it's important to remember that the terms 'independent variable' and 'dependent variable' are used slightly differently from the way that they are used in experimental design. There, they refer to specific variables in an experiment, which have been manipulated in a particular way. In statistical analysis, though, and particularly in multiple regression, the actual variables of the study aren't important. What is important are the sets of scores you are looking at and in what way. So you can call a set of scores the independent variable even if it was obtained in a correlation study.

Sometimes it is obvious which variables you want to include in your analysis. Sometimes, too, the theory that you are investigating will tell you which variables you must include. But sometimes, it isn't so easy to see which ones look most promising. For example, if you have conducted a questionnaire study which has explored several different aspects of the topic, you may want to leave some of the least significant variables out of the analysis, and just concentrate on the ones which seem as though they will account for most of the variation.

In a situation like that, often the best strategy is to get the computer to print out a **correlation matrix**, which shows you how all of the variables that you are analysing correlate with one another (Figure 18.5). You can look through the matrix to locate the dependent variable that you have identified, and it will show you which of the other variables correlate with it most highly. This 'eyeball test' is very useful for identifying relevant variables for a multiple regression.

Figure 18.5 A correlation matrix

Variables	A	B	C	D	E
A	1.0				
B	0.002	1.0			
C	0.84	0.12	1.0		
D	0.37	0.28	0.36	1.0	
E	0.04	0.03	0.17	0.63	1.0

You can include as many variables in a regression analysis as you like (or as your computer's statistics package will bear), but there are disadvantages in including too many. One of them is that you need to have a clear rationale for including each one, and 'it seemed like a good idea at the time' isn't really one which earns you many marks.

Another is the fact that you will need to be able to explain clearly what your findings actually mean, and if you have included too many different variables in your analysis, this could get tricky.

Once you have conducted your regression analysis, you will end up with a computer printout that will give you a general score, known as the **multiple R**. This is the combined correlation of the variables that you have chosen. The printout will also give you R^2, which tells you how much of the variation in your dependent variable can be explained by these variables. And it will usually give you an adjusted R^2 as well, which is an estimate of how these calculations would work in the population as a whole – in other words, which corrects for the fact that you have only obtained a sample of the population and not measured all of it.

Your printout will also give you a breakdown of the amount that each variable contributed to the regression as a whole, and whether its contribution was significant or not. And it will perform an **analysis of variance** to compare the variation which has been identified by this multiple regression, and the leftover, 'residual' variation which is still unaccounted for. We will be looking at analysis of variance in the next chapter, so I won't go into the technical details now; but this analysis of variance will let you know just how significant the variance identified by your multiple regression was.

A multiple regression, as we have seen, can handle just about any number of variables, but if you are analysing a piece of research that you have just carried out, bear in mind that you will always need to understand the result that comes out of the computer. You need to be very clear about your dependent variable, and clear about which of the independent variables you have been investigating, and why. In the next chapter, we will be looking at another statistical test which can deal with several variables at once. The same caution applies to that one, too.

Self-assessment questions

1. *What does a correlation coefficient tell us about the relationship between two variables?*

2. *In what sense is a correlation coefficient both descriptive and inferential?*

3. *What circumstances would result in the choice of a Spearman's rank-order correlation test rather than a Pearson's product-moment test?*

4. *What does the coefficient of determination tell us about the strength of a correlation?*

5. *When would you be likely to use a multiple regression?*

Concepts in use

Which type of test would be most suitable to use for the following tasks?

1. *Comparing measures of body temperature taken during the day with self-ratings of how alert the person felt at the time.*

2. *Comparing the speed of an athlete's reaction time with their heart rate at the same moment.*

3. *Sorting out how much of an overlap there is between reading practice and parental involvement in learning to read.*

4. *Looking at the influence that time spent driving and complexity of traffic might have on driving errors.*

5. *Comparing average daytime temperatures and sales of lettuce in shops.*

19

Analysis of variance

F ratio
One-way ANOVA
Making sense of ANOVA results
Two-way ANOVA tests
Afterword

In Chapter 17, we looked at the *t* test, which provides us with a parametric method for exploring the differences between two sets of scores. The *t* test, as we saw in that chapter, works by comparing the means and the standard deviations of the two groups. If the means seem similar, and the standard deviations overlap, then the test concludes that the two sets of scores are likely to have come from the same population. But if they seem very different, the test statistic tells us that they are likely to have come from different populations.

The only problem with the *t* test – or the main one, anyway – is that it can only deal with two sets of scores at a time. Quite often in modern research, we find that we are actually dealing with several sets of scores, and not just two. Sometimes, this is because we are looking at several different categories of one variable, like having three or four age groups in the study, rather than just two. Sometimes it is because we want to look at the effect of more than one variable at a time. For example, there are many more mature students doing degrees nowadays, and so if we were looking at study skills, we might want to take both age and IQ as variables to be investigated, rather than just looking at one of them on its own.

It's possible, of course, to look at these results by doing lots of different *t* tests. But that has a number of disadvantages. One of them is that it is clumsy, and gets even more so the more variables we include. But a more important one is that doing several tests affects the probabilities. If a test comes out as significant at the level of $p < .05$, that means that the result we have obtained is likely to come about because of chance one time in twenty. What this implies is that if we did twenty tests, then we would be very likely to get these findings by

What do these three terms mean?

parametric statistics

test statistic

Type I error

chance, at least once. This would lead us to a Type I error – rejecting the null hypothesis when in fact it is true. So doing two or more tests on the same data increases the probability of actually hitting that one time in twenty, and getting a Type I error.

What we need to use is a single test which can do the same sort of task as the *t* test, but which can deal with several different conditions or variables at a time. This test is known as the **Analysis of Variance**, or **ANOVA** for short. ANOVA works in much the same way as the *t* test. It looks at means, and how the scores are spread about the mean, and uses that information to judge whether the sets of scores are likely to have come from the same population, or whether they are more likely to have come from different populations. The difference is that ANOVA can deal with a lot more variables at a time.

Essentially, all ANOVA does is compare the means of the various sets of scores to see if they are different enough to have come from different populations. But just looking at the mean on its own wouldn't be enough. If you look back to Chapter 17, and in particular to Figures 17.2 and 17.3, you will see how a difference between the means of two sets of scores might imply that the scores come from separate populations, but it could also imply that they actually come from the same population. The *t* test addresses this problem by looking at how the scores vary around the mean, as well as looking at the mean itself. If the two sets of data overlap a great deal, they could easily have come from the same population. If the variation is small, and there isn't much overlap, that becomes less likely. And that smaller likelihood is reflected in the value of *t* which is obtained from the test.

The *F* ratio

What do these three terms mean?

null hypothesis

groups

factors

Analysis of variance does the same thing. It looks at the means of the data sets (which it refers to as **groups**), and sees how different they are from one another. But it also looks at the variation of scores within each data set, so that it knows what kind of differences should be expected just from random variation or individual differences. By comparing these two kinds of variation – the differences between the means of the data sets, and the variation of scores within the data sets – it provides us with a statistic which we can use to identify whether there are significant differences in the data. That statistic is known as the **variance ratio**, or sometimes the ***F* ratio**, because we use the capital letter *F* to refer to it.

F is called the variance *ratio* because it expresses the ratio between the two different types of variation in the data (see Figure 19.1). It does this by dividing the between-groups variation by the within-groups variation:

$$F = \frac{\text{between-groups variation}}{\text{within-groups variation}}$$

The **between-groups variation** in the formula is the differences between the means in the various data sets. What the F test is looking for is systematic variation between those means – steady variation, which implies that the groups really have come from different populations. But it can only find that sort of systematic variation if it rules out the confounding effect which is produced by the fact that the scores have been obtained from living beings and not robots, so they vary within the groups as well.

Figure 19.1 Between- and within-group variation

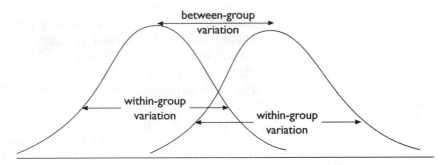

The **within-groups variation** is the variation that we always get within any set of scores. Sometimes this variation is known as the **error variation**, which doesn't mean that it always comes from people making mistakes. It includes those, but it also just means everyday variation caused by random factors or individual differences. ANOVA looks at the within-groups variation, as a whole, and takes that into account when it is looking at how different the means are.

I have been using the term 'variation' here, but what analysis of variance actually uses is the term in its name – the **variance**. We looked at variance in Chapter 15, and if you have forgotten what it is all about, it would be a very good idea to go back and reread that part of the chapter. In summary, though, the variance is a measure of dispersion, like the standard deviation – in other words, it is a way of describing how the scores are scattered around a mean. Mathematically, it is the square of the standard deviation, so we tend to refer to it in writing as s^2.

So if we want to be absolutely accurate in our description of F, we should phrase it like this:

$$\text{variance ratio } (F) = \frac{\text{between-conditions variance}}{\text{error variance}}$$

This is very similar to the way that the t test involves comparing the difference between the means of the two groups, and dividing it by

> **What do these three terms mean?**
>
> *variables*
>
> *between-groups variation*
>
> *within-groups variation*

their standard deviations. They are mathematically related, too, because in numerical terms, F is actually t^2. That similarity isn't just coincidence. As we have seen, analysis of variance and the t test both work in much the same way: they both involve comparing means and taking variance into account. It's just that ANOVA is able to deal with far more conditions and variables.

Using analysis of variance

There is very little need, nowadays, to calculate analysis of variance by hand. If you carry out a study which requires analysis of variance, you should perform the analysis by computer. Doing so leaves much less room for error, and will save you a lot of pointless number-crunching. But you do need to know, in general terms what the computer has done; and you also need to know how to interpret the result.

The most important thing about using ANOVA, whether you calculate it by hand or by computer, is getting to grips with the technical terms. These are important, because you can get lost if you are not sure what's what. I will make sure that they are explained as we go on through this chapter: try not to feel intimidated by them, because it is only a matter of getting used to them.

You may remember from the last chapter that the way that statisticians use the terms 'independent variable' and 'dependent variable' is slightly different from the way that they are used in research methodology. In statistics, as in methodology, the dependent variable is the thing which changes – the measure which provides the scores. But the term 'independent variable' is used more flexibly, to mean one of the types of influence on the scores that we are looking at. In analysis of variance, each of these types of influence is known as a **factor**.

For example, if we were looking at the effects of age and IQ on academic achievement, our dependent variable would be achievement, and measures of achievement would provide the scores for the analysis. We would be interested in two kinds of influence on those scores: one being age, and the other being IQ. We would be looking to see whether the two factors, or independent variables, of age and IQ were influencing our dependent variable of achievement. In another study, we might be interested in age and consumer choice. In that case, we might only have one independent variable, that of age, which we would be exploring to see if it seemed to influence the dependent variable, that of consumer choice. There would be just one factor in that particular analysis of variance.

Even if we only have one factor, though, we can have several different **conditions**. We might have five or six different age groups in our study, for example. Each age group would represent a different

---

What do these three terms mean?

dependent variable

independent variable

degrees of freedom

condition of the independent variable. So we could still end up ana-lysing several different sets of data, even if we only had one factor. In the study of the effects of age and IQ on academic achievement, we would have two factors, as we have seen. But each factor might have several different conditions, because we might like to investigate several different age groups, and several different categories of IQ.

The type of ANOVA we do depends on how many factors we have in our study. If we were looking at something like consumer choice and age, we would have only one factor, age, and so we would perform what is called a **one-way analysis of variance**. In that test, we would be looking for variation between the different age groups – in other words, between the different conditions of a single factor. If we were looking at the influence of age and IQ, we would say we were doing a **two-way analysis of variance**, because we would be looking at the varia-tion produced by two factors (the number of conditions is irrelevant). With five factors, it would be a five-way ANOVA, with three factors we would carry out a three-way ANOVA, and so on.

There isn't really any limit to the number of factors or categories you can have in an analysis of variance, except limitations in com-puting power and limitations in comprehending the implications of the findings. It is an unusual human who can calculate more than a simple three-way ANOVA by hand, without getting lost; but there really is no need to do such a thing anyway. That's what computers are for. Computers usually have an upper limit in the thousands, but if you had a thousand, or even a hundred factors in your analysis, it would be very hard to make sense out of the final result. There's not much point doing an analysis which is so complicated that you don't know what you have found at the end of it!

In this chapter, I will assume that if you want to do ANOVAs you will use a computer. If you really feel you need to do them by hand, look in Greene and d'Oliveira (1999). Here, our exploration of ANOVA will look at general principles, and at the kinds of results you would get from a computer analysis, and not deal with calculation by hand.

One-way analysis of variance

It may seem odd, but the best place to begin if you want to understand what is going on with an analysis of variance is with the final result. When you have completed an analysis of variance, you don't just end up with a single figure. That may be OK for tests which are simply comparing two samples, but when we have several variables being explored, we need more information than that. Instead of a single figure, the results of an ANOVA are presented in a table. Figure 19.2

Figure 19.2 A typical ANOVA table

Source	Degrees of freedom	Sum of squares	Mean squares	F ratio	Probability
Between groups	2	1496.52	748.26	8.65	0.02
Within groups	12	1038.33	86.53		
Total	14	1534.84			

shows a typical table for a one-way analysis of variance for independent measures. It may look complicated, but actually it isn't as bad as it seems.

The way to look at this table is to begin from the right-hand side. The extreme right-hand column is the **probability** of the null hypothesis being true, which should be a familiar concept by now. To regard our results as significant, we want the figure in this column to be lower than the chosen significance level, which is usually $p < .05$ but might vary (see Chapter 14). The second column, reading from the right, gives the value of the **variance ratio**, F, which should also be familiar if you have read this far.

The third column, reading from the right, is headed 'Mean squares'. The term **mean square** is actually just another term for **variance**, and it means exactly the same thing. It just happens to be what variance is called when we are calculating ANOVAs, that's all. You can see that the table contains two mean square values, one for 'Between groups', and one for 'Within groups'. We have already seen how the F ratio is the between-groups variance divided by the within-groups variance, and here it is again. If you divide the lower mean square value in that column into the higher one, you will reach the value of F which is given in the next column.

The fourth column from the right (second from left) is headed 'Sums of squares'. This is the column which tells you how variable the group scores are. A **sum of squares** describes whether a set of scores are clustered tightly around the mean, or whether they are spread out broadly. When we are doing an analysis of variance, we have to calculate sums of squares separately for each data set, which is why it can get so complicated to do by hand. The final table, though, just gives us three sums of squares figures: a between-groups sum of squares, a within-groups sum of squares, and one for the scores as a whole. We use these, together with the degrees of freedom, to calculate the mean squares.

The fifth column in the table, reading from the right, or the first one if you read it in the normal way, describes the **degrees of freedom** in the data. (We looked at degrees of freedom in Chapter 17, so if you have forgotten what they are look back at that chapter to refresh your memory.) Again, it gives you three measures: the between-groups degrees of freedom; the within-groups degrees of freedom, and the degrees of freedom for the total. This column, together with the next one, gives the information that is used to calculate the mean squares. The formula is:

$$MS = \frac{\text{sum of squares}}{\text{degrees of freedom}}$$

The formula is actually used twice – once using the between-groups sums of squares and degrees of freedom, and once using the within-groups sums of squares and degrees of freedom. When each one has been calculated, it gives you the result in the next column.

You can see, then, that the ANOVA table of results gives you quite a lot of information. Reading from left to right, it gives you the degrees of freedom and the sums of squares for the variation between groups, within groups and the total. These are used to calculate the between- and within-groups mean squares, which are given in the next column, and they in turn are used to calculate the variance ratio. The final column gives the probability of those findings happening by chance, or through sampling error.

One-way ANOVA for repeated measures

The example we have just looked at was an analysis of variance for independent measures – in other words, when we have scores from different people in the different conditions. If you have the same people in the various conditions of the study, the analysis of variance looks a little bit different. This is because the independent-measures ANOVA includes both individual differences and experimental errors in its assessment of within-group variance.

When we add up all the scores in each group, to find the total or between-groups sums of squares, each group represents scores from different people. So part of the reason those totals are different lies in the individual differences between the different groups. It all adds up to errors, which is why the independent-measures ANOVA described the within-groups sum of squares as the error sum of squares.

But if we have a repeated-measures design, each group's data have come from the same people. So those scores are likely to be much more similar than ones which have come from an independent-measures design. When the differences between the various data sets are small, then the within-groups variance will be small too. But you can see, I hope, that a small variance from an independent-measures design doesn't mean the same thing as a small variance from a repeated-measures design. The variance from a repeated-measures design might be small purely because it wasn't influenced by individual differences so much.

Having a small within-groups variance for this reason would exaggerate the final F ratio, making it larger than it should be. As we saw earlier, the F ratio is worked out by dividing the between-groups variance by the within-groups variance. So we need to do something about it. This means that ANOVA for repeated measures needs to distinguish more clearly between the within-group variance and the variance which is due to error. It does this by using two extra sums of squares.

One of the new sum of squares represents the variation between the subjects themselves – in other words, the variation between the rows in the data sets. By doing this, the ANOVA for repeated measures is able to get a measure of individual differences. It then uses that measure to calculate the second sum of squares, which represents the amount of variation which is just due to error, and not individual differences. So it ends up with five sums of squares, not three: the total sum of squares (SS_{total}), the between-groups sum of squares ($SS_{betw.cond}$), the within-group sum of squares ($SS_{with.cond}$), the between-subjects sum of squares ($SS_{betw.sub}$), and the error sum of squares (SS_{error}).

> **What do these three terms mean?**
>
> *pairwise comparisons*
>
> *repeated measures*
>
> *mixed conditions*

Making sense of ANOVA results

It's all very well calculating a one-way analysis of variance, but we also need to know how to make sense of the results, once we have got them. Just finding that the F ratio is significant doesn't actually tell us very much. In a study with three conditions, for example, it might mean that all of those conditions were significantly different from one another. But it might not. It might mean that two of them were actually very similar, and only one of them was significantly different. So after we have done an ANOVA, we need to find out what that F ratio actually means.

To do that, we need to perform another test. There are several tests which can be used to find out the implications of a particular ANOVA. They are known, collectively, as **post-hoc tests**, which means tests that we carry out after the event – in other words, after we have done the ANOVA. The test we choose to use, as ever, depends on what we actually want to know; but there are several options available.

The t test

Sometimes all we want to know is whether there is a significant difference between two particular conditions. We can look at that using a straightforward t test, calculated in just the same way as the repeated-measures t test in Chapter 17. The value of t that we obtain will tell us how likely it is that the difference between the two conditions we are interested in could have been obtained purely as a result of sampling error or chance.

As we saw earlier, though, performing more than one t test on the same data increases our chances of making a Type I error. So we can't use the t test if we are interested in the differences between more than one pair of conditions. Instead, there is a special test we can use to make **pairwise comparisons** – that is, to look at the various pairs of conditions in the data. It is known as the Tukey HSD test.

The Tukey HSD test

The HSD in the Tukey test's name stands for 'honestly significant differences', and this should give you an idea of what the test is all about. It is a way of identifying which pairs of conditions in the ANOVA data are the significant ones. It does this by looking at the group means, and particularly at the difference between them. The Tukey test is a slightly conservative test, which means that it is pretty strict about identifying significance, and that reduces your chance of making a Type I error – of assuming that you have found a significant result when you haven't really.

The way that the Tukey test works is by calculating a minimum difference between the group means. That minimum difference is what

---

EXERCISE 19.1   **Understanding ANOVA symbolism**

List A gives a number of common ANOVA symbols. List B gives their definitions. Match up the two lists.

List A	List B
F	the within-groups mean square
SS_{total}	between-groups degrees of freedom
$SS_{with.cond}$	the total sum of squares
MS	the variation ratio
N	the scores
$SS_{betw.cond}$	the within-group sum of squares
$SS_{betw.sub}$	between-groups sum of squares
df_{betw}	the number of scores
MS_{error}	the mean square
X	the between-subjects sum of squares

you need to obtain, in order to conclude that there is a real ('honest') significant difference between two groups in the analysis. Once you have calculated your Tukey HSD statistic, you can simply look at pairs of conditions that you are interested in, and see whether the differences between their means are larger than the HSD figure or not. Incidentally, 'larger' in this case means larger in absolute value. It doesn't matter whether the difference between the means is positive or negative – the Tukey test treats all differences as if they were positive.

The Scheffé test

Sometimes we are not interested in the differences between particular pairs of conditions, but in the differences between one set of conditions and another set. For example, if we had conducted a study of consumer behaviour, which looked at the amount of money spent on recorded music by people in six different age groups, we would want to know if there were significant differences between pairs of age groups, and for that we would use the Tukey test.

But we would also probably want to know whether there were significant differences between groups of scores – say, between older and younger people. Our definition of 'older' might involve combining three different conditions, and so might our definition of 'younger'. Alternatively, we might want to look at 'young' and 'old' people. We might approach that by calling the two youngest categories 'young', and the two oldest categories 'old', and completely ignoring the categories in the middle.

A Tukey test wouldn't be any help in that situation. Instead, we would need to use a Scheffé test. Where the Tukey test is used for pairwise comparisons, the Scheffé test is used for complex comparisons – comparisons which involve combinations of different conditions. It does this by calculating a new value of F, which relates just to the combination of factors that we are interested in. If the value of F that we obtained by doing our Scheffé test is higher than the one we have just worked out, then we are able to say that the difference between those groups of conditions is significant.

There are several other tests which can be used for post-hoc analysis of a one-way ANOVA. However, these three – the t test, the Tukey test, and the Scheffé test – will give you as much as you need to get on with your own analysis most of the time. They can be found in most computer statistics packages which deal with ANOVA, generally under the heading 'post-hoc'. As with so much else when we reach this level of analysis, there's very little point in trying to do them by hand – the machine might as well do them for you. It's what machines are for.

What do these three terms mean?

one-way ANOVA

two-way ANOVA

post-hoc tests

Two-way analysis of variance

The examples we have looked at so far concern analysis of variance which involves just one factor, with several different conditions. But ANOVAs really come into their own when we are doing more complicated research which involves more than one factor. The reason for this is that they are able to look not just at the influence of each of the factors, but also at whether the two factors are interacting with one another.

Figure 19.3 ANOVA without interaction

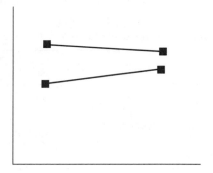

In Chapter 16, we looked at the interaction diagrams which are associated with two-way analysis of variance. These are summary diagrams which show how the two factors interact with one another, and they can take several different forms. If you have conducted a two-way analysis of variance it's useful to draw one up, because it does show some of the most important aspects of your results at a glance. It may show, for example, that there is no interaction at all in your data, as shown in Figure 19.3. Or your diagram may show that the two factors do interact with one another, as shown in Figure 19.4. Both types of illustration – interaction or no interaction – are useful if we are to understand what research data really means.

Figure 19.4 ANOVA with interaction

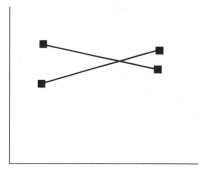

If you are actually conducting a two-way analysis of variance, as I have said repeatedly, it is a good idea to use a computer. Guidance for calculating ANOVAs by hand is given in Hinton (1995), if you really feel you need to do this; but computer analysis is much more practical. What you do need to be very clear about before you begin, though, is the nature of your data. It needs to be equal-interval, as we saw right at the beginning of this section; and you need to be very clear about which data set belongs to which factor, and which condition of that factor. The computer will ask you for this information. So the best thing is to be prepared by laying your data out in a summary sheet which shows the groups very clearly. Figure 19.5 gives an example of how you might do this.

Figure 19.5 Preparing data for ANOVA

An exploration of training systems and diet on sporting performance

TRAINING	DIET		
	No change	New diet A	New diet B
Spaced practice	5	6	4
	9	10	8
	8	6	5
	3	5	12
	4	4	11
Massed practice	4	3	9
	8	10	8
	10	5	4
	11	6	3
	8	7	9

When you have conducted your ANOVA, the computer will give you a summary table, much like the ones you construct for a one-way ANOVA. But it has some important differences. We will begin by looking at the two-way ANOVA summary table for an independent-measures design, which is shown in Figure 19.6.

As you can see, it is very much like the one-way ANOVA table for independent measures. It gives the probability for the first factor, factor A, and the probability for the second factor, factor B. But it also gives a probability for the interaction between the two. In order to calculate this, it obtained a measure of within-conditions error, so that is included in the table as well. If you are familiar with the one-way ANOVA tables, you shouldn't have too much trouble reading this one.

There are two other kinds of two-way analysis of variance. There is, of course, the two-way ANOVA for repeated measures. And there is the two-way ANOVA for mixed conditions, which is when we have independent measures for one factor, and repeated measures for

Figure 19.6 Summary table for a two-way independent-measures ANOVA

Source of variation	Degrees of freedom	Sums of squares	Mean squares	Variance ratio (F)	Probability
Factor A	df_A	SS_A	MS_A	F_A	p_A
Factor B	df_B	SS_B	MS_B	F_B	p_B
Interaction (A × B)	$df_{(A \times B)}$	$SS_{A \times B}$	$MS_{A \times B}$	$F_{A \times B}$	$p_{A \times B}$
Error (within conditions)	$df_{(error)}$	SS_{error}			
Total	$df_{(total)}$	$SS_{(total)}$			

Source: adapted from Hinton (1995).

the other. We will look at the repeated-measures two-way ANOVA table first.

A repeated-measures ANOVA, as you will remember, has the same participants in each condition. We found when we were looking at one-way ANOVAs that this made them slightly more complex, because they needed to separate out the subject effects from other sources of error. This extra complexity is still there with the two-way ANOVA, as you can see from Figure 19.7. It has the familiar elements: the

Figure 19.7 Summary table for a two-way repeated-measures ANOVA

Source of variation	Degrees of freedom	Sums of squares	Mean square	Variance ratio (F)	Probability
Factor A	df_A	SS_A	MS_A	F_A	p_A
Factor B	df_B	SS_B	MS_B	F_B	p_B
Subjects S	df_S	SS_S	(MS_S)	(F_S)	(p_S)
Factor A × B	$df_{(A \times B)}$	$SS_{A \times B}$	$MS_{A \times B}$	$F_{A \times B}$	$p_{A \times B}$
Error for A (A × S)	df_{errorA}	SS_{errorA}	MS_{errorA}		
Error for B (B × S)	df_{errorB}	SS_{errorB}	MS_{errorB}		
Error for A × B (A × B × S)	$df_{errorAB}$	$SS_{errorAB}$	$MS_{errorAB}$		
Total	$df_{(total)}$	$SS_{(total)}$			

Source: adapted from Hinton (1995).

probability for factor A, that for factor B, and that for the interaction between the two, in the same way as the independent-measures two-way ANOVA had. But it also gives the probability for the subject variance, and it gives three separate sets of errors, each of which includes the influence from the subjects in the study. These are the error for factor A, the error for factor B, and the error for the inter-action between them.

It may look more complicated, but if you have got this far, you should be able to interpret these results as well. If you don't remem-ber what they mean, look back at the one-way ANOVA for repeated measures. It's exactly the same apart from the fact that it takes the interaction between the two variables into account. But the way we interpret the table is very similar.

The two-way ANOVA for mixed conditions happens more often than you might think, particularly in experimental research. For example, you might be interested in the way that age and practice affect skill learning. Your dependent variable would be the measure of skill learn-ing that you used; and one of the independent variables would be age. For that, you would use an independent-measures design, unless you had a remarkable degree of patience. But you would be likely to use a repeated-measures design for the different practice conditions, because an independent-measures design would introduce too many problems of individual differences. So you would end up with one independent-measures factor and one repeated-measures factor.

The results table for this type of ANOVA, which is known as a **mixed-design ANOVA**, is illustrated in Figure 19.8. As you can see,

Figure 19.8 Summary table for a two-way mixed-design ANOVA

Source of variation	Degrees of freedom	Sums of squares	Mean squares	Variance ratio (F)	Probability
Factor A	df_A	SS_A	MS_A	F_A	p_A
Error for A	df_{errorA}	SS_{errorA}	MS_{errorA}		
Factor B	df_B	SS_B	MS_B	F_B	p_B
Factor A × B	$df_{(A×B)}$	$SS_{A×B}$	$MS_{A×B}$	$F_{A×B}$	$p_{A×B}$
Error for B & A × B (B × AS)	df_{errorB}	SS_{errorB}	MS_{errorB}		
Error for A × B (A × B × S)	$df_{errorAB}$	$SS_{errorAB}$	$MS_{errorAB}$		
Total	$df_{(total)}$	$SS_{(total)}$			

Source: adapted from Hinton (1995).

it combines some features from the independent-measures ANOVA and some from the repeated-measures ANOVA. When you are putting the data for a mixed-design ANOVA into the computer, remember that the independent-measures factor is the one which comes first – in this case, factor A. The table, as you can see, gives an error for that factor which includes the effect of subjects. It gives the probabilities for factor A, factor B and the interaction between them, as you would expect; but it combines the error for B and the interaction into one figure. There are technical reasons for this, which are to do with the nature of the calculations and I don't propose to go into them here. If you are really interested, check out Hinton (1995) or Greene and d'Oliveira (1999).

As with the one-way ANOVA, there are post-hoc tests that you can conduct on the data to find out some more specific information about your findings. Again, I wouldn't recommend doing these by hand. If you have got this far, it is a relatively straightforward matter to carry out one of these tests by computer, and they are likely to be much more accurate than you would be.

The most important thing of all in this type of analysis is being very clear about where your data have come from and what the factors and conditions are. As long as you understand that, you shouldn't have any trouble interpreting the results of your analysis, or dealing with the computer printout. If you haven't got that clear from the start, it's unlikely that you will be able to make much sense of the result. Remember – 'Garbage In, Garbage Out'!

Afterword

This brings us to the end of our exploration of psychological research methods. As you have seen, the psychologist's tool-kit is a rich and varied one, which spans a tremendously wide range of methods and analytical techniques. You'll also have seen, I hope, that what is important is choosing the right tool for the job. Some types of data lend themselves to certain types of analysis and not others; some kinds of research question can be investigated more effectively using particular research methods.

A psychologist – or any social scientist, for that matter – needs to be able to draw on a wide range of methodological and analytical 'tools' because of the enormous complexity of our subject matter. Human beings are complex and multi-faceted, and never simple. We can focus on just one facet of human behaviour for research purposes, if we want to, but that shouldn't blind us to the fact that we are only ever studying a part of the whole – and that what results when the parts are combined may be something completely unexpected.

EXERCISE 19.2	**Descriptive or inferential?**

The list below contains the names of 14 different statistical techniques. Seven of them represent descriptive statistics, and seven represent inferential tests. Your task is to identify which type of statistic each one represents.

t test
Mann–Whitney *U*
pie chart
chi-square
graph
semi-interquartile range
Wilcoxon Sign test
frequency polygon
Pearson's product-moment correlation
histogram
mode
analysis of variance
Spearman's rho
variation ratio

The research methods and analytical techniques we have looked at in this book are not just different 'tools', though. They span a wide range of philosophical and epistemological approaches. There is no one single way of doing psychology, and no single way of being 'scientific', for that matter. Psychology draws from a number of different philosophical traditions, and each of these has enhanced the discipline. The richness of psychological phenomena is not yet fully reflected by the richness of psychological methodology, but it's beginning to approach it.

Psychology itself draws on insights from all of these types of research, and many more; and it is important for psychology students to have an appreciation of the range of methods, and methodologies, which contribute to modern psychology. You may, in the end, choose to adopt just one type of research method; but you will inevitably come across research reports which have used other methods, so it is necessary to have a reasonably good understanding of the range of different approaches used in psychological research.

It is my hope that this book will have helped you to gain a taste of some of the richness in psychological research methods. It is, of course, only a taste – there is much more detail which could be covered, and many methods and analytical techniques which have had to be omitted. This book is only an introduction, but I hope that it has managed to reflect something of the diversity in modern psychology, and given a guide if you are beginning to explore ways of studying human beings in this particular discipline.

Self-assessment questions

1. *What is the difference between an independent and a dependent variable in experimental design, and an independent and a dependent variable in multiple regression or ANOVA?*

2. *Distinguish between conditions and factors in analysis of variance.*

3. *What is a one-way analysis of variance, and how is it different from a two-way ANOVA?*

4. *Why do we need additional calculations to be included in ANOVA for repeated measures?*

5. *What are the three main post-hoc tests, and what are they used for?*

Concepts in use

Complete the following two tables, putting the name of the appropriate statistical technique in each one.

Descriptive statistics

	nominal data	ordinal data	interval/ ratio data
measure of central tendency			
measure of dispersion			

Two-sample inferential statistics

	nominal data	ordinal data	interval/ ratio data
repeated-measures design			
independent-measures design			i
correlation study	n/a		

Glossary

ABBA design: a research design in which one set of participants is given the first condition (A) and then the second (B), while the other set is given condition B first, followed by A.

action research: a method of undertaking social research which acknowledges that the researcher's presence is likely to influence people's behaviour, and so incorporates the researcher's involvement as a direct and deliberate part of the research, with the researcher consciously acting as change agent.

action research cycle: the circular process of action research, which proceeds from a diagnostic stage to the development of a change strategy, to the action and implementation stage, then to the evaluative stage, and back through the cycle again.

ambiguous questions: questions which have more than one possible meaning.

analysis of variance: a statistical technique which allows researchers to locate significant differences between several different samples.

anecdotal evidence: evidence which is purely based on hearsay and personal experience rather than systematic investigation.

ANOVA: the usual abbreviation for analysis of variance.

ANOVA interaction diagram: a type of diagram which illustrates the relationships between variables identified by an ANOVA.

anti-positivism: an approach to research which emphasises the human interpretation of meanings and implications; introduced as a challenge to hard-line positivism.

artefacts: distortions in data or research findings brought about by artificial situations or uncontrolled variables.

attribution: the process of giving reasons for why things happen.

average: a typical score from a set of data. In everyday use, this term generally refers to the mean.

axis: a vertical or horizontal line used to show distances or amounts on a chart or graph.

bar chart: a graphical representation of a set of data which uses columns or bars to indicate different amounts of each category.

behavioural coding: a method of recording observations which involves using different categories. Each unit of behaviour is observed by checking one of those categories.

behaviourism: a school of thought which holds that the observation and description of overt behaviour are all that is needed to comprehend the human being.

between-groups variation: the general variation which is apparent between different samples of scores, such as the difference in height between, say, Pygmies and Europeans.

bias: systematic distortion in a set of data.

bipolar: having two opposite ends, or poles, with a continuum running between them.

box-plot diagram: diagrams which indicate the medians and semi-interquartile ranges of sets of scores by using a square shape to indicate the median, with lines coming out on either side to indicate the ranges.

bracketing: bringing to consciousness and deliberately setting aside assumptions and presuppositions which might influence a qualitative analysis.

brackets: symbols used in statistical analysis which mean 'do this calculation first'.

calibration: organising a measuring scale, and checking to make sure that it is accurate, or at least appropriate.

case study: a research project which involves the detailed exploration of a single case.

categorisation: grouping data into social categories or sets.

causality: what causes things to happen, or brings about an effect.

change strategy: the method for bringing about change which has been selected by the researcher.

clinical neuropsychology: the branch of psychology concerned with investigating how the brain works by studying the effects of brain damage, disease or injury.

closed questions: questions which have a deliberately limited range of possible answers.

co-ordinates: the numbers which indicate the values of the x and y axes for a particular point on a graph. The co-ordinates therefore indicate exactly where on the graph the point is located.

coefficient of determination: the square of the correlation coefficient obtained from a set of data, which is used to indicate how much of the variance has been accounted for by that particular correlation.

cognitive: to do with mental processes.

comparison groups: groups from which data have been collected, so that they can be used for comparison with the particular groups being studied.

computer aptitude test: a form of psychometric test which explores whether people have the cognitive attributes which will be of use to them in learning to program computers.

confidence levels: another term used to describe significance levels.

confounding: confusing the data by introducing additional factors or influences.

connectionism: an approach to cognitive research which looks at the processing of several strands of data simultaneously.

construct validity: the type of validity which is concerned with whether a particular measure actually reflects the theoretical construct it was designed to evaluate.

consultative register: a form of speech register used when speaking with strangers.

consumer psychologists: psychologists who devote their attention to exploring people's economic and consumer behaviour: the shopping choices that they make, and so on.

content analysis: a form of quantitative analysis which involves identifying categories in a set of data, and counting how often examples of each category occur.

context-specific: relating only to the particular context in which something occurs, and not more generally.

continuous variable: a variable which can have any number of different values, because there is a continuous transition between the values of the scale. This means that it can include fractions and partial amounts and not simply whole numbers.

control condition: a condition in an experiment which is used for comparison with an experimental condition.

conversation analysis: a method of exploring the structures and implications of how people go about conversations.

core analysis: the main analytical process involved in grounded theory, which takes the form of an interactive cycle, exploring concepts which have emerged from the data.

correlated-subjects design: another term used to describe a related-measures design.

correlation: when two variables change together, such that a change in one is likely to be associated with a change in the other.

correlation coefficient: a number between −1 and +1 which expresses how strong the correlation relationship between two variables is.

correlation matrix: a set of correlations arranged as a grid, so correlations between different factors can be easily seen.

cost–benefit analysis: weighing up the advantages (benefits) of a course of action against the disadvantages (costs), and seeing which side of the balance is stronger.

counterbalancing: organising the conditions of an experiment so that the order of presentation is varied, and order effects do not distort the data systematically.

covert research: research in which the people being studied are unaware of it.

criterion validity: a method for assessing whether a psychometric test is valid (i.e. really measures what it is supposed to) by comparing it with some other measure.

critical value: the number which is required in order for the result of a statistical test to be judged significant. Some statistical tests require the result to be equal to or greater than the critical value, while others require the result to be equal to or smaller than the critical value. The size of the critical value is not fixed: it depends on the level of significance required, and either the number of degrees of freedom or the size of the N used in the test.

data: the information obtained as the result of a research study.

data collection: the process of gathering data which can then be analysed to produce research findings.

data-driven technique: a method of analysis which is shaped by the data that have been collected, as opposed to one which imposes a pre-established structure on the material.

data-set: a group of scores or other data which relate to one particular group of research participants.

datum: a single item of information. This term is almost never used.

degrees of freedom: the number of possible options for variation which exist in the data set. For example, if a set of two scores have a given total, then the first score can vary, but the other one must be fixed in order to reach the desired total. This gives one degree of freedom. A set of three scores producing a fixed total would have two degrees of freedom, and so on.

demand characteristics: those aspects of a psychological study (or other artificial situation) which exert an implicit pressure on people to act in ways that are expected of them.

dependent variable: the thing which is measured in an experiment, and which changes, depending on the independent variable. Alternatively, the variable which is taken as the focus of interest in a statistical test.

depth interview: an interview which explores a particular topic in considerable detail, aiming to gather as much information from the interviewee as possible.

descriptive statistics: statistics which summarise or describe data.

diary method: a way of studying what human beings do in everyday life by asking them to note down specific items of information at regular intervals, or on appropriate occasions.

discourse analysis: a method of studying human experience by analysing the things people say to one another, and how they express them, both symbolically and behaviourally.

discursive: to do with discourse.

distribution: the way in which a set of scores is spread across its measuring scale.

distribution-free tests: tests which do not assume that the data fit a particular distribution pattern.

document analysis: a way of conducting psychological research which involves gathering the data from written records or other secondary sources.

double-blind control: a form of experimental control which aims to avoid self-fulfilling prophecies by ensuring that neither the subjects nor the experimenter who carries out the study are aware of the experimental hypothesis.

ecological validity: a way of assessing how valid a measure or test is (i.e. whether it really measures what it is supposed to measure) which is concerned with whether the measure or test is really like its counterpart in the real, everyday world.

elements: the people or objects used to generate constructs in a repertory grid.

emergent properties: the new, additional properties which emerge when several elements are combined into a new whole.

emotively loaded words: words which have strong emotional connotations.

empathy: feeling for someone – understanding how they feel about something by experiencing something of the same emotion oneself.

empiricism: an approach to knowledge which assumes that all knowledge of the world is learned through the input of information from the five external senses.

encoding: changing the form of information in such a way that it can be stored in the brain, or used effectively for analysis.

epistemology: the way that a particular type of knowledge works: what counts as valid reasoning or evidence in different areas of expertise or knowledge.

equal-interval data: data on a measuring scale which has equal gaps between consecutive whole numbers (e.g. money, where £1 represents the same amount regardless of whether it is the fifth or the 61st coin in a pile). Equal-interval data can be added and subtracted.

error variation: the amount of variation which occurs within the groups in an analysis of variance.

ethical: to do with right and wrong.

ethnography: an approach to research which aims to explore experience in terms of its cultural and symbolic contexts.

ethological observation: observing behaviour in the natural environment.

experimenter effects: unwanted influences in a psychological study which are produced, consciously or unconsciously, by the person carrying out the study.

extreme scores: scores which occur at the extreme ends of a distribution or data-set.

eyeball test: scanning the data by looking at it for interesting features.

***F* ratio**: a statistical measure which indicates the nature of the scores in a data set, in terms of how closely they cluster around the mean.

face validity: the surface appearance of validity – whether something looks as though it is probably valid, without that judgement being based on proper criteria.

factors: variables which can exert an influence on research findings or data.

field experiments: experiments conducted in the natural environment – that is, in the real world.

file-drawer problem: the problem caused by the fact that researchers often don't publish the results of studies, so they remain unknown and not included in a meta-analysis.

formula: a symbolic way of expressing a set of statistical calculations.

frequency: how often a score in a particular category occurs.

frequency polygon: a descriptive statistic which shows frequencies as a shape.

funnelling: making a set of questions more specific as they proceed, so that they are eventually narrowed down to a particular topic.

Gaussian distribution: the normal distribution curve.

GIGO: an acronym which stands for 'Garbage In, Garbage Out' – in other words, the quality of what you get depends on the quality of the information you put in.

graph: a descriptive method used for portraying continuous data.

graphical representations: visual images used as descriptive statistics.

grounded theory: an approach to qualitative analysis which seeks to build up theory from the information contained in research data, without imposing external assumptions or ideas.

hermeneutic: to do with meanings and interpretations.

histogram: a bar chart which has been precisely calibrated so that its surface area exactly reflects the proportions of the scores.

hypothesis: a prediction which states the outcome which is likely to take place if a particular theory is true and particular conditions are set up.

hypothetico-deductive research: an approach to research based on evaluating theories by testing hypotheses.

idiographic: describing the individual.

idiosyncratic: personal or unique to a particular individual.

immersion: becoming deeply submerged in the data such that one becomes unaware of other issues.

independent variable: the variable which is manipulated by an experimenter to bring about a result, or investigated by a statistician in terms of its connections with another variable.

independent-measures design: a research design in which different participants are used in the different conditions.

inductive research: an approach to research which is based on exploring data and developing theory from the outcomes.

inferential statistics: statistics which allow the user to make judgements about probability, or the likelihood of getting a particular set of scores by chance.

inter-observer reliability: the extent to which two observers agree.

inter-rater reliability: the extent to which two raters agree.

interpretive repertoires: sets of assumptions or frameworks which people use to interpret or make sense of information.

interquartile range: the spread of a set of scores between the first and third quartiles.

interval data: see equal-interval data.

interview: an approach to collecting data which involves listening to the responses people make when asked questions in a face-to-face situation.

interviewer effects: unwanted influences in an interview study which are produced, consciously or unconsciously, by the person carrying out the interview.

introspection: seeking insight or data by exploring one's own thoughts, feelings, emotions or experiences.

iterative: going through a process repeatedly in order to refine or develop a system or interpretation.

laddering: asking questions which become progressively more personal or intense, with each being based on the response to the previous question.

leading questions: questions which imply what the respondent's answer should be.

levels of analysis: different perspectives for exploring a given phenomenon, such as a human being, organised in sequence, e.g. with lower levels including microbiological or genetic explorations, and higher levels including cultural or socio-economic explorations.

levels of description: see levels of analysis.

levels of measurement: nominal, ordinal, interval or ratio data.

lie scale: a scale included in a questionnaire or psychometric test to identify whether someone is lying or not.

line of best fit: a line which represents the overall shape or size of a correlation.

matched-participant design: a research design in which different people are included in the conditions, but they have been paired up on significant factors, with one from each pair allocated to each condition.

mathematical notation: symbols which describe mathematical operations or unknown quantities.

mean: the arithmetic average of a set of scores.

measures of central tendency: numbers used to express a 'typical' score in a particular set.

measures of dispersion: numbers used to describe the way that the scores in a particular set vary.

median: the middlemost score in a set.

meta-analysis: a research technique which involves examining effects found in a series of studies and calculating the overall probability, as evidence for whether there is an underlying effect or not.

methodology: the assumptions about knowledge and evidence implied by an approach to research, or a school of thought.

mixed conditions: combinations of repeated- and independent-measures designs.

modal: to do with the mode. Modal scores are scores which have the same value as the mode.

mode: the most commonly occurring score in a set.

multiple regression: a statistical technique for looking at how different variables interact together.

multivariate analysis: techniques for analysing data which has several different variables.

narrative review: a literature review which picks out interesting features in the literature and discusses them.

natural science paradigm: a framework for scientific enquiry based on the natural sciences of physics, chemistry and biology.

negative correlation: a correlation in which as one variable increases, the other decreases.

negative skew: a distorted normal distribution curve in which the bulk of the scores have been shifted towards the right of the distribution.

New Paradigm Research: an approach to research which attempts to overcome the manipulative and inhuman aspects of conventional scientific method, and to combine rigour with humanistic values.

nominal data: category data, where the data are simply sorted into different types (e.g. types of building, colours) and all you can do is count how many of each type that there are.

nomothetic tests: tests which are used for comparison between people.

non-modal scores: scores which do not have the same value as the mode.

non-parametric tests: tests which do not make the same set of assumptions as parametric tests. These are generally tests which can be used with ordinal data.

non-verbal cues: information which comes from body language, dress, or the *way* in which things are said rather than from the actual words used.

normal distribution curve: a bell-shaped distribution curve, common in psychological research, which has distinctive mathematical properties.

null hypothesis: the prediction that any results which occur in a study are purely the result of sampling error.

objectivity: an approach which attempts to divorce the self or anything personal from the research process.

observable behaviour: behaviour which can be seen or measured directly.

observational study: a research project based on observation.

one-tailed prediction: a prediction which states the direction of a difference or correlation – that is, which states which will be the larger set of scores, or whether the correlation will be positive or negative.

one-tailed test: a test which is investigating a one-tailed prediction.

one-way ANOVA: analysis of variance in which there is one independent variable, with several conditions.

open questions: questions which the respondent can answer as they choose, in as many words as they like.

open-structure interviewing: a method of carrying out interviews which allows the conversation to roam pretty much as it likes, as long as a set of defined topics are covered.

opportunity sampling: obtaining a research sample by simply getting whatever participants are available.

order effects: experimental problems which occur because of the order in which the conditions have been presented to the participants.

ordinal data: ranked data, where the data can be set in order (e.g. in order of preference), and all you can really say is which one comes after or before another one.

paradigm: the framework of ideas, theories and assumptions within which a scientific community operates.

parametric statistics: statistics for data which conform to three parameters: equal-interval data, equal variance, and normal distribution.

partial correlation: the process of sorting out how much of the variance in a phenomenon results from one particular correlation, and how much from others.

participant observation: observational studies in which the researcher becomes one of the participants, and joins in the action which is being observed.

participants: the people who are studied in a research project.

Pearson's product-moment correlation test: a parametric correlation test.

perfect correlation: a correlation with the value of $+1$ or -1.

personal constructs: individual mini-theories which are ways of making sense of experience.

personality profile: a set of scores on different factors which combine to give an image of personality.

phenomenological: relating to a study or description of experience which aims to represent experience from within the person's own subjective world.

phonetic spelling: spelling which reflects the sounds of words.

pie chart: a circular diagram, divided into slices which represent the proportions of the scores.

pilot test: a practical trial given to a questionnaire, interview schedule or other research tool in order to identify and iron out problems while it is still in the design stage.

polygraph: a device for making multiple measurements of physiological reactions.

population: the total set of scores from which a sample has been drawn.

population norms: sets of scores which represent the typical values obtained from members of a particular population on a particular measure.

positive correlation: a correlation in which the two factors vary in the same direction, so that if one is large, the other is also likely to be large.

positive skew: a distorted normal distribution curve in which the bulk of the scores have been shifted towards the left of the distribution.

positivism: an approach to research which insists that only observable, measurable data should be the subject of study.

post-hoc tests: tests which are carried out after an ANOVA test, in order to make sense of the results.

power: the ability of a test to detect significance if it is present.

primacy effects: experimental influences which have occurred because this is the first time that the participant has encountered the phenomenon.

primer question: a question which introduces a topic and so leads the participant to begin thinking in a certain kind of way.

probability: a statement about how likely it is that something has happened.

probe question: a question which is asked in addition to the main question, in order to elicit more information about a particular topic.

proto-themes: early ideas about themes which may emerge from the data in a grounded theory analysis.

protocols: the verbal reports which people make about what they are doing as they carry out a specific task.

psychometric tests: carefully contructed questionnaire-style measuring instruments which have been designed to measure psychological factors or characteristics.

qualitative analysis: an approach to analysing research data which looks at meanings rather than numbers.

qualitative data: data which consist of non-numerical information, such as words or images.

quantitative analysis: an approach to analysing research data which examines them in terms of numbers and statistics.

quantitative data: data which consist of numbers.

quantitative–qualitative divide: the apparent distinction between qualitative and quantitative data.

quasi-experiments: experiments in which the independent variable has more than one condition, but these have not actually been manipulated by the experimenter.

questionnaire fallacy: the way that people respond to the questions asked at the expense of providing valid information.

quota sampling: a method of sampling in which categories in the population are identified, and the samples obtained aim to reflect the proportions of those categories.

random sampling: a method of sampling in which any member of the population has an equally likely chance of being selected.

randomisation: the distribution of a variable or influence in such a way that it is equally likely to affect any condition of a study.

range: the span of a set of values, from lowest to highest.

ranking: setting scores in order from lowest to highest.

rapport: the sensation of friendship and positive social interaction which facilitates research interviews.

rapport interview: an interview designed in such a way as to foster rapport between the participant and the interviewer.

rating scale: a measuring scale which requires respondents to make value-judgements about a particular object, according to a specified set of values.

ratio data: equal-interval data which also has an absolute zero that you can't go below (e.g. time or length). Money is equal-interval but not ratio, because you can be in debt – i.e. you can have less than no money.

raw data: data which have not been 'cooked' – i.e. subjected to statistical analysis.

RDD: random digit dialling – a method of choosing research participants from the random dialling of telephone numbers.

reactance: when participation in a study changes the participant in some way.

real-world research: research which takes place in everyday settings rather than in the controlled environment of the psychological laboratory.

reflexivity: the interplay of influence and effect, such that the effect becomes the influence, and produces another effect which then again becomes the influence.

regression line: a line which expresses the direction or degree of a particular correlation.

reliability: whether a test or measure is consistent over time in the outcomes that it gives.

reliability coefficient: a correlation coefficient which describes the amount of agreement between two sets of data, representing answers to the same original material.

repeated-measures design: an experimental design in which the same participants take part in both or all conditions of the study.

repertory grid: a technique for identifying and representing data about personal constructs.

replication: repeating a study or research project in such a way as to make sure that all of the important elements are identical, or at least very similar. The term often includes the assumption that the study has produced the same or nearly identical findings.

representative sample: a sample which is typical of its population.

research participant: someone who agrees to take part in a research project.

response bias: the tendency which people have to respond in ways which will make them appear more socially acceptable than they are.

response rate: the proportion of people responding to a questionnaire, by comparison with the full set of people who were approached to do so.

retrospective studies: studies which look back in time and aim to gather data about things that have happened in the past.

rigour: the meticulousness and accuracy of scientific research.

robustness: the ability of a test to detect significance accurately even if it is used with data with inappropriate parameters.

salient quotes: quotations which are relevant to the topic being discussed.

sample: a selection of research participants or scores from a particular population.

sampling technique: a method of obtaining a sample for research or similar purposes.

scaling: the process of adjusting a set of scores such that they can be analysed or represented more easily.

scattergram: a diagram which illustrates a correlation by having one factor as the x axis, the other as the y axis, and the data represented as points scattered between them.

segmentation: dividing the material into sections or segments.

selective perception: the human tendency to perceive what is expected or anticipated.

self-fulfilling prophecies: statements which come true simply because they have been made.

self-report: a report about someone made by themselves.

semi-interquartile range: a version of the range used to represent the variability in ordinal data, and often taken as being roughly equivalent to the standard deviation.

serial processing: processing just one set of information in one way at a given time.

significance level: the degree of probability represented by a test statistic.

significant difference: a difference between two or more sets of scores which has achieved a specified significance level.

single-case experiments: experiments conducted on just one individual or case.

skewed distribution: a distorted normal distribution, such that the bulk of the scores lie either to the right or left of the median rather than being evenly spread on either side.

social responsibility of science: the principle that scientific research occurs within a social context and should reflect ethical and socially responsible values and practices.

Spearman's rank-order correlation test: a non-parametric correlation test used with ordinal data.

speech registers: ways of speaking which vary according to the formality of the setting and the context in which the utterance is being made.

standard deviation: a statistical measure which describes how a set of scores are spread out around a mean.

standard scores: scores which have been produced from a data-set but adjusted so that the form they take is more suitable for analysis.

standardisation: the typical baselines of a psychometric measure in a population; or a preset way of delivering research procedures or instructions.

standardised instructions: a pre-established form of words used by an experimenter in order to minimise potential bias.

standardised procedures: a pre-established way of carrying out an experiment, adopted in all conditions in order to minimise potential bias.

standardised responses: pre-established and regularly patterned ways of responding to questions or situations.

stem and leaf diagram: a form of graphical representation in which a set of numbers is shown with the tens arranged vertically as a 'stem' and the units arranged horizontally as 'leaves'.

stimulus–response learning: a basic form of learning which involves an association between a stimulus and a response, and (in theory at least) does not involve cognitive processing.

structured interview schedule: a pre-established pattern, wording and sequence of questions to be used in a research interview.

structured observation: a form of observing in which the behaviour which is to be observed has been carefully precoded, and the observation takes the form of recording when and how often these precoded behaviours occur.

structured questionnaire: a formal questionnaire in which all of the questions are precisely worded and involve closed questions.

subscales: sets of questions in a psychometric test which contribute to an overall scale, but reflect just one facet of the behaviour or experience which the test is aiming to measure.

subset: a smaller grouping within a set of scores.

sum of squares: a statistical measure used in analysis of variance which indicates the amount of variation in the subgroups of the analysis.

systems analysis: an approach to understanding social behaviour which looks at the ways that whole systems are organised and perpetuate themselves.

tables of results: small charts which summarise the important features of a set of data – usually totals, means and standard deviations.

taxonomy: a set of categories used to summarise and organise more than one data-set.

test items: the individual questions in a psychometric test.

test power: how capable a statistical test is of detecting significance if it is present in the data.

test statistic: the number which is produced when a statistical calculation has been completed, and which then needs to be interpreted using significance tables.

themes: topics or ideas which occur recurrently during the course of a qualitative analysis.

theory-driven analysis: a form of analysis in which the data are organised according to pre-established assumptions about the form it will take, which have been derived from the theory which is being applied.

theory-led investigation: research whose conduct and analysis have been shaped by the theory that it is exploring.

time sampling: a technique used in behavioural observation whereby records of behaviour are collected at set time intervals, e.g. every five minutes.

transcription: the conversion of recorded information such as tapes of interviews into written form.

triangulation: using more than one research method to home in on a particular phenomenon.

two-sample statistical tests: statistical tests which look at the differences or similarities between two sets of data.

two-tailed test: when a statistical test has been applied to the data without any prediction as to the likely direction of the difference or correlation, so it can go either way.

two-way ANOVA: an analysis of variance test which is used to compare two sets of data.

two-way mirror: a mirror used for covert observation, which looks like a mirror from one side, but is transparent from the other.

Type I error: a statistical error in which the null hypothesis is rejected when it should have been retained – that is, a false positive finding.

Type II error: a statistical error in which the null hypothesis is retained when it should have been rejected – that is, a false negative finding.

validity: whether a measuring scale or psychometric test actually measures what it purports to measure.

variable: something which varies – that is, something which can have different values.

variance: a measure describing how much a set of scores are spread out around the mean.

variance ratio: a statistical measure which describes precisely the way that scores are spread out around the mean.

variation ratio: a descriptive statistic which indicates the proportion of modal to non-modal scores in a set of data.

verbal behaviour: words. The term was coined by behaviourists who did not want to imply that what people said might actually reveal any cognitive processing.

vignette: a short description used to summarise a case or situation for qualitative analysis.

visual representations: images or pictures.

within-groups variation: the amount of variation which happens within a single set of scores. In analysis of variance this is known as the error variation.

x **axis**: the horizontal line which indicates amounts on a graph or chart.

y **axis**: the vertical line which indicates amounts on a graph or chart.

z **axis**: the line on a three-dimensional graph or chart which points away from the observer, and indicates amounts on a third scale.

z **scores**: scores which describe how close a single individual's result is to the mean for their particular group. The description is expressed in terms of the number of standard deviations from the mean.

Statistical tables

Table A Critical values for the binomial test (sign test)

N	0.05	0.01
5	–	–
6	0	–
7	0	–
8	0	0
9	1	0
10	1	0
11	1	0
12	2	1
13	2	1
14	2	1
15	3	2
16	3	2
17	4	2
18	4	3
19	4	3
20	5	3
25	7	5
30	9	7
35	11	9

The calculated value must be equal to or less than the critical value shown in the table to achieve that level of significance.

Source: Clegg, F. (1982) *Simple Statistics*. Cambridge: Cambridge University Press.

Table B   Critical values for the chi-square test

Degrees of freedom	0.05	0.01
1	3.84	6.64
2	5.99	9.21
3	7.82	11.34
4	9.49	13.28
5	11.07	15.09
6	12.59	16.81
7	14.07	18.48
8	15.51	20.09
9	16.92	21.67
10	18.31	23.21
11	19.68	24.72
12	21.03	26.22
13	22.36	27.69
14	23.68	29.14
15	25.00	30.58
16	26.30	32.00
17	27.59	33.41
18	28.87	34.80
19	30.14	36.19
20	31.41	37.57
21	32.67	38.93
22	33.92	40.29
23	35.17	41.64
24	36.42	42.98
25	37.65	44.31
26	38.88	45.64
27	40.11	46.97
28	41.34	48.28
29	42.56	49.59
30	43.77	50.89

The value of chi-square obtained from the test must be equal to or higher than the value given in the table to obtain significance.

Source: Fisher, R.A. and Yates, F. (1963) *Statistical Tables for Biological, Agricultural and Medical Research*. Harlow: Pearson Education.

Table C Critical values for the Wilcoxon Signed-ranks test

N	0.05 One-tailed test	0.05 Two-tailed test	0.01 One-tailed test	0.01 Two-tailed test
5	0	–	–	–
6	2	0	–	–
7	3	2	0	–
8	5	3	1	0
9	8	5	3	1
10	10	8	5	3
11	13	10	7	5
12	17	13	9	7
13	21	17	12	9
14	25	21	15	12
15	30	25	19	15
16	35	29	23	19
17	41	34	27	23
18	47	40	32	27
19	53	46	37	32
20	60	52	43	37
21	67	58	49	42
22	75	65	55	48
23	83	73	62	54
24	91	81	69	61
25	100	89	76	68
26	110	98	84	75
27	119	107	92	83
28	130	116	101	91
29	140	126	110	100
30	151	137	120	109
31	163	147	130	118
32	175	159	140	128
33	187	170	151	138
34	200	182	162	148
35	213	195	173	159
36	227	208	185	171
37	241	221	198	182
38	256	235	211	194
39	271	249	224	207
40	286	264	238	220
41	302	279	252	233
42	319	294	266	247
43	336	310	281	261
44	353	327	296	276
45	371	343	312	291
46	389	361	328	307
47	407	378	345	322
48	426	396	362	339
49	446	415	379	355
50	466	434	397	373

The value of T obtained from the test must be equal to or lower than the number given in the table in order to obtain significance.

Source: Siegel, S. (1956) *Nonparametric Statistics for the Behavioural Sciences*. New York: McGraw-Hill. Reproduced with permission of The McGraw-Hill Companies.

Table D   Critical values for the Mann–Whitney U test

One-tailed test 0.05 level of significance

N	1	2	3	4	5	6	7	8	9	10	11	12	13	14	15	16	17	18	19	20
1	–	–	–	–	–	–	–	–	–	–	–	–	–	–	–	–	–	–	0	0
2	–	–	–	–	0	0	0	1	1	1	1	2	2	2	3	3	3	4	4	4
3	–	–	0	0	1	2	2	3	3	4	5	5	6	7	7	8	9	9	10	11
4	–	–	0	1	2	3	4	5	6	7	8	9	10	11	12	14	15	16	17	18
5	–	0	1	2	4	5	6	8	9	11	12	13	15	16	18	19	20	22	23	25
6	–	0	2	3	5	7	8	10	12	14	16	17	19	21	23	25	26	28	30	32
7	–	0	2	4	6	8	11	13	15	17	19	21	24	26	28	30	33	35	37	39
8	–	1	3	5	8	10	13	15	18	20	23	26	28	31	33	36	39	41	44	47
9	–	1	3	6	9	12	15	18	21	24	27	30	33	36	39	42	45	48	51	54
10	–	1	4	7	11	14	17	20	24	27	31	34	37	41	44	48	51	55	58	62
11	–	1	5	8	12	16	19	23	27	31	34	38	42	46	50	54	57	61	65	69
12	–	2	5	9	13	17	21	26	30	34	38	42	47	51	55	60	64	68	72	77
13	–	2	6	10	15	19	24	28	33	37	42	47	51	56	61	65	70	75	80	84
14	–	2	7	11	16	21	26	31	36	41	46	51	56	61	66	71	77	82	87	92
15	–	3	7	12	18	23	28	33	39	44	50	55	61	66	72	77	83	88	94	100
16	–	3	8	14	19	25	30	36	42	48	54	60	65	71	77	83	89	95	101	107
17	–	3	9	15	20	26	33	39	45	51	57	64	70	77	83	89	96	102	109	115
18	–	4	9	16	22	28	35	41	48	55	61	68	75	82	88	95	102	109	116	123
19	0	4	10	17	23	30	37	44	51	58	65	72	80	87	94	101	109	116	123	130
20	0	4	11	18	25	32	39	47	54	62	69	77	84	92	100	107	115	123	130	138

Two-tailed test, 0.05 level of significance

N	1	2	3	4	5	6	7	8	9	10	11	12	13	14	15	16	17	18	19	20
1	–	–	–	–	–	–	–	–	–	–	–	–	–	–	–	–	–	–	–	–
2	–	–	–	–	–	–	–	0	0	0	0	1	1	1	1	1	2	2	2	2
3	–	–	–	–	0	1	1	2	2	3	3	4	4	5	5	6	6	7	7	8
4	–	–	–	0	1	2	3	4	4	5	6	7	8	9	10	11	11	12	13	13
5	–	–	0	1	2	3	5	6	7	8	9	11	12	13	14	15	17	18	19	20
6	–	–	1	2	3	5	6	8	10	11	13	14	16	17	19	21	22	24	25	27
7	–	–	1	3	5	6	8	10	12	14	16	18	20	22	24	26	28	30	32	34
8	–	0	2	4	6	8	10	13	15	17	19	22	24	26	29	31	34	36	38	41
9	–	0	2	4	7	10	12	15	17	20	23	26	28	31	34	37	39	42	45	48
10	–	0	3	5	8	11	14	17	20	23	26	29	33	36	39	42	45	48	52	55
11	–	0	3	6	9	13	16	19	23	26	30	33	37	40	44	47	51	55	58	62
12	–	1	4	7	11	14	18	22	26	29	33	37	41	45	49	53	57	61	65	69
13	–	1	4	8	12	16	20	24	28	33	37	41	45	50	54	59	63	67	72	76
14	–	1	5	9	13	17	22	26	31	36	40	45	50	55	59	64	67	74	78	83
15	–	1	5	10	14	19	24	29	34	39	44	49	54	59	64	70	75	80	85	90
16	–	1	6	11	15	21	26	31	37	42	47	53	59	64	70	75	81	86	92	98
17	–	2	6	11	17	22	28	34	39	45	51	57	63	67	75	81	87	93	99	105
18	–	2	7	12	18	24	30	36	42	48	55	61	67	74	80	86	93	99	106	112
19	–	2	7	13	19	25	32	38	45	52	58	65	72	78	85	92	99	106	113	119
20	–	2	8	13	20	27	34	41	48	55	62	69	76	83	90	98	105	112	119	127

Table D *continued*

One-tailed test, 0.01 level of significance

N	1	2	3	4	5	6	7	8	9	10	11	12	13	14	15	16	17	18	19	20
1	–	–	–	–	–	–	–	–	–	–	–	–	–	–	–	–	–	–	–	–
2	–	–	–	–	–	–	–	–	–	–	–	–	0	0	0	0	0	0	1	1
3	–	–	–	–	–	–	0	0	1	1	1	2	2	2	3	3	4	4	4	5
4	–	–	–	–	0	1	1	2	3	3	4	5	5	6	7	7	8	9	9	10
5	–	–	–	0	1	2	3	4	5	6	7	8	9	10	11	12	13	14	15	16
6	–	–	–	1	2	3	4	6	7	8	9	11	12	13	15	16	18	19	20	22
7	–	–	0	1	3	4	6	7	9	11	12	14	16	17	19	21	23	24	26	28
8	–	–	0	2	4	6	7	9	11	13	15	17	20	22	24	26	28	30	32	34
9	–	–	1	3	5	7	9	11	14	16	18	21	23	26	28	31	33	36	38	40
10	–	–	1	3	6	8	11	13	16	19	22	24	27	30	33	36	38	41	44	47
11	–	–	1	4	7	9	12	15	18	22	25	28	31	34	37	41	44	47	50	53
12	–	–	2	5	8	11	14	17	21	24	28	31	35	38	42	46	49	53	56	60
13	–	0	2	5	9	12	16	20	23	27	31	35	39	43	47	51	55	59	63	67
14	–	0	2	6	10	13	17	22	26	30	34	38	43	47	51	56	60	65	69	73
15	–	0	3	7	11	15	19	24	28	33	37	42	47	51	56	61	66	70	75	80
16	–	0	3	7	12	16	21	26	31	36	41	46	51	56	61	66	71	76	82	87
17	–	0	4	8	13	18	23	28	33	38	44	49	55	60	66	71	77	82	88	93
18	–	0	4	9	14	19	24	30	36	41	47	53	59	65	70	76	82	88	94	100
19	–	1	4	9	15	20	26	32	38	44	50	56	63	69	75	82	88	94	101	107
20	–	1	5	10	16	22	28	34	40	47	53	60	67	73	80	87	93	100	107	114

Two-tailed test, 0.01 level of significance

N	1	2	3	4	5	6	7	8	9	10	11	12	13	14	15	16	17	18	19	20
1	–	–	–	–	–	–	–	–	–	–	–	–	–	–	–	–	–	–	–	–
2	–	–	–	–	–	–	–	–	–	–	–	–	–	–	–	–	–	–	0	0
3	–	–	–	–	–	–	–	0	0	0	1	1	1	2	2	2	2	2	3	3
4	–	–	–	–	–	0	0	1	1	2	2	3	3	4	5	5	6	6	7	8
5	–	–	–	–	0	1	1	2	3	4	5	6	7	7	8	9	10	11	12	13
6	–	–	–	0	1	2	3	4	5	6	7	9	10	11	12	13	15	16	17	18
7	–	–	–	0	1	3	4	6	7	9	10	12	13	15	16	18	19	21	22	24
8	–	–	–	1	2	4	6	7	9	11	13	15	17	18	20	22	24	26	28	30
9	–	–	0	1	3	5	7	9	11	13	16	18	20	22	24	27	29	31	33	36
10	–	–	0	2	4	6	9	11	13	16	18	21	24	26	29	31	34	37	39	42
11	–	–	0	2	5	7	10	13	16	18	21	24	27	30	33	36	39	42	45	48
12	–	–	1	3	6	9	12	15	18	21	24	27	31	34	37	41	44	47	51	54
13	–	–	1	3	7	10	13	17	20	24	27	31	34	38	42	45	49	53	56	60
14	–	–	1	4	7	11	15	18	22	26	30	34	38	42	46	50	54	58	63	67
15	–	–	2	5	8	12	16	20	24	29	33	37	42	46	51	55	60	64	69	73
16	–	–	2	5	9	13	18	22	27	31	36	41	45	50	55	60	65	70	74	79
17	–	–	2	6	10	15	19	24	29	34	39	44	49	54	60	65	70	75	81	86
18	–	–	2	6	11	16	21	26	31	37	42	47	53	58	64	70	75	81	87	92
19	–	0	3	7	12	17	22	28	33	39	45	51	56	63	69	74	81	87	93	99
20	–	0	3	8	13	18	24	30	36	42	48	54	60	67	73	79	86	92	99	105

The calculated value of U must be lower than or equal to the critical value given in the table to obtain significance.

Source: Siegel, S. (1956) *Nonparametric Statistics for the Behavioural Sciences*. New York: McGraw-Hill. Reproduced with permission of The McGraw-Hill Companies.

Table E Critical values for the t test

df	0.05 One-tailed test	0.05 Two-tailed test	0.01 One-tailed test	0.01 Two-tailed test
1	6.314	12.706	31.821	63.657
2	2.920	4.303	6.965	9.925
3	2.353	3.182	4.541	5.841
4	2.132	2.776	3.747	4.604
5	2.015	2.571	3.365	4.032
6	1.943	2.447	3.143	3.707
7	1.895	2.365	2.998	3.499
8	1.860	2.306	2.896	3.355
9	1.833	2.262	2.821	3.250
10	1.812	2.228	2.764	3.169
11	1.796	2.201	2.718	3.106
12	1.782	2.179	2.681	3.055
13	1.771	2.160	2.650	3.012
14	1.761	2.145	2.624	2.977
15	1.753	2.131	2.602	2.947
16	1.746	2.120	2.583	2.921
17	1.740	2.110	2.567	2.898
18	1.734	2.101	2.552	2.878
19	1.729	2.093	2.539	2.861
20	1.725	2.086	2.528	2.845
21	1.721	2.080	2.518	2.831
22	1.717	2.074	2.508	2.819
23	1.714	2.069	2.500	2.807
24	1.711	2.064	2.492	2.797
25	1.708	2.060	2.485	2.787
26	1.706	2.056	2.479	2.779
27	1.703	2.052	2.473	2.771
28	1.701	2.048	2.467	2.763
29	1.699	2.045	2.462	2.756
30	1.697	2.042	2.457	2.750
40	1.684	2.021	2.423	2.704
60	1.671	2.000	2.390	2.660
120	1.658	1.980	2.358	2.617
∞	1.645	1.960	2.326	2.576

The test value must be equal to or larger than the critical value given in the table in order to be significant.

If the number of degrees of freedom you want is not given in the table, use the next lowest value. If it is very large, use the values in the row marked ∞.

Table F Critical values for Spearman's rank-order correlation test

N	0.05		0.01	
	One-tailed test	*Two-tailed test*	*One-tailed test*	*Two-tailed test*
5	0.900	1.000	1.000	–
6	0.829	0.886	0.943	1.000
7	0.714	0.786	0.893	0.929
8	0.643	0.738	0.833	0.881
9	0.600	0.683	0.783	0.833
10	0.564	0.648	0.746	0.794
12	0.506	0.591	0.712	0.777
14	0.456	0.544	0.645	0.715
16	0.425	0.506	0.601	0.665
18	0.399	0.475	0.564	0.625
20	0.377	0.450	0.534	0.591
22	0.359	0.428	0.508	0.562
24	0.343	0.409	0.485	0.537
26	0.329	0.392	0.465	0.515
28	0.317	0.377	0.448	0.496
30	0.306	0.364	0.432	0.478

The value of rho obtained from the calculations must be equal to, or larger than, the critical value given in the table to obtain that level of significance.

Source: Siegel, S. (1956) *Nonparametric Statistics for the Behavioural Sciences*. New York: McGraw-Hill. Reproduced with permission of The McGraw-Hill Companies.

Table G   Critical values for Pearson's product-moment correlation test

	0.05		0.01	
df	*One-tailed test*	*Two-tailed test*	*One-tailed test*	*Two-tailed test*
1	0.9877	0.9969	0.9995	0.9999
2	0.9000	0.9500	0.9800	0.9900
3	0.8054	0.8783	0.9343	0.9587
4	0.7293	0.8114	0.8822	0.9172
5	0.6694	0.7545	0.8329	0.8745
6	0.6215	0.7067	0.7887	0.8343
7	0.5822	0.6664	0.7498	0.7977
8	0.5494	0.6319	0.7155	0.7646
9	0.5214	0.6021	0.6851	0.7348
10	0.4973	0.5760	0.6581	0.7079
11	0.4762	0.5529	0.6339	0.6835
12	0.4575	0.5324	0.6120	0.6614
13	0.4409	0.5139	0.5923	0.6411
14	0.4259	0.4973	0.5742	0.6226
15	0.4124	0.4821	0.5577	0.6055
16	0.4000	0.4683	0.5425	0.5897
17	0.3887	0.4555	0.5285	0.5751
18	0.3783	0.4438	0.5155	0.5614
19	0.3687	0.4329	0.5034	0.5487
20	0.3598	0.4227	0.4921	0.5368
25	0.3233	0.3809	0.4451	0.4869
30	0.2960	0.3494	0.4093	0.4487
35	0.2746	0.3246	0.3810	0.4182
40	0.2573	0.3044	0.3578	0.3932
45	0.2428	0.2875	0.3384	0.3721
50	0.2306	0.2732	0.3218	0.3541
60	0.2108	0.2500	0.2948	0.3248
70	0.1954	0.2319	0.2737	0.3017
80	0.1829	0.2172	0.2565	0.2830
90	0.1726	0.2050	0.2422	0.2673
100	0.1638	0.1946	0.2301	0.2540

The value of r obtained must be equal to, or higher than, the critical value given in the table to obtain significance.

Source: Fisher, R.A. and Yates, F. (1963) *Statistical Tables for Biological, Agricultural and Medical Research*. Harlow: Pearson Education.

References

Anderson, N.R. and West, M.A. (1994) *The Team Climate Inventory: Manual and User's Guide*. Windsor: ASE, NFER-Nelson.

Banister, P. (1994) Observation, in P. Banister, E. Burman, I. Parker, M. Taylor and C. Tindall, *Qualitative Methods in Psychology: A Research Guide*. Buckingham: Open University Press.

Beloff, H. (1997) Making and un-making identities: a psychologist looks at art-work, in N. Hayes (ed.) *Doing Qualitative Analysis in Psychology*. Hove: Psychology Press.

Benewick, R. and Holton, R. (1987) The peaceful crowd: crowd solidarity and the Pope's visit to Britain, in G. Gaskell and R. Benewick (eds) *The Crowd in Contemporary Britain*. London: Sage.

Bettelheim, B. (1943) Individual and mass behaviour in extreme situations, *Journal of Abnormal & Social Psychology*, 38: 417–52.

Bower, G.H. (1981) Mood and memory, *American Psychologist*, 36: 129–48.

Breakwell, G.M. and Wood, P. (1995) Diary techniques, in G. Breakwell, S. Hammond and C. Fife-Schaw (eds) *Research Methods in Psychology*. London: Sage.

Breakwell, G.M., Hammond, S. and Fife-Schaw, C. (1995) *Research Methods in Psychology*. London: Sage.

British Psychological Society (1990) Revised ethical principles for research with human subjects, *The Psychologist*, 3: 269–72.

Bromley, D.B. (1977) *Personality Descriptions in Ordinary Language*. New York: Wiley.

Brown, J. and Canter, D. (1985) How people behave in fires, in M. Brenner, J. Brown and D. Canter (eds) *The Research Interview: Uses and Abuses*. London: Academic Press.

Bryant, P. and Bradley, L. (1985) *Children's Reading Problems*. Oxford: Blackwell.

Cook, T.D. and Campbell, D.T. (1979) *Quasi-experimentation: Design and Analysis Issues for Field Settings*. Chicago: Rand McNally.

Craik, I.F.M. and Lockhart, R.S. (1972) Levels of processing: a framework for memory research, *Journal of Verbal Learning and Verbal Behavior*, 11: 671–84.

Curtiss, S. (1977) *Genie: A Psycholinguistic Study of a Modern-Day 'Wild Child'*. New York: Academic Press.

Dawes, R.M. and Smith, T. (1985) Attitude and opinion measurement, in G. Lindzey and E. Aronson (eds) *The Handbook of Social Psychology*. New York: Random House.

Doise, W., Clemence, A. and Lorenzi-Cioldi, F. (1993) *The Quantitative Analysis of Social Representations*. Hemel Hempstead: Harvester-Wheatsheaf.

Dunn, J. (1988) *The Beginnings of Social Understanding*. Oxford: Blackwell.

Edwards, D. (1997) *Discourse and Cognition*. London: Sage.

Eiser, J.R. (1975) Attitudes and the use of evaluative language: a two-way process, *Journal for the Theory of Social Behaviour*, 5: 235–48.

Ericsson, K.A. and Simon, H.A. (1984) *Protocol Analysis: Verbal Reports as Data*. Cambridge, MA: MIT Press.

Eysenck, H.J. (1978) An exercise in mega-silliness, *American Psychologist*, 33: 517.

Farr, R.M. (1987) Social representations: a French tradition of research, *Journal for the Theory of Social Behaviour*, 17: 343–69.

Festinger, L., Riecken, H.W. and Schachter, S. (1956) *When Prophecy Fails*. Minneapolis: University of Minneapolis Press.

Fife-Schaw, C. (1995) Levels of measurement, in G. Breakwell, S. Hammond and C. Fife-Schaw (eds) *Research Methods in Psychology*. London: Sage.

Finn, G.P.T. (1997) Qualitative analysis of murals in Northern Ireland: paramilitary justification for political violence, in N. Hayes (ed.) *Doing Qualitative Analysis in Psychology*. Hove: Psychology Press.

Foster, J. (1993) *Starting SPSS/PC & SPSS for Windows: A Beginner's Guide to Data Analysis*, 2nd edn. Wilmslow: Sigma Press.

Garfinkel, H. (1967) *Studies in Ethnomethodology*. Englewood Cliffs, NJ: Prentice Hall.

Ghiselin, B. (1952) *The Creative Process*. Berkeley: University of California Press.

Gilbert, G.N. and Mulkay, M. (1984) *Opening Pandora's Box: A Sociological Analysis of Scientists' Discourse*. Cambridge: Cambridge University Press.

Gilhooly, K.J., Wood, M., Kinnear, P.R. and Green, C. (1988) Skill in map reading and memory for maps, *Quarterly Journal of Experimental Psychology*, 40A: 87–107.

Gilhooly, K.J., McGeorge, P., Hunter, J. *et al.* (1995) Biomedical knowledge in diagnostic thinking: the case of electrocardiogram (ECG) interpretation. Unpublished manuscript, University of Aberdeen, cited by K.J. Gilhooly and C. Green, Protocol analysis: theoretical background, in J.T.E. Richardson (ed.) *Handbook of Qualitative Research Methods*. Leicester: BPS Books.

Gill, R. (1996) Discourse analysis: practical implementation, in J.T.E. Richardson (ed.) *Handbook of Qualitative Research Methods*. Leicester: BPS Books.

Glaser, B.G. and Strauss, A.L. (1967) *The Discovery of Grounded Theory: Strategies for Qualitative Research*. New York: Aldine.

Glass, G. (1976) Primary, secondary and meta-analysis of research, *Educational Research*, 5: 3–8.

Glass, G., McGraw, B. and Smith, M.L. (1981) *Meta-analysis in Social Research*. Beverley Hills, CA: Sage.

Gould, S.J. (1981) *The Mismeasure of Man*. New York: Norton.

Gould, S.J. (1996) *The Mismeasure of Man*, 2nd edn. Harmondsworth: Penguin.

Green, C. and Gilhooly, K.J. (1996) Protocol analysis: practical implementation, in J.T.E. Richardson (ed.) *Handbook of Qualitative Research Methods*. Leicester: BPS Books.

Greene, J. and d'Oliveira, M. (1999) *Learning to Use Statistical Tests in Psychology*, 2nd edn. Buckingham: Open University Press.

Gribbin, J. (1995) *Schrödinger's Kittens*. London: Weidenfeld and Nicolson.

Guilford, J.P. (1956) *Fundamental Statistics in Psychology and Education*, 4th edn. New York: McGraw-Hill.

Hammersley, M. (1992) *What's Wrong with Ethnography?* London: Routledge.

Hayes, N. (1995) *Psychology in Perspective*. Basingstoke: Macmillan.

Hayes, N. (1997a) Theory-led thematic analysis: social identification in small companies, in N. Hayes (ed.) *Doing Qualitative Analysis in Psychology*. Hove: Psychology Press.

Hayes, N. (ed.) (1997b) *Doing Qualitative Analysis in Psychology*. Hove: Psychology Press.

Hayes, N. (1997c) *Successful Team Management*. London: International Thomson Business Press.

Hayes, N. (1998) Psychological processes in organisational cultures I: Social representations and organisational semiotics, *Human Systems*, 9: 59–65.

Hayes, N. (2000) *Foundations of Psychology*, 3rd edn. London: Thomson Learning.

Hayes, N. and Lemon, N. (1990) Stimulating positive cultures in growing companies, *Leadership & Organisational Change Management*, 11(7): 17–21.

Heath, C. and Luff, P. (1993) Explicating face-to-face interaction, in N. Gilbert (ed.) *Researching Social Life*. London: Sage.

Hinton, P. (1995) *Statistics Explained*. London: Routledge.

Holdaway, S. (1982) 'An inside job': a case study of covert research on the police, in M. Bulmer (ed.) *Social Research Ethics*. Basingstoke: Macmillan.

Hunter, J.E., Schmidt, F.L. and Jackson, G.B. (1982) *Meta-analysis: Cumulating Research Findings across Studies*. Beverley Hills, CA: Sage.

James, W. (1890) *Principles of Psychology*. New York: Holt.

Johnson, C.E., Wood, R. and Blinkhorn, S.F. (1988) Spriouser and spriouser: the use of ipsative personality tests, *Journal of Occupational Psychology*, 61: 153–62.

Kuhn, T. (1962) *The Structure of Scientific Revolutions*. Chicago: University of Chicago Press.

Lemon, N. and Taylor, H. (1997) Caring in casualty: the phenomenology of nursing care, in N. Hayes (ed.) *Doing Qualitative Analysis in Psychology*. Hove: Psychology Press.

Lewin, K. (1946) Action research and minority problems, *Journal of Social Issues*, 2: 34–46.

Lewin, K. (1947) Feedback problems of social diagnosis and action, *Human Relations*, 1: 147–53.

Lewin, K. (1952) *Field Theory in Social Science*. London: Tavistock.

Linton, M. (1975) Memory for real-world events, in D.A. Norman and D.E. Rumelhart (eds) *Explorations in Cognition*. San Francisco: Freeman.

Manstead, A.S.R. and McCulloch, C. (1981) Sex-role stereotyping in British television advertisements, *British Journal of Social Psychology*, 20: 171–80.

Marsh, P., Rosser, E. and Harré, R. (1978) *The Rules of Disorder*. London: Routledge & Kegan Paul.

Massarik, F. (1981) The interviewing process re-examined, in P. Reason and J. Rowan (eds) *Human Inquiry: A Source Book of New Paradigm Research*. Chichester: Wiley.

Milgram, S. (1973) *Obedience to Authority*. London: Tavistock.

Miller, T., Velleman, R., Rigby, K., Orford, J., Tod, A., Copello, A. and Bennett, G. (1997) The use of vignettes in the analysis of interview data: relatives of people with drug problems, in N. Hayes (ed.) *Doing Qualitative Analysis in Psychology*. Hove: Psychology Press.

Neisser, U. (1976) *Cognition and Reality*. New York: W.H. Freeman & Co.

Nisbett, R.E. and Wilson, T.D. (1977) Telling more than we can know: verbal reports on mental processes, *Psychological Review*, 84: 231–59.

Orne, M.T. (1962) On the social psychology of the psychological experiment: with particular reference to demand characteristics and their implications, *American Psychologist*, 17: 276–83.

Osgood, C.E. (1952) The nature and measurement of meaning, *Psychological Bulletin*, 49: 197–237.

Parker, I. (1994) Discourse analysis, in P. Banister, E. Burman, I. Parker, M. Taylor and C. Tindall, *Qualitative Methods in Psychology: A Research Guide*. Buckingham: Open University Press.

Pidgeon, N. and Henwood, K. (1997) Using grounded theory in psychological research, in N. Hayes (ed.) *Doing Qualitative Analysis in Psychology*. Hove: Psychology Press.

Pomerantz, A. and Fehr, B.J. (1997) Conversation analysis: an approach to the study of social action as sense making practices, in T.A. van Dijk (ed.) *Discourse Studies: A Multidisciplinary Introduction*. London: Sage.

Popper, K.R. (1959) *The Logic of Scientific Discovery*. London: Hutchinson.

Potter, J. (1996) Discourse analysis and constructionist approaches: theoretical background, in J.T.E. Richardson (ed.) *Handbook of Qualitative Research Methods*. Leicester: BPS Books.

Radin, D.I. (1997) *The Conscious Universe: The Scientific Truth of Psychic Phenomena*. New York: HarperEdge.

Reason, J.T. (1979) Actions not as planned: the price of automatisation, in G. Underwood and R. Stevens (eds) *Aspects of Consciousness Vol. I*. London: Academic Press.

Reason, P. and Rowan, J. (eds) (1981) *Human Inquiry: A Sourcebook of New Paradigm Research*. Chichester: Wiley.

Reynolds, P.D. (1982) Moral judgements: strategies for analysis with application to covert participant observation, in M. Bulmer (ed.) *Social Research Ethics*. London: Macmillan.

Rosenhan, D.L. (1973) On being sane in insane places, *Science*, 179: 250–8.

Rosenthal, R. (1979) The 'file-drawer problem' and tolerance for null results, *Psychological Bulletin*, 86: 638–41.

Rosenthal, R. and Fode, K.L. (1963) The effect of experimenter bias on the performance of the albino rat, *Behavioural Science*, 8: 183–9.

Rosenthal, R. and Jacobsen, L. (1968) *Pygmalion in the Classroom: Teacher Expectations and Pupil Intellectual Development*. New York: Holt, Rinehart & Winston.

Searle, A. (1999) *Introducing Research and Data in Psychology: A Guide to Methods and Analysis*. London: Routledge.

Sherrard, C. (1997) Repertoires in discourse: social identification and aesthetic taste, in N. Hayes (ed.) *Doing Qualitative Analysis in Psychology*. Hove: Psychology Press.

Silverman, I. (1977) *The Human Subject in the Psychological Laboratory*. New York: Pergamon.

Sloboda, J.A. (1985) *The Musical Mind: The Cognitive Psychology of Music*. Oxford: Clarendon Press.

Smith, J.A. (1997) Developing theory from case studies: self-reconstruction and the transition to motherhood, in N. Hayes (ed.) *Doing Qualitative Analysis in Psychology*. Hove: Psychology Press.

Sommer, R. (1983) Action research is formative: research at the Saskatchewan hospital, *Journal of Applied Behavioural Science*, 19(4): 427–38.

Sommer, R. (1987) An experimental investigation of the action research approach, *Journal of Applied Behavioural Research*, 23(2): 185–99.

Spearman, C. (1907) Demonstration of formulae for true measures of correlation, *American Journal of Psychology*, 18: 161–9.

Stevens, S.S. (1946) On the theory of scales of measurement, *Science*, 103: 677–80.

Strauss, A.L. and Corbin, J. (1990) *Basics of Qualitative Research: Grounded Theory Procedures and Techniques*. Newbury Park, CA: Sage.

Taylor, M. (1994) Ethnography, in P. Banister, E. Burman, I. Parker, M. Taylor and C. Tindall, *Qualitative Methods in Psychology: A Research Guide*. Buckingham: Open University Press.

Ten Have, P. (1999) *Doing Conversation Analysis: A Practical Guide*. London: Sage.

Uzzell, D. (1995) Ethnographic and action research, in G. Breakwell, S. Hammond and C. Fife-Schaw (eds) *Research Methods in Psychology*. London: Sage.

Van Dijk, T.A. (1987) *Communicating Racism: Ethnic Prejudice in Thought and Action*. Newbury Park, CA: Sage.

Wood, D.J. (1981) Problem-solving and creativity, in C.I. Howarth and W.E.C. Gillham (eds) *The Structure of Psychology: An Introductory Text*. London: George Allen & Unwin.

Wood, P. (1995) Meta-analysis, in G. Breakwell, S. Hammond and C. Fife-Schaw (eds) *Research Methods in Psychology*. London: Sage.

Wright, R.L.D. (1976) *Understanding Statistics*. New York: Harcourt Brace Jovanovich.

Wundt, W. (1862) *Beiträge zur Theorie der Sinneswahrnehmung*. Leipzig: C.F. Winter.

Index